Advances and Controversies in Hematopoietic Transplantation and Cell Therapy

Series Editors

Syed A. Abutalib
Deerfield, Illinois, USA

James O. Armitage
Omaha, Nebraska, USA

Each volume will focus on different aspects of blood and marrow transplantation or cellular therapy and presents up-to-date data and concepts as well as controversial aspects.

More information about this series at http://www.springer.com/series/13907

Syed A. Abutalib
Anand Padmanabhan
Huy P. Pham • Nina Worel
Editors

Best Practices of Apheresis in Hematopoietic Cell Transplantation

Springer

Editors
Syed A. Abutalib
Cancer Treatment Centers of America
Dept Hematology & Bone Marrow
Transplantation
Deerfield, IL
USA

Huy P. Pham
Department of Pathology
Keck School of Medicine of USC
Los Angeles, CA
USA

Anand Padmanabhan
BloodCenter of Wisconsin
Milwaukee, WI
USA

Nina Worel
Department of Blood Group Serology
and Transfusion Medicine
Medical University of Vienna
Vienna
Austria

ISSN 2569-1376 ISSN 2569-135X (electronic)
Advances and Controversies in Hematopoietic Transplantation and Cell Therapy
ISBN 978-3-319-55130-2 ISBN 978-3-319-55131-9 (eBook)
https://doi.org/10.1007/978-3-319-55131-9

This Springer imprint is published by the registered company Springer Nature Switzerland AG
The registered company address is: Gewerbestrasse 11, 6330 Cham, Switzerland

Contents

Introduction and Rationale 1

Anand Padmanabhan, Nina Worel, Huy P. Pham, and Syed A. Abutalib

With great pleasure, we present this inaugural edition of *Best Practices of Apheresis in Hematopoietic Cell Transplantation* as part of the handbook series on *Advances and Controversies in Hematopoietic Cell Transplantation and Cellular Therapy*. This project is a collaborative effort that spanned a time period of more than 2 years and included more than 20 experts, many whom are national leaders in their respected fields.

Hematopoietic progenitor cell (HPC) transplantation has been used increasingly in the treatment of both nonmalignant and neoplastic conditions. There are many critical steps to ensure a successful transplantation and obtaining an adequate amount of HPCs is one of them. Currently, HPCs can be obtained from related or unrelated donors (allogeneic HPC collections), the patient him/herself (autologous HPC collections), or cord blood. Similar to the source, there are various methods of obtaining HPCs. Typically, they are harvested either from the bone marrow or from the peripheral blood after mobilization. At this time, especially for the treatment of

A. Padmanabhan
Transfusion Medicine, Versiti Wisconsin & Medical College of Wisconsin, Milwaukee, WI, USA
e-mail: anand.padmanabhan@bcw.edu

N. Worel
Department of Blood Group Serology and Transfusion Medicine, Medical University of Vienna, Vienna, Austria
e-mail: nina.worel@meduniwien.ac.at

H. P. Pham
Department of Pathology, Keck School of Medicine of the University of Southern California, Los Angeles, CA, USA
e-mail: phamh@usc.edu

S. A. Abutalib (✉)
Hematology and BMT Program, Clinical Apheresis Program, Hematology Program Development, Cancer Treatment Centers of America, Zion, IL, USA

S. A. Abutalib et al. (eds.), *Best Practices of Apheresis in Hematopoietic Cell Transplantation*, Advances and Controversies in Hematopoietic Transplantation and Cell Therapy, https://doi.org/10.1007/978-3-319-55131-9_1

neoplastic diseases, the majority of HPCs are obtained from peripheral blood by apheresis due to the ease of collection and other clinical benefits for the donor/recipient discussed in the following chapters. Additionally, apheresis procedures may also be used to treat complications arising from allogeneic hematopoietic cell transplantation (allo-HCT), such as extracorporeal photopheresis (ECP) for the treatment of acute or chronic graft-versus-host disease, or in preparation of the patient for the transplant, such as therapeutic plasma exchange for recipient's isoagglutinin reduction (in major mismatched) or red blood cell exchange for decreasing host's red blood cells that would be the target for passenger lymphocyte syndrome (in minor mismatched) in patients undergoing ABO mismatched allo-HCT. Hence, apheresis plays an important role in the field of HCT. However, although the common goal is to get the patient to transplant, apheresis practices to achieve this goal may vary between institutions. This handbook seeks to provide readers with "Best Practices in Apheresis" with an emphasis on using this technique in the field of hematopoietic cell transplantation (HCT).

Since HPC product collections and HCT are highly regulated, this handbook begins with a chapter discussing various administrative and regulatory considerations. Accreditation by the Foundations for Accreditation in Cellular Therapy (FACT) or Joint Accreditation Committee ISCT and EBMT (JACIE) is an important benchmark of quality assurance used by many transplant programs; thus, a chapter on the topic of FACT/JACIE inspections and practical tips on how to avoid common citations is helpful and, therefore, is included. The next several chapters outline the process of donor selection and evaluations and different mobilization strategies commonly used in both allogenic and autologous transplant settings. A brief summary of the technical aspects and principles of different apheresis devices utilized in the collection process, including lymphocyte collection for donor lymphocyte collection (DLI), as well as information on cellular processing, such as in bone marrow harvests, along with prediction algorithms for HPC collection are provided. The remainder of the handbook discusses different apheresis procedures and their indications in the field of HPC transplantation. Specifically, anticoagulation and peri-procedural considerations are discussed along with different indications for the use of therapeutic plasma exchange/immunoadsorption, red blood cell exchange, and extracorporeal photopheresis. Furthermore, there are risks associated with apheresis procedures and thus, a chapter on how to recognize and provide care for apheresis complications is provided. Finally, recommendations and guidance on handling common challenges in apheresis medicine, such as in children or apheresis practice in a limited resource setting, are provided.

The main focus of this book is to provide readers with best practices as implemented by experts in the apheresis field. The book may appeal to a broad range of providers involved in different aspects of care in HCT, from a variety of different medical specialties. We also believe this book may be a valuable resource to transplant practitioners who may not be very familiar with apheresis techniques as applied in the area of HCT.

Although the authors and editors have aimed for perfection in content, grammar, and syntax, we are realistic enough to know that there will be errors in our book.

Therefore, we created an email for the readers to alert us such mistakes or criticisms and to discuss different viewpoints, as well as to provide suggestions for the next edition of the book. Please email us at: abutalib110@gmail.com.

In conclusion, we are very grateful for the opportunity given to us by Springer Publishers. We are also deeply indebted to the expert contributors who made this book possible. We hope that this handbook will help enhance knowledge of HPC transplant practitioners and trainees.

Administrative and Regulatory Considerations for Apheresis Collection Facilities

2

Joseph (Yossi) Schwartz and Jörg Halter

2.1 Introduction

Autologous mononuclear cells, collected by leukocytapheresis and cryopreserved, have virtually replaced marrow as a source of CD34^{+} cells for autologous hematopoietic cell rescue after myeloablative therapy for myeloma and lymphomas. Furthermore, the recent introduction of chimeric antigen receptor T-cell (also known CAR T-cell) therapy involves removal of T-cells from the patient via leukocytapheresis and subsequently their modification so that they express receptors specific to the patient's particular cancer. As such, apheresis facilities, which perform those collections, are an integral and critical part such therapeutic modalities including allogeneic peripheral blood hematopoietic progenitor cell collections.

The field of cellular therapy which includes apheresis facilities as the cellular product collection facility is a highly regulated discipline. Over the world, different regulatory bodies are providing oversight at various levels. While in most countries, national regulations are in place provided by governmental authorities, for example, the Food and Drug Administration (FDA); there might be additional regulations at a state level. Furthermore, national regulations may follow directives from a state union (e.g., EU directives being obligatory for EU member states) or might be supplemented by standards published from nongovernmental organizations (see below). Although the latter are not legally binding, they might be regarded to represent the standard of care in legal cases where no laws apply.

J. (Y.) Schwartz (✉)
Transfusion Medicine and Cellular Therapy, Pathology and Cell Biology, Columbia University Medical Center, New York Presbyterian Hospital, New York, NY, USA
e-mail: js2745@cumc.columbia.edu

J. Halter
Hematology, University Hospital Basel, Basel, Switzerland
e-mail: jhalter@hin.ch; joerg.halter@usb.ch

S. A. Abutalib et al. (eds.), *Best Practices of Apheresis in Hematopoietic Cell Transplantation*, Advances and Controversies in Hematopoietic Transplantation and Cell Therapy, https://doi.org/10.1007/978-3-319-55131-9_2

The FDA and Centers for Medicare and Medicaid Services (CMS) are the primary regulatory agencies providing federal oversight in the United States. In addition, state health departments and other agencies may provide some degree of regulatory oversight. In the European Union, the European Council and Commission provides oversight for those facilities, releasing directives that translate into national laws and regulations while oversight is provided by health authorities of the EU member states. In addition, individual countries might have their own regulatory frame. Individuals and apheresis facilities involved with cellular therapies should be familiar with the different requirements of these agencies.

Apheresis facilities also should be familiar with all relevant state/country and local laws and regulations, including professional licensure requirements for medical and laboratory personnel, as many states/countries (in the United States and worldwide) have regulations which apply to apheresis professionals. Further laws and regulations may cover equipment (apheresis instruments, collection sets, additive solutions, etc.). Furthermore, in some situations, apheresis facilities providing cell therapy products in other states/countries must comply with local regulations in the final destination.

It is important to distinguish between regulation and accreditation. Regulations have the force of law while accreditation standards are not legally binding. Cellular therapy facilities must follow the rules set by regulatory agencies. In contrast, accreditation agencies such as FACT-JACIE, AABB, or the Joint Commission (the United States only) publish specific sets of standards that need to be met in order to provide accreditation. Some regulatory agencies will grant deeming authority to selected accreditation agencies. For example, the CMS regulates laboratory testing through the Clinical Laboratory Improvement Amendments (CLIA). CMS accepts certain accreditation agency inspections. Table 2.1 summarizes agencies and organizations involved in regulation and accreditation of cellular therapy facilities including apheresis facilities. The scope of their regulatory oversight and/or accreditation is detailed on these organizations' respective websites.

Table 2.1 Regulatory or accreditation agencies involved in cellular therapies

Regulatory agencies	Accreditation organizations
The Food and Drug Administration (FDA)	AABB
Centers for Medicaid and Medicare Services (CMS)	Foundation for the Accreditation of Cellular Therapy (FACT)
Department of Homeland Security	The Joint Accreditation Committee—ISCT and EBMT (JACIE)
Nuclear Regulatory Commission (NRC)	National Marrow Donor Program (NMDP)
Environmental Protection Agency (EPA)	World Marrow Donor Association (WMDA)
Occupational Safety and Health administration (OSHA)	College of American Pathologists (CAP)
Council of Europe/European Commission	

2.2 Human Cells, Tissues, and Cellular- and Tissue-Based Products (HCT/Ps)

In the United States, human cells, tissues, and cellular- and tissue-based products (HCT/Ps) are defined as articles containing or consisting of human cells or tissues that are intended for implantation, transplantation, infusion, or transfer into a human recipient (Code of Federal Regulations 2015). HCT/Ps can be derived from deceased or living donors (Table 2.2). The FDA established a comprehensive, tiered, risk-based regulatory framework applicable to HCT/Ps. These regulations, which were published in three parts (referred to as the "tissue rules") and contained in the code of federal regulation (CFR), more specifically in 21 CFR 1271, became fully effective on May 25, 2005, and are applicable to all HCT/Ps, including hematopoietic progenitor cells (HPCs), that are recovered on or after this date (Code of Federal Regulations 2014; FDA Tissue Guidances n.d.). This risk-based framework authorizes the FDA to establish and enforce regulations necessary to prevent the introduction, transmission, or spread of communicable diseases in HCT/Ps which are regulated solely under section 361 of the Public Health Service (PHS) Act [42 USC 264] (United States Code n.d.) (Table 2.3).

In the European Union, the EU directives 2004/23/EC, 2015/566, 2006/17/EC, 2006/86/EG, and 2015/565 currently apply (for updates, please consult www.eur-lex.europa.eu), while for advanced therapy medicinal products (ATMP) further regulations from the European Medicines Agency apply (www.ema.europa.eu).

The AABB, The Foundation for the Accreditation of Cellular Therapy (FACT), and the Joint Accreditation Committee ISCT and EBMT (JACIE) set voluntary cellular therapy standards (Table 2.4) including collection, processing, and administration (Allickson 2015; FACT 2015) with accreditation cycles of two, three, and four years, respectively. The principles of these standards and accreditation are based on a peer-based review process incorporating both medical and laboratory practice which is best suited to protect patient safety, improve cellular therapy practices, and protect the research environment. College of American Pathologists (CAP) transfusion medicine checklist (College of American Pathologists, Commission on Laboratory Accreditation 2015) includes cellular therapy and apheresis-specific requirements. The World

Table 2.2 Examples of HCT/Ps

From deceased donors[a]	From living donors[a]
Skin	Hematopoietic stem/progenitor cells from bone marrow, peripheral and cord blood
Dura mater	Other cell therapy products (e.g., pancreatic islets, mesenchymal stem/stromal cells, fibroblasts)
Cardiovascular tissues	Reproductive cells and tissues
Ocular tissues	
Musculoskeletal tissues	

[a]In general, but there are exceptions

Table 2.3 US regulations for manufacturers of hematopoietic progenitor cells

Type of HPC product	Regulatory category/oversight	Key regulations (21 CFR except as noted)	FDA premarket licensure, approval, or clearance?
Minimally manipulated bone marrow, not combined with another article (with some exceptions) and for homologous use	Health Resources and Services Administration oversight	42 US Code 274(k)	Not applicable
Autologous or allogeneic related (1st or 2nd degree blood relative)-donor HPCs	PHS Act Section 361: HCT/Ps[a]	1271.10(a)[b] (must meet all criteria); 1271 Subparts A–F	No
Minimally manipulated Unrelated-donor peripheral blood HPCs, not combined with another article (with some exceptions) and for homologous use	PHS Act Sections 361 and 351: HCT/Ps regulated as drugs and/or biological products	1271 Subparts A–D Applicable biologics/drug regulations	Delayed implementation
Minimally manipulated unrelated-donor umbilical cord blood cells	PHS Sections 361 and 351: HCT/Ps regulated as drugs and/or biological products	1271 Subparts A–D	Yes (after October 20, 2011): BLA or IND application
HPCs that don't meet all the criteria in 21 CFR 1271.10(a)	PHS Sections 361 and 351 HCT/Ps regulated as drugs and/or biological products	1271 subparts A–D Applicable drugs/biologics regulations	Yes: IND and BLA

HPC hematopoietic progenitor cell, *CFR* code of federal regulations, *FDA* Food and Drug Administration, *PHS* public health service, *HCT/Ps* human cells, tissues, and cellular- and tissue-based products, *IND* investigational new drug, *BLA* biologics license application

[a]As defined by 2005 tissue regulations [21 CFR 1271.3(d)]

[b]21 CFR 1271.10(a) as applied to Section 361 (see full rule for details) requires that HPCs be (1) minimally manipulated, (2) for homologous use only, (3) not combined with another article (except water; crystalloids; or sterilizing, preserving, or storage agents with no new safety concerns), and (4) for autologous use or for allogeneic use in a first- or second-degree blood relative

Table 2.4 Cellular therapy accreditation

Organization	Standards review cycle
AABB	Two years
FACT	Four years
JACIE	Four years
NMDP	Two years
WMDA	Five years
CAP	Not set (yearly published updated check list)

Marrow Donor Association (WMDA) fosters international collaboration to facilitate the exchange of high-quality hematopoietic stem cells for clinical transplantation worldwide and to promote the interests of donors. WMDA is also accrediting and qualifying donor registries who follow its global standards that cover all aspects of unrelated hematopoietic stem/progenitor cell registry operations. The National Donor Marrow Program (NMDP) Standards set forth basic guidelines and requirements for programs working with the NMDP. The Standards encompass network participation criteria with requirements for transplant centers, recruitment centers, and product collection centers. The NMDP standards are designed to ensure that donors and patients receive high-quality care and that government standards are met (Table 2.4).

The Circular of Information for the Use of Cellular Therapy Products is jointly written by the AABB and multiple organizations involved in cellular therapy for users of certain minimally manipulated unlicensed cellular therapy products (AABB et al. 2016). It is getting revised periodically with representatives from all relevant organizations and many of the standard setting organizations require it will be included with the collected cellular therapy product when being shipped or transported.

In addition, the Alliance for Harmonization of Cellular Therapy Accreditation (AHCTA), which is under the umbrella of WBMT, encompasses all the above-mentioned accreditation organizations. AHCTA is working toward creating a global comprehensive single set of quality, safety, and professional standards which cover all aspects of the process from assessment of donor eligibility to transplantation and clinical outcomes of HCTs and related cellular therapies. AHCTA provides helpful documents to navigate the different sets of participating organizations' standards. Moreover, crosswalk documents comparing the different set of cellular therapy standards were created and are available on the AHCTA website (http://www.ahcta.org/documents.html). AHCTA also published a document on essential elements as a resource for new or developing programs, identifying the most important quality system elements for cells and tissues for administration.

Of note, the FDA regulations in 21 CFR Part 1271 require HCT/P manufacturers to have a tracking and labeling system that enables tracking each product from the donor to the recipient and from the recipient back to the donor. The HCT/P manufacturers are also required to inform the facilities that receive the products of the tracking system that they have established. ISBT 128 and equivalent systems in Europe, such as Eurocode, are considered an acceptable labeling system for those purposes.

2.3 Expert Opinion

Cellular therapy regulations and standards such as the FACT-JACIE cellular therapy standards ensure high-quality cellular therapy products as they standardize processes related to collection, processing and administration. Those standards are based on scientific literature, clinical practice, governmental regulations, and community inputs. Based on these standards, the accreditation agency offer accreditation to transplant programs in order to encourage health institutions and facilities performing bone marrow and peripheral blood transplantation to establish and maintain quality management systems impacting on all aspects of their activities and to engage in continuous improvement. In order to be in compliance with the current edition of the standards, apheresis facilities need to review the new edition of the standards and use the accompanying guidance to understand the intent of the standards and how the change is different than their current process. In addition, each accreditation organization is providing tools to help make the transition smooth including a comprehensive summary of changes and a crosswalk comparing the previous edition to the new one.

2.4 Future Directions

Ideally, one set of standards which are comprehensive and acceptable by all organizations involved in regulating and accrediting apheresis facilities should be the goal. This will achieve a global comprehensive single set of quality, safety, and professional standards which cover all aspects of the process from assessment of donor eligibility to transplantation and clinical outcomes of HCTs and related cellular therapies and decrease the burden of apheresis facilities to be familiar with different sets of standards.

References

AABB, America's Blood Centers, American Association of Tissue Banks, American Red Cross, American Society for Apheresis, American Society for Blood and Marrow Transplantation, College of American Pathologists, Foundation for the Accreditation of Cellular Therapy, ICCBBA, International Society for Cellular Therapy, Joint Accreditation Committee, National Marrow Donor Program, and Netcord (2016) Circular of information for the use of cellular therapy products. AABB, Bethesda, MD. http://www.aabb.org/. Accessed 17 June 2016

Allickson J (ed) (2015) Standards for cellular therapy services, 7th edn. AABB, Bethesda, MD

Code of Federal Regulations (2014) Title 21, CFR Part1271. US Government Printing Office, Washington, DC. http://www.accessdata.fda.gov/scripts/cdrh/cfdocs/cfcfr/CFRSearch.cfm?CFRPart=1271

Code of Federal Regulations (2015) Title 21, CFR Part 1271.3(d). US Government Printing Office, Washington, DC. http://www.accessdata.fda.gov/scripts/cdrh/cfdocs/cfcfr/cfrsearch.cfm?fr=1271.3. Accessed 4 Feb 2016

College of American Pathologists, Commission on Laboratory Accreditation (2015) Transfusion medicine checklist. July 28, 2015 edition. College of American Pathologists, Northfield, Ill

FACT (2015) International standards for hematopoietic cellular therapy: product collection, processing and administration, 6th edn. Foundation for Accreditation for Cellular Therapy (FACT), Omaha, NE

FDA Tissue Guidances. http://www.fda.gov/BiologicsBloodVaccines/GuidanceCompliance RegulatoryInformation/Guidances/Tissue/

http://www.ahcta.org/documents.html. Accessed 4 Feb 2016

United States Code. Title 42, USC Part 264 (Regulations to Control Communicable Diseases)

FACT-JACIE Standards: Common Citations and How Best to Avoid Them

3

Dennis A. Gastineau and Kara K. Wacker

3.1 Introduction

This chapter will examine the evolution of the most common citations during inspections for accreditation under the FACT-JACIE Hematopoietic Cellular Therapy Standards, in its seventh edition as of this writing (FACT-JACIE n.d.). For each area of citations, methods to address these citations to perform high-quality collection of hematopoietic progenitor cell (HPC) products will be discussed. The trends discussed in this chapter reflect inspections performed by the Foundation for Accreditation of Cellular Therapy (FACT).

Blood and marrow transplantation is a highly complex process requiring a coordinated team from many disciplines all contributing to the treatment and outcome of the transplant recipient. The focus of this highly specialized community has been to improve outcomes and widen the field of candidates for this often life-saving but high-risk procedure.

The average number of citations for the programs undergoing their sixth accreditation cycle as of 2017 was over 20, demonstrating that citations are not rare, and has actually increased coincidence with more extensive quality management standards and with increased inspector training.

D. A. Gastineau (✉)
Human Cellular Therapy Laboratory, Department of Laboratory Medicine and Pathology, Mayo Clinic, Phoenix, AZ, USA
e-mail: Gastineau.dennis@mayo.edu

K. K. Wacker
Foundation for the Accreditation of Cellular Therapy, University of Nebraska, Omaha, NE, USA
e-mail: kwacker@unmc.edu

S. A. Abutalib et al. (eds.), *Best Practices of Apheresis in Hematopoietic Cell Transplantation*, Advances and Controversies in Hematopoietic Transplantation and Cell Therapy, https://doi.org/10.1007/978-3-319-55131-9_3

Part C Apheresis Collection Facility Standards contains the requirements for apheresis collection facilities. This chapter will examine common citations in each section of this part and explore options of avoiding these. As this chapter is based upon these standards, there will be phrases and sentences essentially identical to those in the standards.

3.2 Standards

FACT was founded in 1996 by a group of clinicians and laboratorians who saw an opportunity for the blood and marrow transplant field to improve care for all patients through a process of self-assessment and inspection by peers active in the field. These visionaries represented FACT's parent organizations, the American Society for Cellular Therapy and Transplantation (ASTCT) and the International Society for Cell and Gene Therapy (ISCT). Two years later, the Joint Accreditation Committee ISCT & EBMT (JACIE) was founded by the European division of ISCT and the European Society for Blood and Marrow Transplantation (EBMT). FACT and JACIE have partnered in the development of the last several editions of the standards.

At the time of this writing, more than 180 blood and marrow transplant programs throughout the world are accredited by FACT and JACIE, many on their seventh cycle of accreditation. It is rare for a program to not be cited for at least some deficiencies. Examining the pattern of the deficiencies may be instructive and allow programs to concentrate development in these areas for greatest impact on quality and outcomes.

3.3 Common Citation Areas

The ten most common areas of citations are in quality management in all three sectors: processing, apheresis, and clinical. In apheresis, labeling and standard operating procedures (SOPs) also had a high incidence for citation. Historically, quality management citations increased as quality management system expectations rose and the emphasis on proactive management replaced reactive event management. It is encouraging that, overall, the citations in these main areas have declined over the last several cycles, suggesting that clinical medicine is successfully introducing quality management to its highly complex care, and in many areas blood and marrow transplantation has led the rest of medicine in this effort. FACT's 3-year accreditation cycle means that programs are continuously engaged in activities related to the standards, and as the standards have evolved, the changes have begun to slow as important standards are identified and less important standards deleted.

Two definitions should always be kept in mind when interpreting standards: "shall" means a requirement must be met and "should" means it is highly recommended (and often becomes a "shall" in the next set of standards).

3.4 Sections of the Standards and the Common Citations

3.4.1 C1: General

Few citations occur in this section as they are broad descriptions, but there is the potential for more citations as divided responsibility for cellular product manufacturing occurs with local collection, shipping to a third-party facility, and receipt after manufacturing for distribution to the patient. The relationships among the parties are crucial and must be defined in writing and periodically reviewed. Appropriate registration and licensure according to applicable laws is required, and these vary from state to state and country to country. Regulatory compliance does not alone ensure compliance with FACT.

3.4.2 C2: Apheresis Collection Facility

The citations in this section dealing with facilities has increased as more attention has been paid to the appropriately designated areas for not only collection, but temporary storage of the product as well as the proper storage of supplies, reagents, and equipment.

Common citations in this area include lack of controls on temperature and humidity, or the determination of what the limits of these conditions (i.e., acceptance criteria) should be. In general, all reagents, supplies, and equipment will have storage and operating temperatures, and many will have specific humidity requirements. Knowing what these limits are and knowing, with data, whether the facility air conditioning is able to ensure that the temperature and humidity levels are always in these ranges is important. A table tracking these storage requirements will help the program comply with these standards.

Critical is the maintenance of the facility in a manner designed to minimize health risks to patients, visitors, and staff. In addition, medical support for patients, particularly in the event of a site away from a hospital, must be rapidly available in emergencies. Although rare, these may happen during HPC collection.

3.4.3 C3: Personnel

Requirements for all the managing personnel are described. One issue for the medical director can be the requirement of 2-years experience (7th edition) performing and/or supervising cellular therapy product collection procedures, so succession planning is very important for any program. A possible solution is to appoint associate directors who share the responsibilities, perhaps cross-covering each program in cell processing and apheresis. A more recent challenge has been the requirement of 10 h of educational activities for management personnel and providers. Commonly misunderstood is that this standard does NOT require certified educational hours, only the tracking of topics, dates and hours to comply. The following are required:

1. Title of activity
2. Type of activity (e.g., webinar, meeting, grand rounds)
3. Topic (hematology, stem cell transplantation, immunology)
4. Date of activity
5. Approximate duration of the activity

ASBMT offers practice improvement modules, and other groups offer similar modules that qualify for these hours of educational activity.

Qualifications for quality managers have become more detailed, but one situation often found wanting is the oversight of the quality manager's work. Sometimes the quality manager is performing work that he or she then is the signatory for review, which may not be in compliance with the standards.

Lastly, for collection services providing services for both adult and pediatric populations, age-appropriate training must be demonstrated; for example, red cell priming of machines for low-weight donors.

3.4.4 C4: Quality Management (QM)

The QM section remains the section with highest proportion of citations in the apheresis section, although somewhat lower than in earlier editions of the standards. In this section, there is a standard requiring annual review of the effectiveness of the quality program by the apheresis collection facility director or designee, and this review must be provided to the clinical program director. If it is a designee performing these functions, that designee should be identified in the quality management plan. Documentation of each of these steps is required, by signature or by the minutes of a meeting where the report is reviewed.

In small programs, it may be necessary to engage another individual knowledgeable in quality activities to review the work performed by the quality manager to avoid bias; although some reviews, such as the annual summation or audits of overall procedures that may include procedures performed by the designated quality manager, may be performed by the quality manager as long as the reports are then reviewed by the director.

The assignment of responsibility is a common area of confusion and citation. These responsibilities should be defined in a clear organizational chart. In very large programs, two versions of the chart may be helpful, one of the high-level relationships and another that includes all the individuals in an area.

Staff job descriptions are required for all positions, and one often overlooked is that of the director, who may have been in place for decades and for whom no description was ever written. From these job descriptions, critical competencies can be derived, and these critical competencies must have not only initial qualification but annual competency evaluation. It is easy to fall behind in these competency evaluations, especially for a program in a rapid growth phase.

Document control must be defined in the QM plan. Where there is an overriding departmental or institutional document control system, that system should be referenced and be available to the inspectors. There must be a listing of the documents specific to the apheresis collection area. A common problem is document approval; programs need to ensure both initial approval and review and re-approval at least every 2 years. Furthermore, a coversheet for all procedures is insufficient; each procedure must be reviewed and signed.

There must be a method to ensure that documents are not altered by mistake. Word processing documents are difficult to fully lock, and other formats should be sought. The current electronic version is the best document to reference. If documents are printed, there must be a date of printing and a policy or a statement on the printed document that states expiration occurs at the end of that day. This is a common deficiency in many electronic policy systems. A document format showing initial date of introduction and all the versions should be present, and a commendable practice is a short statement of the primary change or changes in each version of the document.

Agreements with any third parties, including environmental services, contracted personnel, and external clinical and manufacturing facilities, must define the limits of responsibility of each party and must be reviewed regularly, at least every 2 years. Demonstration of that review is a common deficit, and should be clear and available to the inspector.

3.4.4.1 Outcome Analysis

There is a requirement that data for each type of HPC product collected or procedure be analyzed, both individually and in aggregate. This means that products that fall outside expected ranges are assessed for procedural deviations and equipment function. Time to engraftment must also be followed, although it is not required that the apheresis group be the primary recorder or reporter of those data.

3.4.4.2 Audits

A common deficiency is the completion of either no audits or audits that are not true audits (such as aggregating total nucleated cells collected with each procedure without further analysis). Audits should be undertaken with a specific goal, and should be performed by someone who is not responsible for the majority of the work being done. An outside individual, such as quality staff from the processing laboratory, would be a good solution for the apheresis unit with a small number of staff. Each edition of the standards has specified required audits, such as donor eligibility determination. A very common deficiency is a failure to perform a follow-up audit when a corrective action has been implemented to solve an identified problem.

3.4.4.3 Positive Microbial Products

Unlike blood products where a positive culture from the product results in immediate discard, HPC products are sometimes irreplaceable, either due to the time frame or because donor/patients may not mobilize again. FACT-JACIE standards are specific about how this situation should be handled, and the program should have SOP(s) addressing this issue that must include(s) who contacts the providers, how donors are assessed for possible bacteremia, and investigation of other possible causes for the positive culture. If it is determined that there is no reasonable choice but to infuse the positive-culture HPC product, this infusion must be reported to the FDA and the SOP(s) should define the person in the facility to make such report. Each part of this description may be missing in a program's SOPs and result in citation(s), so carefully following the standards and organizing the interaction of apheresis, processing, and clinical portions of the program is critical to the best care of the donor and patient.

3.4.4.4 Event Management

Events can range from leaving a blank on a form for cleaning the facility to taking the wrong product over to the hospital floor. These are quite different in severity and require different analytical pathways. If every forgotten blank on a form were investigated in the same manner of a wrong product, the quality system would be paralyzed. However, how the events are assessed, aggregated and reported must be specifically noted, including evidence that there has been review up to the level of the Clinical Program Director. A Quality Handbook published by FACT on its website may be helpful in constructing an event management program. There are events noted by the apheresis unit and then there are events noted externally which can be classified as "complaints." This could be a patient complaint about communication or it could be a notice from the processing laboratory that a unit had, for example, 75 mL of red cells in the product. There should be tracking and analysis of both types of complaints. Lastly, the results of event management activities should be communicated not only to leadership but, where appropriate and in the right format, to the entire staff.

3.4.4.5 Interruption of Operations

There have been numerous weather-related disasters that have interrupted hospital services, and there should be plans specific to the collection services, as an allogeneic recipient may have already received myeloablative conditioning and require the planned fresh product donation. While the institutional disaster plan may be a reference for the majority of issues, some portion specific to apheresis should be in the quality plan. Where programs refer to the institutional disaster plan, they often fail to have plans specific to the blood and marrow transplant program.

3.4.4.6 Validation

Although the concepts of validation of processes are increasingly understood, a common deficiency is the failure to have an approved validation plan specifying the particular process and expected outcomes signed by the director and the quality manager. There is then a second signature set from the same people demonstrating that the plan, results, and analysis are accepted. Anytime there is a change in the process, including critical supplies, a revalidation must be done. This is often focused and not as extensive as the initial validation.

3.4.5 C5: Policies and Procedures

There is a very specific list of policies and procedures in the standards that must be addressed as a core set. If the program does not have an SOP with that title, it is critical that topic is covered in another SOP. There should be an SOP that defines all the elements of the working SOPs and provides a structure for the staff to follow in writing new SOPs (i.e., SOP for SOP). Each SOP is required to have a specific structure, and a common shortfall is the lack of specific endpoints and range of expected results. In addition, there must be a reference section with current references.

3.4.6 C6: Allogeneic and Autologous Donor Evaluation and Management

Written criteria for evaluation of donors is required. For allogeneic donors, this evaluation must be performed by someone other than the recipient's physician. Programs can comply with this standard either by using another transplant physician or using internal medicine physicians specifically trained in evaluating donors.

Donor eligibility and suitability are different. A donor, to be eligible, must be free from all risk factors for relevant communicable diseases and have infectious disease markers that are negative or nonreactive. A donor can be ineligible due to positive travel history, for example. However, if this donor is still the best donor in the clinical judgement of both the donor and recipient physicians, the decision to use an ineligible donor must be clearly documented including the consent of the recipient. Some programs use specific consent forms for this; others rely on clinical note documentation. There is a guidance document relevant to this from the FDA (see US FDA Final Guidance (Eligibility Determination for Donors of Human Cells, Tissues, and Cellular and Tissue-based Product [HCT/Ps], August 2007).

Donor (either allogeneic or autologous) suitability is the medical fitness of the donor to undergo the collection procedure. Blood and marrow transplant programs must have initial documentation and then evidence of interim assessment prior to each procedure. Pregnancy testing within seven days of starting the donor mobilization is required and, as applicable, within seven days prior to the initiation of the recipient's preparative regimen.

3.4.6.1 Consents to Donate

Common deficiencies of the consents to donate include specifically addressing the donor's right to refuse, alternative means of donation, and what could happen to the recipient if the donor rescinds consent after the recipient has received conditioning, and specific consent to release the donor information to the recipient.

3.4.6.2 Communication of Results Between Apheresis and the Processing Laboratory

There are several sections addressing how results must be communicated in writing. If all parts of the program share the same medical record, shared laboratory results and communication within the medical record suffice.

3.4.7 C7: Coding and Labeling of Cellular Therapy Products

Facilities have often been cited for not having ISBT 128 labeling either implemented or in the state of "active implementation," meaning there was evidence of planning that demonstrate actual implementation will be completed. The standards now require full implementation of ISBT 128, and facilities have been cited for not completing implementation.

There are extensive descriptions of labeling requirements, essentially all covered in ISBT 128 labeling, but the other common citations in this section have been for the label content at the end of collection requiring that the primary product container and concurrent plasma container bear all the required information in the Labeling Table in Appendix II of the FACT-JACIE standards. This labeling is required by many organizations and regulators in addition to FACT.

3.4.8 C8: Process Controls

3.4.8.1 Inventory Control

The second most common apheresis citation concerns the receipt of supplies and reagents. Each supply or reagent must be visually examined for evidence of acceptable condition. The SOP describing this required inspection must cover acceptable visual properties (such as the expectation that fluid must be clear) and there must be logs documenting the receipt and the individual acknowledging receipt and performing the inspection. In addition, there must be a system to track each of these supplies or reagents to the collection of a specific product.

For the receipt of a product, a form with a table documenting the receipt with personnel initials may be of help. A more sophisticated approach might be an electronic system that the person uses to enter the supply into inventory, and as part of the entry process, the condition of the material is documented.

The trackability can be as laborious as writing down the lot number of each supply used during the process, a date and time range that the lot was in use, or the use of barcoding to document the supply with its relevant data recorded on the record. These are examples of three different but acceptable means of satisfying this requirement. It demonstrates that there is flexibility in the standards.

3.4.8.2 Equipment Calibration and Inspection Prior to Use

Equipment must be clean and verified to be within its calibration period. There must also be documentation of those assessments prior to daily use. Equipment must also be standardized and calibrated regularly using a traceable standard where available. The first can be addressed by a form on each piece of equipment or on the collection record. Equipment must be calibrated either by the manufacturer, by trained individuals from within the institution, or by the collection personnel themselves using proper calibration reference equipment. This requires a fairly high level of training and it is most common to outsource calibration and preventive maintenance (PM) outside of the apheresis area.

3.4.8.3 Documentation of Donor Assessment

A written interim assessment by a qualified person must be entered prior to each collection procedure demonstrating that the person is assessed to be fit for that day's collection. This assessment must be performed by a physician or registered nurse to assure there have been no relevant changes in the health of the donor. A daily note entered in the record noting any laboratory values required according to the SOP, as well as vital signs and a general assessment, would satisfy this standard. The initial assessment is almost always documented but these interim assessments are sometimes missed.

3.4.8.4 Central Venous Catheters

Placement and use of a central venous catheter poses a risk to the donor. After the central venous catheter is placed by a licensed health care professional, the adequacy of placement must be documented prior to use. This could be a declaration by the radiologist or a note in the chart by a provider confirming the location of the catheter. Reviewing the image prior to use is optimal, but the interpretation is sufficient. Failure to have this documentation consistently present is a common citation.

3.4.8.5 Distribution of Products from Apheresis

Before the product leaves the collection unit, it must pass specific release criteria designated by the program, and, if not, there must be specific procedures defining how and by whom the assessment and decision to release the product will be made.

There is additional responsibility when products leave the apheresis unit and go directly to a patient. In that event, SOPs describing the collection procedure and the expected outcomes must include methods to assure that the product meets those release criteria for clinical administration before the product is distributed.

In cooperation with the cell processing laboratory, the apheresis facility should assure that consistent cell collections are occurring, and one method would be to compare the collected CD34 positive cell number with the peripheral blood CD34 result to see if a proportionate collection occurred. Aggregated data should also be reviewed for a set of endpoints (e.g., volume of blood processed, length of procedure, product volume, condition of the collection container, and visual inspection of the product for clumping or clotting). A worksheet and checklist would facilitate this documentation.

3.4.8.6 Extra corporeal Photopheresis (ECP)

A written plan prior to the initiation of ECP is required, and the target of the therapy including grade of graft-versus-host disease (GVHD) and involved organs must be identified. These are not always found during inspections. There should then be an SOP indicating the usual schedule to be followed, particularly in the first 4 weeks as response to ECP may be delayed. A standardized initial treatment plan should be followed to assure comparability of outcomes. Determination of the tapering schedule and length of treatment is based on assessment of response, and thus, there should be documented periodic assessments of the response to the therapy. At the end, a summary of the treatment must be documented, and there may be cooperation between the apheresis provider and the transplant provider to complete this assessment.

3.4.9 C9: Cellular Therapy Product Storage

There is common misunderstanding of what constitutes storage of a product once it has been collected. The product is always doing something, and storage is occurring once the product is taken off the machine and until the product is either taken directly to the processing laboratory or handed directly to processing laboratory personnel in a validated transportation vessel (or the product is taken or handed directly to the clinical program). Defined storage areas separate from other work must be defined, and the temperature of storage, humidity, and the security of storage must be addressed. For short-term storage, room temperature may be elected, but then in the storage area there should be monitoring of the temperature to assure it remains in a defined range (such as 20–24 °C). Longer-term storage will likely be in a refrigerator, and that temperature must be defined and monitored. The security of the storage area must be addressed, and the refrigerator, if unattended, must be in a restricted access area or locked.

Transportation of the product to the processing laboratory must be in a container validated to maintain temperature for a time sufficient for delayed delivery and at the extremes of temperature that could be experienced locally. Continuous monitoring of the temperature may be appropriate. The continuous monitoring device must be periodically calibrated to assure proper monitoring. A label at the end of collection must include storage temperature.

3.4.10 C10: Cellular Therapy Product Transportation and Shipping

Transportation and shipping are two different methods of distributing a product to another entity. Transportation means that the product is accompanied at all times by trained personnel (such as a courier); shipping means that the product is not accompanied by trained personnel (such as a commercial shipping company). If the product remains within a campus, such as inside continuous structures, or is hand-carried on an airplane by trained personnel, it is considered transported. Shipping and transportation on public roads require additional container characteristics and information. The transportation and shipping temperatures must be defined and the process and container must be validated. Of note, when defining transportation and storage temperature, it is important to use only the least restrictive temperature range necessary to maintain integrity of the product. Defining tighter temperature ranges will only make it more difficult to comply.

Furthermore, agreements between the facilities must define the limits of responsibility for each participant, including chain of custody. A process with a checklist or examples of completed paperwork may suffice.

3.4.11 C11: Records

Records are commonly cited for not being complete, legible or indelible. A record of initials and signatures helps identify written attestations, but, where possible, check boxes and electronic records should be used. Error correction must preserve the initial entry, and there must be methods to prevent loss or destruction of both paper and electronic records. The inspector is instructed to review storage of recent records and the system for archiving records for accessibility and confidentiality.

Records must be retained for at least 10 years after distribution or administration, or as required by applicable laws and regulations. Regulatory bodies may require a more lengthy maintenance period. The complexity of meeting the different requirements of different entities makes it difficult to meet all requirements; thus, it may be easier to retain all records indefinitely. Included in this documentation are the records of products; patients and donors; and facilities, equipment, supplies, reagents and personnel. Electronic versions may be retained with appropriate backup, and one approach is to retain current supply records (including certificates of analysis) in paper form and then scan for long-term retention.

3.5 Summary

Completely avoiding citations may not be possible and there are many more standards than this chapter could possibly mention; however, standards that present the most frequent citations were outlined and potential strategies to assure compliance were delineated.

It is important to always carefully use the FACT Hematopoietic Cellular Therapy Accreditation Manual which is filled with helpful suggestions and interpretations, and to monitor the FACT website for updates to the standards, such as new editions and interim requirements.

Reference

FACT-JACIE International Standards for Hematopoietic Cellular Therapy Product Collection, Processing, and Administration, Seventh Edition, March 2018

Donor Evaluation for Hematopoietic Stem and Progenitor Cell Collection

4

Laura S. Connelly-Smith

4.1 Introduction

Hematopoietic cell transplantation (HCT) remains a potentially curative treatment for life-threatening hematological and non-hematological diseases. Over the last several years, the total number of HCTs performed worldwide has exceeded 60,000 a year (Niederwieser et al. 2016; Gratwohl et al. 2010). Autologous hematopoietic cell transplantation (auto-HCT) accounts for the majority of all procedures performed, and in the United States, the number continues to increase at a fast rate, mainly from transplants performed for plasma cell and lymphoproliferative disorders extending to older patients (Gratwohl et al. 2010; Center for International Blood and Marrow Transplant Research (CIBMTR) 2016). Allogeneic HCTs (allo-HCT) have exceeded 30,000 per year worldwide with the number of transplant recipients surpassing 8000 a year in the United States (Center for International Blood and Marrow Transplant Research (CIBMTR) 2016). Approximately 70% of allogeneic transplants use hematopoietic progenitor cells (HPCs) from volunteered unrelated donors (URDs). Advances in HLA typing, new immunosuppressive protocols, improved supportive care, and the administration of nonmyeloablative (NMA) or reduced-intensity conditioning (RIC) regimens contribute to the increased frequency of HCT. The observed continuous annual increase of around 10% is mainly because of a rise in allo-HCT from URDs (Gratwohl et al. 2010, 2013). There has also been an increase in alternate donor sources with HLA-haploidentical donors now exceeding umbilical cord blood transplants (Center for International Blood and Marrow Transplant Research (CIBMTR) 2016).

L. S. Connelly-Smith (✉)
Apheresis and Cellular Therapy, SCCA, Seattle, WA, USA

Division of Hematology, UW Medical Center, Seattle, WA, USA

Fred Hutch, Seattle, WA, USA
e-mail: Lauracs1@seattlecca.org

S. A. Abutalib et al. (eds.), *Best Practices of Apheresis in Hematopoietic Cell Transplantation*, Advances and Controversies in Hematopoietic Transplantation and Cell Therapy, https://doi.org/10.1007/978-3-319-55131-9_4

Although CD34^{+} cell donation by apheresis is considered a relatively safe procedure with very low rates of serious adverse events (Schmidt et al. 2017), the risk of both physical and psychological harm exists. At the same time, there is also potential harm to any recipient through the infusion of the graft, especially by communicable diseases. For allogenic donors, it is important to optimize the whole donation experience as these donors will undergo a procedure for which they will not be receiving any direct benefit. There is however a potential sense of satisfaction derived from this altruistic act (Boo et al. 2011). Therefore, for URD, an excellent reputation of a safe and efficient process is needed to ensure adequate number of donors being maintained and joining the national registries (Billen et al. 2014).

Pretransplant donor evaluation is an essential process to safeguard the quality and safety of donation. The primary goals of allo-HCT donor evaluation are to ensure that a) there is minimal risk to the health of the donor from the collection procedure and b) to protect the recipient from transmissible diseases.

4.2 Regulatory Guidance, National Registries, and Accreditation Agencies

On May 25, 2005, the US Food and Drug Administration (FDA) implemented comprehensive regulations governing the collection and manufacture of human products for transplantation and immune modulation, as well as a variety of other cellular- and tissue-based human products (Food and Drug Administration 2005). These regulations are based on the FDA's responsibility to limit the transmission of infectious diseases through the administration of these products and apply to peripheral blood stem cells, cord blood, and donor lymphocytes. The responsibility for bone marrow regulations has been assigned to the Health Resources and Services Administration (HRSA).

The FDA regulations include the requirements for establishing donor eligibility and apply not only to products collected or manufactured within the country, but also to those imported from outside the United States (Food and Drug Administration 2005). Other international regulatory bodies, for example, European Directives for Donation of Tissues and Cellular Therapy Products (Human Tissue Authority (HTA) Regulations 2007) also have detailed requirements for donor evaluation to ensure the safety of the product for the recipient; however, unlike FDA regulations, they do not address donor safety issues.

Given the extensive international collaboration and exchange of HPC products, most regulatory agencies work closely with national registries, such as the National Marrow Donor Program (NMDP) and the World Marrow Donor Association (WMDA). These national registries develop and establish appropriate guidance to ensure HPC donation is performed safely and ethically in volunteer URDs and have published their recommendations for donor evaluation (Sacchi et al. 2008; Lown et al. 2014; National Marrow Donor Program (NMDP) n.d.-a). Donors are assessed as to their suitability and eligibility to donate HPCs. Donor suitability refers to the general health or medical fitness of any autologous or allogeneic HPC donor to undergo the collection procedures. Donors are evaluated as to their risk and overall safety to donate. Donor eligibility refers to issues that relate to an allogeneic donor for who all screening and testing has been completed in accordance with applicable laws and regulations and who has been determined to be free of risk factors for relevant communicable diseases. URDs are only eligible if they are unrestrictedly healthy. Often however, physicians struggle with decision making as to the suitability of a relative as a donor that would not otherwise meet the suitability criteria for unrelated donation. The suitability criteria for related donors (RDs) is often less strict and with considerable variability between transplant centers. Differences between RDs and URDs may exist in mobilization and collection practices (Sacchi et al. 2008; Confer et al. 2011; O'Donnell et al. 2010; Clare et al. 2010). Published data suggest that the risks for serious adverse events and reactions might be higher for RDs than for URDs, but the amount of adequate prospective data in the RD setting is still limited (Halter et al. 2009; Kodera et al. 2014). Many institutions have developed their own processes for the evaluation of RDs; historically, there had been no national guidance available. In 2015, the Worldwide Network for Blood and Marrow Standing Committee on Donor Issues developed a consensus document with recommendations for donor workup and final clearance of family donors that would otherwise not be able to serve as URD because of age or preexisting diseases (Worel et al. 2015).

The FACT-JACIE (Foundation for the Accreditation of Cellular Therapy/Joint Accreditation Committee ISCT and EBMT) international standards were founded in 1994 to address obstacles faced when transplantation involves donors and recipients in different countries. This voluntary organization establishes international guidelines for the collection and transfer of hematopoietic stem cells. Members include donor registries, cord blood registries, and numerous individuals working together to advance HCT. FACT/JACIE addresses issues, including donor evaluation criteria, a donor follow-up policy, and the requirement that "Allogeneic donor suitability should be evaluated by a physician who is not the physician of the recipient." Accreditation is the means which a center can demonstrate that it is performing a required level of practice in accordance with agreed standards of excellence. Essentially it allows a center to certify that it operates an effective quality management system. In many countries, however, accreditation is not mandatory for centers assessing RDs. Improved compliance with internationally recognized donor care paradigms have been seen in centers with FACT-JACIE accreditation; however, important practice gaps in all centers irrespective of accreditation continue to be seen (Anthias et al. 2016a, b). Other organizations that provide additional insight into US regulations regarding donor evaluation include the AABB, the American Society for Blood and Marrow Transplant (ASBMT), the International Society for Cellular Therapy (ISCT), and the Center for International Blood and Marrow Transplant Research (CIBMTR).

4.3 Donor Assessment

4.3.1 Donor Eligibility

Similar to blood transfusion, HPC donation has the potential to transmit a wide range of blood-borne diseases. For example, hepatitis B (Lau et al. 1999), hepatitis C (Strasser and McDonald 1999; Shuhart et al. 1994), human T-lymphotrophic virus type 1 (HTLV-1) and type 2 (HTLV-2) (Kikuchi et al. 2000; Ljungman et al. 1994), Chagas disease (Villalba et al. 1992), malaria (Mejia et al. 2012), syphilis (Naohara et al. 1997), and brucellosis (Ertem et al. 2000) have all been reported to be transmitted by HPCs. In the United States, strict federal regulations regarding the evaluation of HPC donors are laid out in Title 21 of the Code of Federal regulations; Part 1271 (Human cells, Tissues and Cellular- and Tissue-Based Products). Subpart C is Donor Eligibility Determination and lays out the requirements for donor screening and testing for "relevant" communicable disease agents and diseases (RCDAD) (Table 4.1). Relevant communicable disease agents and diseases (RCDADs) are identified by the FDA as having the potential to cause significant pathogenicity to recipients of human cells, tissues, and cellular- and tissue-based products and are defined as infections that

Table 4.1 Current relevant communicable disease agents and diseases (RCDADs) for viable leukocyte rich human cells, tissues, and cellular- and tissue-based products

RCDAD	Evaluation	
Specifically listed in CFR	Screening	Testing
HIV types 1 and 2	X	X
Hepatitis B	X	X
Hepatitis C	X	X
HTLV types 1 and 2	X	X
Creutzfeldt-Jakob disease (CJD)/ variant CJD	X	
Treponema pallidum (syphilis)	X	X
Risks associated with xenotransplant	X	
CMV		X
Not specifically listed		
WNV (June 1–October 31)[a]	X	X
ZIKV	X	
Trypanosoma cruzi (Chagas)[b]	X	X
Sepsis	X	
Vaccinia virus infection	X	

HIV human immunodeficiency virus, *HTLV* human T-cell lymphotropic virus, *CMV* cytomegalovirus, *WNV* west nile virus, *ZIKV* zika virus

[a]In US FDA requires NAT testing for WNV between the months of June 1 and October 31

[b]Evaluation for Chagas disease in draft guidance

1. Bring risk of transmission to the recipient
2. Have a severe effect on the recipient if transmitted
3. Have available appropriate screening measures or tests to identify the potential donor's risks of exposure to and/or possible infection with the disease

The FDA identifies specific RCDADs by listing them either specifically in the CFR or by publishing a guidance document to communicate any changes. Some institutions and accreditation bodies may choose to include evaluation of other agents or diseases such as malaria.

To determine eligibility, donors need to be screened and tested for RCDADs. Assessing the risk of disease transmission involves three components (Food and Drug Administration 2005):

1. Targeted screening history
2. Examination for physical signs of disease
3. Laboratory testing for specific pathogens or traits

A **screening history** involves interviewing the donor about their medical history and relevant social behavior. It includes the review of relevant medical records for clinical evidence of RCDADs. The FDA recommends that the screening interview be a documented dialogue, administered by phone or in person, with appropriate follow-up or verification by a trained individual if the donor health history is self-administered. Various registries have developed HPC donor-screening questionnaires and their use recommended, to elicit medical history and to identify high-risk behaviors associated with risk of disease transmission (AABB n.d.-a; National Marrow Donor Program 2002). The screening history should also include communicable disease risks associated with xenotransplantation. One such questionnaire that is freely available is the hematopoietic progenitor cell (HPC), Apheresis and HPC, Marrow Donor History Questionnaire (DHQ) (Appendix 4.1) developed by the AABB Inter-organizational DHQ-HPC Task Force to provide establishments with a standardized tool to screen allogeneic HPC donors for communicable disease risk factors in accordance with requirements of the FDA, AABB, FACT, and the NMDP (AABB n.d.-a).

These DHQ materials are periodically reviewed to ensure continued compliance with regulatory and accrediting agencies. Companion documents provide rationale for the questioning and recommendations for evaluation of responses (AABB n.d.-b). Institutions are notified of any changes as well as the timeline for implementation through existing publications and websites maintained by members of the task force. When a new version of the documents is posted, the previous version is maintained for a period of time to allow facilities to transition to the new version. The NMDP has developed similar medical history questionnaires to support its work with unrelated donors (https://network.bethematchclinical.org/workarea/downloadasset n.d.).

In the process of completing the DHQ, clinical staff must verbally interact with the donor to review and verify donor's responses to the DHQ and to ensure the DHQ was signed and dated. All donors should have appropriate age-related donor health questionnaires with a parent or legal guardian (proxy) when required for age. Appropriate arrangements must be made for donors with developmental delays, appropriate interpreters for nonnational-speaking patients. Donors who are not English or native speaking in the country of assessment should have a medical interpreter who is not a family member or friend of the family.

A **physical examination** should be performed to identify any signs or stigmata that may indicate high-risk behavior for or infection with RCDAD(s). The examination should include recent tattoos, piercings, or signs of intravenous drug use, as well as signs of significant illnesses to determine eligibility for the donation procedure. Several institutions have developed a supplemental examination checklist (Appendix 4.2) to ensure a thorough examination for signs or stigmata of RCDADs.

In accordance with FDA regulation, **laboratory testing** using FDA-approved assays must be performed on the donor' blood for, at least, the following infectious disease agents: human immunodeficiency virus 1 and 2 (HIV 1 and 2), hepatitis B virus (HBV), hepatitis C (HCV), *Treponema pallidum* (syphilis), human T-cell lymphotrophic virus I and II (HTLV I and II), and cytomegalovirus (CMV). The FDA has provided core requirements for laboratory testing (Table 4.2). For emerging infectious diseases including the Zika virus (ZIKV), severe acute respiratory syndrome (SARS), and West Nile virus (WNV), additional screening questions were emergently added to the donor qualification process in the United States, based upon recommendations from the FDA. WNV is only infectious during the viremic phase and NAT testing must be performed concomitantly with product collection (or within 7 days before or after collection). While it might not be possible to prevent the infusion of an infected product, knowing that a product was infected with WNV would provide an opportunity to develop a preemptive treatment strategy. In the United States, WNV testing is to be performed specifically between June 1 and October 31 of each year. For all other establishments and intending to import human cells, tissues, and cellular- and tissue-based products into the United States, testing of human cells, tissues, and cellular- and tissue-based products donors for WNV should be performed year-round.

It is also desirable to perform testing for prior infections with varicella zoster virus (VZV) and Epstein-Barr virus (EBV) and possibly others, such as

Table 4.2 FDA core requirements for laboratory testing

– Use appropriate FDA-licensed, FDA-approved, or FDA-cleared donor-screening tests (Table 4.3)
– Laboratories used for laboratory testing must be certified under the Clinical Laboratory Improvement Amendments of 1988 (42 U.S.C. 263a) and 42 CFR part 493, or equivalent requirements as determined by the Centers for Medicare and Medicaid Services (CMS)
– Testing must be performed in accordance with the manufacturer's instructions for use (IFU)
– For Hematopoietic Stem/Progenitor Cell (HSPC) Donors the laboratory specimen to be used for donor testing may be collected up to 30 days prior to or within 7 days after human cells, tissues, and cellular- and tissue-based products recovery. For all other cells or tissue from the donor, laboratory testing must be performed at or up to 7 days before or after recovery

Table 4.3 Examples of FDA-licensed donor-screening tests

Pathogen	FDA-licensed screening test
HIV-1	• Anti-HIV-1 or combo test for anti-HIV-1 and anti-HIV-2, **AND** • NAT test for HIV-1 or combination NAT testHIV-2
HIV-2	• Anti-HIV-2 or combo test for anti-HIV-1 and HIV-2
HTLV-I/II	• Anti-HTLV-I/II
HBV	• Hepatitis B surface antigen (HBsAg), **AND** • Total antibody to hepatitis B core antigen (IgG & IgM; anti-HBc) • NAT test for HBV
HCV	• Anti-HCV • NAT test for HCV or combination test
WNV	• NAT test for WNV
Treponema pallidum	• Nontreponemal or treponemal
CMV	• Anti-CMV, total IgG, and IgM

HIV human immunodeficiency virus, *HTLV* human T-cell lymphotropic virus, *CMV* cytomegalovirus, *WNV* west nile virus, *ZIKV* zika virus

toxoplasmosis. Positive tests for exposure to these agents may not preclude donation or make the donor ineligible but may modify the transplant approach or post-transplant surveillance strategies.

All RCDAD screening results should be communicated effectively to the collection center as well as to the physician responsible for accepting the human cells, tissues, and cellular- and tissue-based products. This notification should be part of a standard procedure and clearly documented. Any human cells, tissues, and cellular- and tissue-based products donor whose specimen tests positive (or reactive) using any of the assays is considered ineligible (exception syphilis and CMV screening). Confirmatory tests should be considered when a positive (or reactive) screening test result is received for such purposes as donor counseling or investigating discordant test results. If a confirmatory test is performed and is negative or nonreactive, these results would not override a positive or reactive screening test and the donor still remains ineligible. Screening tests for syphilis are the exception. Because of the potential for false-positive results in nontreponemal testing, if a specific treponemal confirmatory test is negative, the donor will be deemed eligible from syphilis standpoint. A donor who tests positive or reactive for CMV is not necessarily ineligible to donate human cells, tissues, and cellular- and tissue-based products. A positive or reactive (past or recent exposure (IgG or IgM)) CMV test result should also be communicated to the physician responsible for accepting the human cells, tissues, and cellular- and tissue-based products. In case of a positive IgM CMV, it is best to exclude CMV seroconversion.

After completion of donor eligibility screening history, physical examination, and laboratory tests, written donor eligibility determination is required for all human cells, tissues, and cellular- and tissue-based products donors, except for autologous use. All human cells, tissues, and cellular- and tissue-based products must not be transplanted, infused, or transferred until the donor has been determined to be eligible, unless (1) there is no other appropriate donor and the proposed donor poses less risk to the recipient than not using the donor and (2) approval is obtained from the recipient to proceed with transplantation using these cells. This often poses concern because information about donor health is strictly confidential and can only been released with explicit permission from the donor. If HPC collection proceeds with an ineligible donor, written justification is needed and shall be documented.

The results of these RCDAD screening tests must be reviewed prior to initiating preparative conditioning therapy in the recipient. If the time between initial donor evaluation and collection is delayed, repeat testing may be necessary. In the event of missing or incomplete screening test results at the time of HPC collection, the product should be labeled clearly by the collection center that the product has not been evaluated for infectious disease markers. Donors are declared as ineligible, with processing centers having policies and procedures in place for the storage and release of "ineligible donor" products.

4.3.2 Donor Suitability

All donors must be medically evaluated to detect conditions that might significantly increase donor risk to unacceptable levels and to ensure their safety to donate. Peripheral blood hematopoietic progenitor cell (HPC) donation typically involves the administration of 4 or 5 daily injections of granulocyte-colony stimulating factor (G-CSF) and/or other mobilizing agent followed by apheresis collection. For autologous patients, mobilization commonly includes G-CSF +/− plerixafor or chemotherapy. Side effects of HPC mobilization with G-CSF or other mobilization agent(s) and apheresis collection should be taken into consideration when assessing donor suitability. The designated physician (or appropriately licensed supervised advanced practitioner) performs a medical history and physical examination according to standard medical practice. Medical records should also be reviewed as part of the assessment. The history not only provides an additional opportunity to review/affirm questions provided on donor screening health questionnaire but looks to evaluate current health. Typical questions to be covered during history taking are seen in Table 4.4. The physical examination will also include assessment of signs/stigmata of RCDADs (Appendix 4.2). Vital sign testing, height, weight, noting Karnofsky- or Lansky- performance scores, and assessment of venous access are an essential part of the physical examination. Laboratory testing and other investigations are also required to evaluate a donor's suitability (Table 4.5).

The NMDP has developed several tools or lists of clinical disorders/diseases to assess an URD donor's health and RCDAD risk (National Marrow Donor Program (NMDP) n.d.-a). Several centers often use these tools as guidance for their RDs. Donors with atypical responses to screening questions, history, and physical examination must be evaluated on a case-by-case basis to determine the donor's eligibility and suitability. The individual performing or evaluating the health screening, history, and PE should be knowledgeable by training or experience to accept or defer donors. In general, donors with moderate or severe organ impairment should be deferred; this includes donors with coronary artery disease and renal or hepatic impairment. Occasionally, a medical condition is identified that does not warrant

Table 4.4 Typical questions asked on taking a donor history

History of heparin allergy, heparin intolerance, heparin-induced thrombocytopenia
History of requirement for therapeutic anticoagulation
Immunization history
Blood product transfusions and donation(s)
Allergies
Current medication (prescription and nonprescription)
Previous exposure to anesthetics and family history of problems to anesthesia
Infectious disease risk including recent upper and lower respiratory tract infections within the last 30 days, risk of tuberculosis exposure
Pulmonary and upper airway disease
Cardiovascular disease including treatment
Diabetes mellitus
Arthritis including back problems
Autoimmune diseases
Abnormalities of the spine
Possibility of pregnancy for all biological female donors with reproductive potential
Travel history
Cancer
Inherited disease(s)

Table 4.5 Typical laboratory and other investigations performed in donor evaluation

Complete blood count (CBC) with differential and reticulocyte count
Electrolytes (Na, K, CO_2, chloride), blood urea nitrogen (BUN) and creatinine, alkaline phosphatase, lactate dehydrogenase (LDH), alanine aminotransferase (ALT, SGPT), glucose, serum total protein plus albumin, or serum protein electrophoresis
ABO, Rh typing, antibody screening
Infectious disease markers (IDMs) (see above)
CMV antibody screening (see text)
Serum beta-HCG pregnancy (if female of child-bearing potential)
Malarial testing if donors travelled to malaria endemic areas
Screening for hemoglobinopathy (e.g., SickleDex or equivalent)
If donating for Thalassemia patient, thalassemia screening for hemoglobin A, A2, and F
urinalysis
Tuberculosis testing as clinically indicated
Oxygen saturation
Chest X-ray and EKG as clinically indicated. Chest X-ray and EKG are not routinely required However, they may be performed at the discretion of the examining medical professional or the collection facility/donor center physicians based on medical assessment Criteria for whom to perform an EKG may include • History of diabetes mellitus (DM) • History of cardiovascular disease (CVD) • Treatment with digoxin or diuretics • Pulmonary disease (room air $O_2 < 90\%$) • Smoking >20 pack years • Age over 40 (males) and over 50 (females) • If a delay in donor collection of more than 30 days repeat EKG may be required in certain cases such as history of DM, CVD, and treatment with digoxin or diuretics. Otherwise for other donors this can be repeated if more than 6 months since the last EKG Criteria for who to perform a chest X-ray may include • History of pulmonary disease • Oxygen saturation <90%

immediate deferral, but may require further investigation. Any referral to a specialist or additional workup required should be expedited and the recipients team should be informed as soon as possible so that the transplant clinicians can determine whether or not the donor, if found to be suitable, would be available in a timely manner.

If a donor is deemed unsuitable but a decision is made that there is no other suitable donor available and the donor is prepared to take a reasonable risk, a justification must be documented.

In the event that the transplant procedure is delayed, collection or transplant facilities may require repeat donor assessment within a specified time. The NMDP requires that donor assessment is always current to within 12 weeks (3 months) of the proposed collection date. This includes a repeat administration of a screening questionnaire with additional tests to ensure continuing medical suitability based on updated information provided. There are no mandatory tests and NMDP does not require any extended testing when less than 6 months have passed since the original physical examination date. Laboratory markers for RCDADs however will need to be repeated within 30 days from collection of HPCs (Table 4.2).

Additional risks for recipient safety following donation, other than infectious diseases, that need to be assessed during evaluation of the donor include autoimmune diseases (ADs), inherited diseases, and malignancy. The development of an AI disorder from a donor with the same condition has been reported and includes thyroid disease (Olivares et al. 2002; Thomson et al. 1995), diabetes mellitus (Lampeter et al. 1998), psoriasis (Snowden and Heaton 1997), and vitiligo (Campbell-Fontaine et al. 2005). Inherited diseases within the hematopoietic system that will be transmitted include hemoglobinopathies such as sickle cell disease, thalassemia, congenital platelet disorders, and inherited bone marrow failure syndromes.

Transmissions of malignant diseases from donors to patients have been reported in the past, most of them inadvertently from subclinical malignant disease or diseases not recognized by the current screening methods. The risk for transmission of tumors is assumed to be of a very low incidence. These rates do not include secondary malignancies of donor cell origin arising in the recipient after allo-HCT.

In addition, patients with a history of heparin allergy, heparin intolerance, or heparin-induced thrombocytopenia are at increased risk for complications with infusion of heparin-containing products. This is essentially important if heparin is used as part of the anticoagulant during the apheresis collection process. Donor evaluation provides an ideal opportunity to get full informed consent. The donor would require a comprehensive discussion of potential risks and "theoretical donor safety" issues. The donor should be aware that they are not obliged to donate, even if for a family member. There should be no coercion and it is essential that allogeneic donor suitability should be evaluated by a physician who is not the physician of the recipient. If the donor consents to donation and then chooses to pull out of their decision after the recipient has started conditioning treatment, the potential risks to the recipient should be discussed fully with the donor.

4.4 Children as Donors

The most suitable donor for younger patients who undergo allo-HCT is often a minor sibling. In rare cases, children may also be considered as potential donors for an adult sibling, parent, or other family member. Worldwide data indicate that more than 30% of children undergoing HCT receive allografts from siblings under the age of 18 (Miano et al. 2007). The use of minors as HPC donors is considered medically safe (Pulsipher et al. 2005) and legally accepted given that no alternative approach of comparable effectiveness exists; however, donation of HPCs is not without risk (Pulsipher et al. 2013; Styczynski et al. 2012; Grupp et al. 2006) and appropriate medical evaluation of the donor is essential.

The source of the graft (peripheral blood vs. bone marrow) has the greatest influence on the type of adverse events that may present. It is important to note that in children majority of grafts are of bone marrow origin. Side effects include pain, either from G-CSF treatment, placement of central venous catheter (CVC), or the puncture wounds made when harvesting bone marrow. Most young donors will require a CVC for apheresis, thus, exposing them to potential risks such as bleeding, infection, pneumothorax, and complications of sedation or general anesthesia (Pulsipher et al. 2005; Styczynski et al. 2012). Collection of peripheral blood graft requires special attention in children, with the use of growth factors being the main issue. Long-term adverse effects from a brief treatment course with G-CSF for the harvest of HPCs via apheresis continues to be studied in ongoing investigations, but to date, no convincing evidence has shown significant health risks (Pulsipher et al. 2006). The worldwide network for blood and marrow transplantation (WBMT) recommends G-CSF is used with caution and only when needed and emphasize the need for long-term follow-up for these donors (Halter et al. 2013). Several published findings suggest that pediatric donors may experience psychosocial issues around the time of and following donation including higher anxiety and lower self-esteem than non-donors (Packman et al. 2008), moderate levels of post-traumatic stress, depression, behavioral problems, identity problems, guilt, and resentment (Packman et al. 1997, 2008; Wiener et al. 2007). Young donors may also fear the medical aspects and pain involved in donation and experience anxiety and ambivalence about donation (Kinrade 1987; MacLeod et al. 2003).

Although parents for the majority consent to medical interventions on behalf of their children, respecting a child's autonomy and obtaining a child's assent or appropriately regarding his or her dissent or refusal—is generally thought to be of paramount ethical importance. Decision makers are burdened with great responsibility: their choice will have life-and-death consequences for another vulnerable child.

Recognizing that HPC donation has no physical benefit to these young donors and its associated with potential risks, the American Academy of Pediatrics Committee on Bioethics (AAPCOB) (Committee on Bioethics 2010) has published guidelines specifying when minors may ethically serve as HPC donors. The AAPCOB has deemed that children may ethically serve as hematopoietic stem cell donors if five criteria are fulfilled (Table 4.6).

Table 4.6 The 5 AAPCOB criteria for minors to ethically serve as hematopoietic progenitor cell donors (Committee on Bioethics 2010)

1. There is no medically equivalent histocompatible adult relative who is willing and able to donate
2. There is a strong personal and emotionally positive relationship between the donor and recipient
3. There is a reasonable likelihood that the recipient will benefit
4. The clinical, emotional, and psychosocial risks to the donor are minimized and are reasonable in relation to the benefits expected to accrue to the donor and to the recipient
5. Parental permission and, where appropriate, child assent have been obtained

A donor advocate with expertise in pediatric development (second physician or a child life specialist) should be appointed for all children who have not reached the age of majority (age at which a person is recognized by state law to be an adult) and who are being evaluated as hematopoietic graft donors. The donor advocate must be independent of the team responsible for direct care of the recipient to ensure that the AAPCOB recommendations are met. He or she should ideally be involved from the onset, starting with the decision about whether the minor should undergo HLA testing so that potential family or sibling donors with medical or psychological reasons not to donate would not be HLA typed. Donors with medical conditions should be carefully examined by skilled professionals, and if their risks of complications with collection are increased, they should be deferred.

In the advancement of the effectiveness of different hematopoietic stem cell transplants, research is often needed to be performed on donors and/or recipients. When the donor is a minor, the research must conform to the federal regulations governing pediatric subjects. This may require national review when the research imposes more than minimal risk without prospect of direct benefit to donor subjects. Several publications have addressed this area and should be considered before donors are evaluated for research (Wendler et al. 2016; Shah et al. 2015).

4.5 Older Adults as Donors

With the increased availability of NMA conditioning over the last two decades (Pingali and Champlin 2015; Alyea et al. 2005), and improvement in supportive care, the ability of many older patients to tolerate allo-HCT has now become apparent. For older patients, an HLA-matched sibling is often a donor. Unlike URD registries, there are no strict age limits recommended for related allogeneic donors. There is experience available in the literature for donors up to the age of 75 years.

Many health disorders are more prevalent with increasing chronological age, including cardiovascular, cerebrovascular and peripheral vascular disease, chronic airways diseases, diabetes mellitus, malignancies, etc., and must be taken into consideration by any provider assessing the suitability of an older individual to donate. In some reports, HPC collection by apheresis seems to be a safe procedure for donors ≥60 including those with significant comorbidities (Ghada et al. 2006). However, certain complications are more frequent in the older donors and have demonstrated more procedure related complications than younger donors (Lysák et al. 2011). For example, one study demonstrated higher complications associated with hypocalcemia, thrombocytopenia, and problems with venous access in donors ≥55 years of age compared with younger donors (29% vs. 15%, $P = 0.0096$). Venous access complications were also more frequently present in donors with circulatory system diseases (arterial hypertension, chronic venous insufficiency) compared with the donors without this medical history (11% vs. 3%, $P = 0.006$) (Lysák et al. 2011). A recent related-donor safety study, looking at health-related quality of life issues among older related HCT donors (>60 years) compared to younger adult counterparts, showed very few differences in indicators in physical and mental health donation-related experiences (Switzer et al. 2017). This may suggest that older sibling donors do not experience the donation process as significantly more physically or psychologically impactful than their younger counterparts and, in some aspects, their experiences were more positive—for example, less donation-related pain and less anxiety about donation. There was less conclusive evidence supporting the procedure in sibling donors as old as mid-70s (Switzer et al. 2017).

Regarding graft composition, some authors have found that in older donors may be different from that obtained in younger donors (Al-Ali et al. 2011; Richa et al. 2009; Miller 1996) with $CD34^+$ cells in the peripheral blood and apheresis yield being lower in older donors (Richa et al. 2009; Suzuya et al. 2005). One study noted the failure of mobilization (collection of less than $2 \times 10^6 CD34^+$cells/kg of recipient body weight) rate at 7% in the older donor group (≥55 years) versus 0.8% in the younger donor group. It was noted, however, that in donors younger than 50 years, the relationship is not statistically significant and is no longer an independent prognostic factor, also seen by other studies (Ings et al. 2006). Several studies have however reported contradictory results regarding donor-predicting factors for mobilization and yield and cannot confirm an independent influence of age on mobilization (Bagnara et al. 2000; Miflin et al. 1996; Rinaldi et al. 2012). There is some suggestion that the conflicting results are likely due to often small sample sizes and heterogeneous treatment with mobilizing regimens (Lysák et al. 2011).

In autologous transplantation, elderly patients can have a high risk of poor mobilization (Goker et al. 2015). Some studies reported that $CD34^+$ cell mobilization in patients of advanced age (70 years and older) with multiple myeloma was poor but still possible (Morris et al. 2003). This is contrary to that reported suggesting no differences in the mobilization kinetics between younger (<65 years) and older (≥65 years) myeloma patients (Jantunen et al. 2006). Other investigations into whether age affects mobilization in autologous transplantation has also been contradictory in donors <70 years old (Bensinger et al. 1994, 1995). Therefore, age can be a confounding factor in autologous stem cell mobilization. Several donor factors predict outcome after allo-HCT and age is one of the important non-HLA factors affecting the survival rates after transplantation (Kollman et al. 2001). Clinical practice often prefers "HLA-matched siblings" as first-line donors for transplantation despite donor's age; however, the survival rates for unrelated donor transplants with young fully HLA compatible donors are similar to those using older sibling donors (Kollman et al. 2016). Allo-HCT from older adults have been associated with higher nonrelapse mortality (NRM) but donor age was not associated with relapse (Kollman et al. 2016). Observed higher rates of grade II to IV acute GvHD after transplantation of grafts from older donors may be explained by replacement of naïve T-cells with memory T-cells as the immune system ages in the older donors (Miller 1996).

4.6 Donors with Psychological/Psychiatric Disorders

On occasion, the only matched related donor identified may be an individual who has a known psychological/psychiatric disorder, and the decision for any physician to deem this prospective donor suitable may be very difficult indeed. In 2013, the WBMT standing committee on donor issues held an international workshop to develop a consensus document with recommendations of suitability criteria for final donor workup in family donors and included donors with psychological-psychiatric disorders (Worel et al. 2015). These recommendations as well as recruitment assessment tools such as those used by NMDP registries may be helpful for physicians who have concerns about suitability in these donors (National Marrow Donor Program (NMDP) n.d.-a, n.d.-b).

Donors with a history of substance abuse may not be automatically deferred, but require a careful history and medical assessment. Donors should be assessed for risk factors for infectious diseases or underlying psychiatric disorders. Compulsive dependence on a chemical can cause various physical ailments such as liver damage secondary to alcohol abuse. In the case of infrequent substance abuse with marijuana alone, individuals are mostly suitable but may require cessation of use before donation or initiating G-CSF. Donors with a previous history (and not currently using) of cocaine, crack, and methamphetamine (intranasal/oral) abuse might also be suitable; however, the use of these drugs has been associated with an increased risk of cardiovascular disorders, and careful assessment of the donor is required. In intravenous drug abusers, donation is generally not recommended due to the increased risk of communicable diseases such as HIV, hepatitis B, and hepatitis C with contaminated needles. Individuals who are on a substitution program but otherwise healthy may be suitable.

Donors with eating disorders (anorexia and/or bulimia) are suitable only if their disease is stable under appropriate treatment and their BMI is >16.0 in adults (Worel et al. 2015). These potential donors should be deferred if their overall physical status (including body size, demeanor, skin color, etc.) indicates serious health concerns.

HPC donation in individuals with multiple personality disorders and psychosis is generally not recommended. Subjects with obsessive-compulsive, attention deficit, or attention-deficit hyperactivity disorders are suitable if their disease is well controlled. However, the donor's capacity to follow through the donation process may be affected.

In donors with underlying psychiatric disorders such as anxiety, depression, and bipolar disorders or in donors where there is concern that donors may not follow-through with donation, bone marrow harvest procedures may be questionable and apheresis collection and cryopreservation should be considered in advance before the conditioning regimen is started.

4.7 Medication

Certain medication may potentially defer a donation or render a donor ineligible (Table 4.7) due to concern for potential RCDAD transmitted by transfusions and HCT. Donors would be declared ineligible but may be able to donate dependent on institutional practice.

For the majority of potential donors, it is not usually the medication that they are taking that is likely to be a concern, but rather the underlying medical condition for which that treatment was prescribed, that may make a donor unsuitable to donate. Certain medications would potentially increase donor or recipient risk, but these are often also required to treat a medical condition that would likely defer the donor as well (Table 4.8). For certain medication for which the donor's medical conditions are well controlled, the donor may be suitable to proceed with donation (Table 4.8). For donors on lithium, due to its interaction with GCSF, HPC collection using apheresis is generally not allowed and these donors may be considered and evaluated for marrow donation.

If a donor or a recipient has a past allergic reaction to heparin or a history of heparin-induced thrombocytopenia (HIT), the donor may donate by apheresis; however, the anticoagulant use for both circuit and product should be with ACD-A (i.e., citrate) alone.

Table 4.7 Medication rendering donor ineligibility (AABB Medication Deferral List n.d.)

- Human growth hormone. Concern for Creutzfeldt-Jakob disease (CJD)
- Donors with diabetes previously receiving bovine insulin. Concern for new variant CJD the same agent responsible for bovine spongiform encephalopathy (BSE) or "Mad Cow Disease"
- Hepatitis B immune globulin (HBIG) used to prevent infection following an exposure to HBV. HBIG does not prevent HBV infection in every case and if a donor has taken it in the last 12 months HBV can still be transmitted
- Unlicensed vaccine is usually associated with a research protocol and the effect with regard to stem cell recipients is unknown

Table 4.8 Recommendations for suitability to donate based on medication (National Marrow Donor Program (NMDP) 2016)

Accept	Evaluate for suitability	Defer related donor (author's practice)	Defers unrelated donor (NMDP practice)
Oral contraceptives	Short term oral steroids (taking <3 months) such as prednisone, hydrocortisone, cortisone	Uncontrolled diabetes	Insulin
Medications that have fetal risk (i.e. category X), such as isotretinoin, etretinate, finasteride, dutasteride, if underlying condition is acceptable	Anti-inflammatory or pain medications taken on daily/ frequent basis to control chronic pain such as ibuprofen, indomethacin, meperidine, celecoxib, hydrocodone	Chemotherapy including tamoxifen unless taking for cancer prevention	Chemotherapy including tamoxifen unless taking for cancer prevention

(continued)

Table 4.8 (continued)

Accept	Evaluate for suitability	Defer related donor (author's practice)	Defers unrelated donor (NMDP practice)
Thyroid hormone replacement medication (not for cancer), if well-controlled	Oral diabetic medications including chlorpropamide, tolbutamide, tolazamide, glipizide, glyburide, glimepiride	Patient on cardiac medications for angina or uncompensated CHF	Cardiac medications such as nitrates, nitroglycerin and digoxin
Prescription eye drops, if underlying condition is acceptable	Injected non-insulin medication such as exenatide or lyraglutide for treatment of diabetes	Immunosuppressive medication such as azathioprine, tacrolimus, MMF, cyclosporine, cyclophosphamide and methotrexate	Immunosuppressive medication such as azathioprine, tacrolimus, MMF, cyclosporine, cyclophosphamide and methotrexate
Topical medications (i.e., for acne) including topical steroids	Medications used as part of a clinical trial or investigation[a]	TNF Blockers	TNF Blockers
Allergy medications such as antihistamines or allergy shots		Long-term oral steroids (>3 months) such as prednisone, hydrocortisone, cortisone	Long-term oral steroids (>3 months) such as prednisone, hydrocortisone, cortisone
Antibiotic or antiviral, if treating current infection that is resolving or for treatment of acne		Treatment of a condition requiring antiplatelet agents for TIA or unmanaged cardiac disease. Treatment with anticoagulation for venous thromboembolism	Treatment of a condition requiring anticoagulant or antiplatelet medication
Anti-anxiety and anti-depression medications, such as diazepam and fluoxetine (selective serotonin reuptake inhibitors), if underlying condition is well-controlled		Lithium (Defer PB HPC donation, can collect donor by bone marrow harvest)	Lithium (Defer PB HPC donation, can collect donor by bone marrow harvest)
Hypertension medications, if blood pressure is well-controlled and there is no underlying cardiac disease			

Table 4.8 (continued)

Accept	Evaluate for suitability	Defer related donor (author's practice)	Defers unrelated donor (NMDP practice)
Over-the-counter vitamins, mineral, and herbal products			
Antacid or acid reflux medications such as proton pump inhibitors (PPIs), H2 receptor antagonists, if underlying condition is well controlled			

[a]Accept if participation in an investigational study that does not involve receipt of an experimental medication

4.8 Zika Virus

Zika virus (ZIKV) became a notifiable condition in the United States in January 2016 (Centers for Disease Control and Prevention 2016) and, by February of the same year, was declared a Public Health Emergency of International Concern by the World Health Organization (WHO 2005). Although infections are frequently asymptomatic or mildly symptomatic, deaths have been reported. Associations with severe neurologic complications in infants born to mothers infected with ZIKV during pregnancy as well as neurologic complications in adults (e.g., Guillain-Barre Syndrome) have made ZIKV a high-priority pathogen. There are currently no licensed vaccines or therapeutics against ZIKV (Food and Drug Administration 2017); however, there are numerous vaccine candidates currently in development. As of February 2016, local mosquito-borne transmission had not been reported in the continental United States, but only multiple travel-associated cases had been reported. In July 2016, Florida was added to the list of areas of risk of ZIKV transmission (Table 4.9). By February 2017, up to 200 documented cases of mosquito-borne transmission of ZIKV to a human had occurred in the continental United States in southern Florida and the Brownsville, Texas, area.

The FDA identified ZIKV as a RCDAD. The potential risk of transmission of ZIKV by HCT/Ps was supported by evidence that ZIKV has been detected in tissues such as semen and placenta. In March 2016, no FDA-cleared diagnostic tests for ZIKV were available and the FDA provided donor screening recommendations to reduce the risk of transmission of ZIKV by HCT/Ps (Food and Drug Administration 2016). All donors of HCT/Ps should be considered ineligible if they have had a medical diagnosis of ZIKV infection in the past 6 months and resided in, or travelled to, an area with active ZIKV transmission within the past 6 months. Donors were also declared ineligible if they had sex within the past 6 months with a male who was known to have either of the risk factors.

Table 4.9 List of areas with risk of ZIKV transmission (Centers for Disease Control and Prevention 2017)

Americas		
Anguilla	Dominican Republic	Panama
Antigua	Ecuador	Paraguay
Argentina	El Salvador	Peru
Aruba	Florida, state of*	Saba
Barbados	French Guiana	Saint Barthélemy
Belize	Grenada	Saint Lucia
Bolivia	Guadeloupe	Saint Martin
Bonaire	Guatemala	Saint Vincent and the
Brazil	Guyana	Grenadines
Colombia	Haiti	Saint Eustatius
Commonwealth of Puerto	Honduras	Saint Maarten
Rico, US territory	Jamaica	Suriname
Costa Rica	Martinique	Trinidad and Tobago
Cuba	Monserat	Turks and Caicos Islands
Curacao	Mexico	U.S Virgin Islands
Dominica	Nicaragua	Venezuela
Oceana/Pacific Islands	**Africa**	
American Samoa	Angola	Guinea-Bissau
Fiji	Benin	Kenya
Kosrae, Federated States of	Burkina-Faso	Liberia
Micronesia	Burundi	Mali
Marshall Islands	Cameroon	Niger
New Caledonia	Cape Verde	Nigeria
Palau	Central African Republic Chad	Rwanda
Papua New Guinea	Congo (Congo-Brazzaville)	Senegal
Samoa	Côte d'Ivoire Democratic	Sierra Leone
Solomon Islands	Republic of the Congo	South Sudan
Tonga	(Congo-Kinshasa)	Sudan
Asia	Equatorial Guinea Gabon	Tanzania
Bangladesh	Gambia	Togo
Burma (Myanmar)	Ghana	Uganda
Cambodia	Guinea	
India		
Indonesia		
Laos		
Malaysia		
Maldives		
Pakistan		
Philippines		
Singapore		
Thailand		
Timor-Leste (East Timor)		
Vietnam		

The first few blood transfusion transmissions that have been reported were in Brazil, where four transmissions occurred from three donors. On August 26, 2016, FDA issued revised guidance, recommending that blood centers in all states and the United States territories screen individual units of donated whole blood and blood components with a blood-screening test authorized for use by FDA under an investigational new drug (IND) application, or with a licensed test when available. In late 2016, blood centers began implementing investigational blood tests with nucleic acid testing (Goodnough and Marques 2017).

As of April 2017, there remained no commercially available diagnostic test cleared by FDA for the detection of ZIKV. Current tests with IND include serologic tests (to assess whether individuals who may have recently been exposed to ZIKV were actually infected) and PCR or NAT tests (to diagnose acute/active ZIKV infection).

There is currently no mandate to perform laboratory testing for ZIKV in HCT/Ps; however, several centers are currently using IND serological or NAT tests available to them. In the event that laboratory testing is performed, attention should be given to the following:

1. Results must be included in the donor's relevant medical records.
2. A reactive/positive test is considered a risk factor, even if an investigational test was used.
3. A nonreactive/negative test does not override any risk factors identified in the March 2016 ZIKV guidance (Food and Drug Administration 2016).

4.8.1 Expert Point of View

The donation of HPC is a well-recognized and regulated procedure that is performed on thousands of patients and donors throughout the world annually. Donation of autologous HPC is part of a treatment plan with high-dose therapy in these patients aiming for potential cure or at least prolonged remission from their underlying malignancy. The aim of their donated HPCs is to "rescue" the patients' marrows from the myeloablative chemotherapy received at the time of transplant for which a patient needs to be reasonably medically fit to receive. In these patients, suitability for HPC collection is often determined at the time of deeming the patient a suitable candidate for auto-HCT. The majority of severe complications are often associated with the pancytopenia accompanying chemomobilization. As a result of this as well as the predictability of cytokine only mobilized collections, several centers now collect autologous donor HPCs from using G-CSF with/without plerixafor as mobilization agent(s) only. These patients need to be assessed for suitability to donate; however, as the HPCs infused are their own, there is less concern for transmission of communicable diseases and eligibility to donate is not needed (Food and Drug Administration 2005).

Allogeneic HPC donation is a safe procedure with very low rates of serious adverse events. The side effects commonly faced during donation are transient for the majority of both related and unrelated donors. However, there have been several donation-related deaths (Halter et al. 2009), mostly in the related donor setting. As the majority of fatal and serious adverse events have occurred in donors with preexisting medical issues, it is suspected that robust donor assessment procedures will reduce fatal complications. Therefore, all donors must be carefully evaluated and fully informed prior to HPC donation by clinicians with good understanding of the potential physical and psychological complications and factors that may increase risk. As discussed, donors must also be able to provide informed consent without coercion or pressure and for this the medical evaluation of any allogeneic donor should never be conducted by a physician in the same transplant team caring for the recipient.

In addition to suitability determination, donor eligibility determination is also essential and physicians evaluating allogeneic donors should be up to date with regulations and laws governing screening requirements for RCDADs. These are important particularly with the emergence of new diseases such as that seen with WNV, SARS, and ZIKV.

Several regulatory agencies, registries, and accreditation bodies ensure steps taken to improve donor and patient safety alike. National and international registries continue to provide updated recommendations for the safe selection of unrelated donors and provide tools and recent guidance that could be extrapolated and used in the related donor setting (Sacchi et al. 2008; Lown et al. 2014; Worel et al. 2015). Donor and collection centers should be encouraged to enroll in accreditation bodies, such as FACT/JACIE and AABB, to enable potential improvements in the standard of donor evaluation and collection as well as to ensure continuous improvements in their own quality management system.

4.8.2 Future Directions

Despite 3–5-year survival rates being nearly similar between matched URD and sibling RD HCT (Horowitz 2012), the higher incidence of GvHD often assumes a matched sibling as the transplant physician's first choice for the majority of transplant indications. In light of this as well as the notable increase in the use of related HLA-haploidentical transplants (Center for International Blood and Marrow Transplant Research (CIBMTR) 2016), RD will continue to need appropriate evaluations as to their medical suitability to donate. There continues to be concern about the heterogeneity in the care of related HPC donors (O'Donnell et al. 2010). Changes to FACT standards (The Foundation for the Accreditation of Cellular Therapy (FACT) 2017) addressed some of these issues and there has since been some improvement in the practice of adult related-donor care (Anthias et al. 2016a, b). However, there still appears to be particular concerns including counseling and assessment of donors before HLA typing, with the use of unlicensed mobilization agents, and the absence of long-term donor follow-up (O'Donnell et al. 2010).

The World Marrow Donor Association (WMDA) brings forward a compelling argument for the management of RD to be performed by donor registries by offering an established structure for donor care, and extensive experience in the medical evaluation of donors. In particular, they suggest there should be significant consideration for registry provision of centralized donor follow-up (Anthias et al. 2015). Donor long-term follow-up is an important aspect of donor evaluation and further development of follow up of donors should be an integral part of a donor program to allow vigilance and surveillance of donations and improve knowledge of the risks of donation.

At the end of 2011, a US appeals court ruled that it was now legal to pay apheresis donors for their HPC (Medpage Today 2012). Unlike bone marrow tissue, it was felt that peripheral blood HPC are no different from other body fluids like semen and plasma where national organ transplant act (NOTA) does not prohibit paid donors. In a concession to the spirit of NOTA, it was deemed that the compensation could not be in the form of cash but rather a voucher that can be applied to things such as scholarships, education, housing, or donation to a charity. In 2011, the WMDA put out a position statement why HPC donors should not be paid (Boo et al. 2011). Reasons included ethical concerns raised by remuneration, potential to damage the public will to act altruistically, the potential for coercion and exploitation of donors, increased risk to patients, and harm to local transplantation programs and international stem cell exchange, and the povssibility of benefiting some patients while disadvantaging others.

Appendix 4.1: Example of Donor History Questionnaire[a]

Donor history questionnaire-HPC, apheresis and HPC, marrow	**Yes**	**No**	
Are you			
1. Currently taking an antibiotic?			
2. Currently taking any other medication for an infection?			
Please read the Medication Deferral List			
3. Are you now taking or have you ever taken any medications on the Medication List?			
4. Have you read the educational materials?			
In the past **12 weeks** have you			
5. Had any vaccinations or other shots?			
6. Had contact with someone who had a smallpox vaccination?			
In the past **12 months** have you			
7. Been told by a healthcare professional that you have West Nile Virus infection or any positive test for West Nile Virus?			
8. Had a blood transfusion?			
9. Come into contact with someone else's blood?			
10. Had an accidental needle-stick?			
11. Had a transplant or graft from someone other than yourself, such as organ, bone marrow, stem cell, cornea, sclera, bone, skin or other tissue?			
12. Had sexual contact with anyone who has HIV/AIDS or has had a positive test for the HIV/AIDS virus?			
13. Had sexual contact with a prostitute or anyone else who takes money or drugs or other payment for sex?			
14. Had sexual contact with anyone who has ever used needles to take drugs or steroids, or anything *not* prescribed by their doctor?			
15. Female donors: Had sexual contact with a male who has ever had sexual contact with another male? (Males: check "I am male.")			I am male ☐

16. Had sexual contact with a person who has hepatitis?		
17. Lived with a person who has hepatitis?		
18. Had a tattoo?		
19. Had ear or body piercing?		
20. Had or been treated for syphilis or other sexually transmitted infections?		
21. Been in juvenile detention, lockup, jail, or prison for more than 72 h?		
In the past **3 years** have you		
22. Been outside the United States or Canada?		
In the past **5 years**, have you		
23. Received money, drugs, or other payment for sex?		
24. Male donors: Had sexual contact with another male, even once? (Females: check "I am female.")		I am female ☐
25. Used needles to take drugs, steroids, or anything *not* prescribed by your doctor?		
From **1980 through 1996**		
26. Did you spend time that adds up to three (Center for International Blood and Marrow Transplant Research (CIBMTR) 2016) months or more in the United Kingdom? (Review list of countries in the UK)		
27. Were you a member of the U.S. military, a civilian military employee, or a dependent of either a member of the U.S. military or civilian military employee?		
From **1980 to the present**, did you		
28. Spend time that adds up to five (Schmidt et al. 2017) years or more in Europe? (Review list of countries in Europe.)		
29. Receive a transfusion of blood or blood components in the United Kingdom or France? (Review list of countries in the UK.)		
Have you **EVER**		
30. Had a positive test for the HIV/AIDS virus?		
31. Had hepatitis or any positive test for hepatitis?		
32. Had malaria?		
33. Had Chagas disease and/or a positive test for *T. cruzi*?		
34. Had babesiosis?		
35. Tested positive for HTLV, had adult T-cell leukemia, or had unexplained paraparesis (partial paralysis affecting the lower limbs)?		
36. Received a dura mater (or brain covering) graft?		
37. Had sexual contact with anyone who was born in or lived in Africa?		
38. Been in Africa?		
39. Been diagnosed with any neurological disease?		
40. Had a transplant or other medical procedure that involved being exposed to live cells, tissues, or organs from an animal?		
41. Has your sexual partner or a member of your household ever had a transplant or other medical procedure that involved being exposed to live cells, tissues, or organs from an animal?		
42. Have any of your relatives had Creutzfeldt-Jakob disease?		

Additional Questions	Yes	No
March 2016 Final Guidance "Donor Screening Recommendations to Reduce the Risk of Transmission of Zika Virus by Human Cells, Tissues, and Cellular and Tissue-Based Products"		
In the past **6 months** have you		
Zika Additional Question: 1. **For Living Donors**—Had a Zika virus infection?		
Zika Additional Question: 2. **For Living Donors**—Lived in or traveled to an area with active Zika virus transmission? (Review the list of ZIKA virus areas of transmission)		
Zika Additional Question: 3. **For Living Donors**—Had sexual contact with a man, who in the **6 months prior to sexual contact**, has had a Zika virus infection or lived in or traveled to an area with active Zika virus transmission?		
May omit question number 4 if this type of donation is not applicable to your program		
Zika Additional Question: 4. **For Non-Heart-Beating (Cadaveric) Donors**—In the past **6 months** has the donor had a medical diagnosis of a Zika virus infection?		

[a]AABB HPC, Apheresis and HPC, Marrow DHQ Version 1.6, December 2016—with permission

Appendix 4.2: Example of Physical Examination Supplemental Checklist

Areas to be evaluated and documented during history and physical examination (H&P) of potential allogeneic/syngeneic donors of peripheral blood stem cells or marrow. Note in Comments location, severity, and/or physical findings.

Yes No

[ ] [ ] Physical evidence of non-medical percutaneous drug use such as needle tracks, including examination of tattoos, which may be covering needle tracks
Comments:

[ ] [ ] Physical evidence of recent tattooing, ear piercing, or body piercing
Comments:

[ ] [ ] Disseminated lymphadenopathy
Comments:

[ ] [ ] Oral thrush
Comments:

[ ] [ ] Blue or purple spots consistent with Kaposi's sarcoma
Comments:

[ ] [ ] Unexplained jaundice, hepatomegaly, or icterus
Comments:

[ ] [ ] Physical evidence of sepsis, such as unexplained generalized rash
Comments:

[ ] [ ] Large scab consistent with recent smallpox immunization
Comments:

[ ] [ ] Eczema vaccinatum
Comments:

[ ] [ ] Generalized vesicular rash (generalized vaccina)
Comments:

[ ] [ ] Severely necrotic lesion consistent with vaccina necrosum
Comments:

[ ] [ ] Corneal scarring consistent with vaccinial keratitis
Comments:

References

AABB (n.d.-a) AABB HPC, Apheresis and HPC, Marrow DHQ Version 1.6, December 2016. http://www.aabb.org/tm/questionnaires/Documents/dhqhpc/v1-6/DHQ-HPC_A-M%20 v1.6.pdf. Accessed 1 May 2017

AABB (n.d.-b) AABB HPC, Apheresis and HPC, Marrow DHQ Version 1.6, December 2016. Flow Charts. http://www.aabb.org/tm/questionnaires/Documents/dhqhpc/v1-6/Flowcharts%20 A-M%20v1.6.pdf. Accessed 1 May 2017

AABB Medication Deferral List (n.d.). http://www.aabb.org/tm/questionnaires/Documents/dhq/v2/DHQ%20Medication%20Deferral%20List%20v2.0.pdf. Accessed 1 May 2017

Al-Ali HK, Bourgeois M, Krahl R et al (2011) The impact of the age of HLA-identical siblings on mobilization and collection of PBSCs for allogeneic hematopoietic cell transplantation. Bone Marrow Transplant 46:1296–1302

Alyea EP, Kim HT, Ho V et al (2005) Comparative outcome of nonmyeloablative and myeloablative allogeneic hematopoietic cell transplantation for patients older than 50 years of age. Blood 105(4):1810–1814

Anthias C, van Walraven SM, Sørensen BS (2015) Related hematopoietic cell donor care: is there a role for unrelated donor registries? Bone Marrow Transplant 50(5):637–641

Anthias C, O'Donnell PV, Kiefer DM et al (2016a) European Group for Blood and Marrow Transplantation Centers with FACT-JACIE accreditation have significantly better compliance with related donor care standards. Biol Blood Marrow Transplant 22(3):514–519

Anthias C, Shaw BE, Kiefer DM et al (2016b) Significant improvements in the practice patterns of adult related donor care in US transplantation centers. Biol Blood Marrow Transplant 22(3):520–527

Bagnara GP, Bonsi L, Strippoli P et al (2000) Hemopoiesis in healthy old people and centenarians: well-maintained responsiveness of CD34+ cells to hemopoietic growth factors and remodeling of cytokine network. J Gerontol A Biol Sci Med Sci 55(2):B61–B70

Bensinger W, Longin K, Appelbaum F et al (1994) Peripheral blood stem cells (PBSCs) collected after recombinant granulocyte colony stimulating factor (rhG-CSF): an analysis of factors correlating with the tempo of engraftment after transplantation. Br J Haematol 87:825–831

Bensinger W, Appelbaum F, Rowley S et al (1995) Factors that influence collection and engraftment of autologous peripheral-blood stem cells. J Clin Oncol 13:2547–2555

Billen A, Madrigal JA, Shaw BE (2014) A review of the haematopoietic stem cell donation experience: is there room for improvement? Bone Marrow Transplant 49(6):729–736

Boo M, van Walraven SM, Chapman J et al (2011) Remuneration of hematopoietic stem cell donors: principles and perspective of the World Marrow Donor Association. Blood 117:21–25

Campbell-Fontaine A, Coad JE, Kovach R et al (2005) Adoptive transfer of vitiligo after allogeneic peripheral blood stem cell transplant. Bone Marrow Transplant 36(8):745–746

Center for International Blood and Marrow Transplant Research (CIBMTR) (2016) Summary Slides . http://www.cibmtr.org/ReferenceCenter/SlidesReports/SummarySlides/pages/index.asp. Accessed 1 May 2017

Centers for Disease Control and Prevention (n.d.) Areas with risk of Zika Virus. https://www.cdc.gov/zika/geo/index.html. Accessed 15 Aug 2017

Centers for Disease Control and Prevention (2016) National Notifiable Diseases Surveillance System (NNDSS). https://wwwn.cdc.gov/nndss/conditions/zika/. Accessed May 2017

Clare S, Mank A, Stone R et al (2010) Management of related donor care: a European survey. Bone Marrow Transplant 45:97–101

Committee on Bioethics (2010) Children as hematopoietic stem cell donors. Pediatrics 125:392–404

Confer DL, Shaw BE, Pamphilon DH et al (2011) WMDA guidelines for subsequent donations following initial BM or PBSCs. Bone Marrow Transplant 46:1409–1412

Ertem M, Kurekci AE, Aysev D et al (2000) Brucellosis transmitted by bone marrow transplantation. Bone Marrow Transplant 26:225–226

Food and Drug Administration (2016) Donor Screening Recommendations to Reduce the Risk of Transmission of Zika Virus by Human Cells, Tissues, and Cellular and Tissue-Based Products. Guidance for Industry. . https://www.fda.gov/downloads/biologicsbloodvaccines/guidancecomplianceregulatoryinformation/guidances/tissue/ucm488582.pdf. Accessed 1 May 2017

Food and Drug Administration (2017) Zika virus response updates from the FDA. https://www.fda.gov/EmergencyPreparedness/Counterterrorism/MedicalCountermeasures/MCMIssues/ucm485199.htm. Accessed 1 May 2017

Food and Drug Administration, HHS (2005) Human cells, tissues, and cellular and tissue-based products; donor screening and testing, and related labeling. Fed Regist 70(100):29949–29952

Ghada A, Guthrie KA, Sorror ML et al (2006) Apheresis safety and product yield among elderly donors for allogeneic sibling hematopoietic stem cell transplantation (HST). Blood 108:abstract 5223

Goker H, Etgul S, Buyukasik Y (2015) Optimizing mobilization strategies in difficult-to-mobilize patients: the role of plerixafor. Transfus Apher Sci 53:23–29

Goodnough LT, Marques MB (2017) Zika virus and patient blood management. Anesth Analg 124(1):282–289

Gratwohl A, Baldomero H, Aljurf M et al (2010) Hematopoietic stem cell transplantation A Global Perspective. JAMA 303(16):1617–1624

Gratwohl A, Baldomero H, Passweg J (2013) Hematopoietic stem cell transplantation activity in Europe. Curr Opin Hematol 20:485–493

Grupp SA, Frangoul H, Wall D et al (2006) Use of G-CSF in matched sibling donor pediatric allogeneic transplantation: a consensus statement from the Children's Oncology Group (COG) Transplant Discipline Committee and Pediatric Blood and Marrow Transplant Consortium (PBMTC) Executive Committee. Pediatr Blood Cancer 46:414–421

Halter J, Kodera Y, Ispizua AU et al (2009) Severe events in donors after allogeneic hematopoietic stem cell donation. Haematologica 94:94–101

Halter JP, van Walraven SM, Worel N et al (2013) Allogeneic hematopoietic stem cell donation-standardized assessment of donor outcome data: a consensus statement from the Worldwide Network for Blood and Marrow Transplantation (WBMT). Bone Marrow Transplant 48:220–225

Horowitz MM (2012) Does matched unrelated donor transplantation have the same outcome as matched sibling transplantation in unselected patients? Best Pract Res Clin Haematol 25(4):483–486

https://network.bethematchclinical.org/workarea/downloadasset

Human Tissue Authority Regulations (2007) . https://www.hta.gov.uk/policies/eu-tissue-and-cells-directives. Accessed 1 May 2017

Ings SJ, Balsa C, Leverett D et al (2006) Peripheral blood stem cell yield in 400 normal donors mobilised with granulocyte colony-stimulating factor (G-CSF): impact of age, sex, donor weight and type of G-CSF used. Br J Haematol 134(5):517–525

Jantunen E, Kuittinen T, Penttilä K et al (2006) High-dose melphalan (200 mg/m^2) supported autologous stem cell transplantation is safe and effective in elderly (>or =65 years) myeloma patients: comparison with younger patients treated on the same protocol. Bone Marrow Transplant 37:917–922

Kikuchi H, Ohtsuka E, Ono K et al (2000) Allogeneic bone marrow transplantation-related transmission of human T lymphotropic virus type I (HTLV-I). Bone Marrow Transplant 26:1235–1237

Kinrade LC (1987) Preparation of sibling donor for bone marrow transplant harvest procedure. Cancer Nurs 10:77–81

Kodera Y, Yamamoto K, Harada M et al (2014) PBSC collection from family donors in Japan: a prospective survey. Bone Marrow Transplant 49:195–200

Kollman C, Howe CW, Anasetti C et al (2001) Donor characteristics as risk factors in recipients after transplantation of bone marrow from unrelated donors: the effect of donor age. Blood 98(7):2043–2051

Kollman C, Spellman SR, Zhang MJ et al (2016) The effect of donor characteristics on survival after unrelated donor transplantation for hematologic malignancy. Blood 127(2):260–267

Lampeter EF, McCann SR, Kolb H (1998) Transfer of diabetes type 1 by bone-marrow transplantation. Lancet 351(9102):568–569

Lau GK, Lee CK, Liang R (1999) Hepatitis B virus infection and bone marrow transplantation. Crit Rev Oncol Hematol 31:71–76

Ljungman P, Lawler M, Asjo B et al (1994) Infection of donor lymphocytes with human T lymphotrophic virus type 1 (HTLV-I) following allogeneic bone marrow transplantation for HTLV-I positive adult T-cell leukaemia. Br J Haematol 88:403–405

Lown RN, Philippe J, Navarro W et al (2014) Unrelated adult stem cell donor medical suitability: recommendations from the World Marrow Donor Association Clinical Working Group Committee. World Marrow Donor Association Clinical Working Group Committee. Bone Marrow Transplant 49(7):880–886

Lysák D, Kořístek Z, Gašová Z et al (2011) Efficacy and safety of peripheral blood stem cell collection in elderly donors; does age interfere? J Clin Apher 26(1):9–16

MacLeod KD, Whitsett SF, Mash EJ et al (2003) Pediatric sibling donors of successful and unsuccessful hematopoietic stem cell transplants (HCST): a qualitative study of their psychosocial experience. J Pediatr Psychol 28:223–231

Medpage Today. Ruling on Paying Stem Cell Donors Stands 2012. https://www.medpagetoday.com/hematologyoncology/hematology/31908. Accessed 1 May 2017

Mejia R, Booth GS, Fedorko DP et al (2012) Peripheral blood stem cell transplant-related Plasmodium falciparum infection in a patient with sickle cell disease. Transfusion 52:2677–2682

Miano M, Labopin M, Hartmann O et al (2007) Haematopoietic stem cell transplantation trends in children over the last three decades: a survey by the paediatric diseases working party of the European Group for Blood and Marrow Transplantation. Bone Marrow Transplant 39:89–99

Miflin G, Charley C, Stainer C (1996) Stem cell mobilization in normal donors for allogeneic transplantation: analysis of safety and factors affecting efficacy. Br J Haematol 95(2):345–348

Miller RA (1996) The aging immune system: primer and prospectus. Science 273(5271):70–74

Morris CL, Siegel E, Barlogie B et al (2003) Mobilization of CD341 cells in elderly patients (>/5 70 years) with multiple myeloma: influence of age, prior therapy, platelet count and mobilization regimen. Br J Haematol 120:413–423

Naohara T, Suzuki G, Masauzi N et al (1997) Positive seroconversion syphilis in a patient with acute lymphocytic leukemia after allogeneic bone marrow transplantation. Rinsho Ketsueki 38:228–230

National Marrow Donor Program (2002) National marrow donor program standards, 18th edn. National Marrow Donor Program, Minneapolis

National Marrow Donor Program (NMDP) (2016). Assessment Tool At Recruitment. https://network.bethematchclinical.org/workarea/downloadasset.aspx?id=5090. Accessed 1 May 2017

National Marrow Donor Program (NMDP) (n.d.-a) Be the Match. Donor Assessment. https://network.bethematchclinical.org/apheresis-and-collection-centers/donor-assessment/. Accessed 1 May 2017

National Marrow Donor Program (NMDP) (n.d.-b) Assessing Non-Medical Factors Affecting Donor Suitability. https://network.bethematchclinical.org/workarea/downloadasset.aspx?id=5082. Accessed 1 May 2017

Niederwieser D, Baldomero H, Szer J et al (2016) Hematopoietic stem cell transplantation activity worldwide in 2012 and a SWOT analysis of the Worldwide Network for Blood and Marrow Transplantation Group including the global survey. Bone Marrow Transplant 51(6):778–785

O'Donnell PV, Pedersen TK, Confer DL et al (2010) Practice patterns for evaluation, consent, and care of related donors and recipients at hematopoietic cell transplantation centers in the United States. Blood 115:5097–5101

Olivares JL, Ramos FJ, Olivé T et al (2002) Autoimmune thyroiditis after bone marrow transplantation in a boy with Wiskott-Aldrich syndrome. J Pediatr Hematol Oncol 24(9):772–776

Packman W, Crittenden MR, Schaeffer E et al (1997) Psychosocial consequences of bone marrow transplantation in donor and nondonor siblings. J Dev Behav Pediatr 18:244–253

Packman W, Crittenden MR, Rieger Fischer JB et al (2008) Sibling perceptions of the bone marrow transplantation process. J Psychosoc Oncol 4615:81–105

Pingali SR, Champlin RE (2015) Pushing the envelope—nonmyeloablative and reduced intensity preparative regimens for allogeneic hematopoietic transplantation. Bone Marrow Transplant 50(9):1157–1167

Pulsipher MA, Levine JE, Hayashi RJ et al (2005) Safety and efficacy of allogeneic PBSC collection in normal pediatric donors: the pediatric blood and marrow transplant consortium experience (PBMTC) 1996–2003. Bone Marrow Transplant 35:361–367

Pulsipher MA, Nagler A, Iannone R et al (2006) Weighing the risks of G-CSF administration, leukopheresis, and standard marrow harvest: ethical and safety considerations for normal pediatric hematopoietic cell donors. Pediatr Blood Cancer 46:422–433

Pulsipher MA, Chitphakdithai P, Logan BR et al (2013) Acute toxicities of unrelated bone marrow versus peripheral blood stem cell donation: results of a prospective trial from the National Marrow Donor Program. Blood 121:197–206

Richa E, Papari M, Allen J et al (2009) Older age but not donor health impairs allogeneic granulocyte colony-stimulating factor (G-CSF) peripheral blood stem cell mobilization. Biol Blood Marrow Transplant 15:1394–1399

Rinaldi C, Savignano C, Pasca S et al (2012) Efficacy and safety of peripheral blood stem cell mobilization and collection: a single-center experience in 190 allogeneic donors. Transfusion 52(11):2387–2394

Sacchi N, Costeas P, Hartwell L (2008) Haematopoietic stem cell donor registries: World Marrow Donor Association recommendations for evaluation of donor health. Bone Marrow Transplant 42(1):9–14

Schmidt AH, Mengling T, Hernández-Frederick CJ et al (2017) Retrospective analysis of 37,287 observation years after peripheral blood stem cell donation. Biol Blood Marrow Transplant 17:30302–30306

Shah NN, Wayne AS, Grady C et al (2015) Children as hematopoietic cell donors in research: when is it approvable? Bone Marrow Transplant 50(1):15–19

Shuhart MC, Myerson D, Childs BH et al (1994) Marrow transplantation from hepatitis C virus seropositive donors: transmission rate and clinical course. Blood 84:3229–3235

Snowden JA, Heaton DC (1997) Development of psoriasis after syngeneic bone marrow transplant from psoriatic donor: further evidence for adoptive autoimmunity. Br J Dermatol 137(1):130–132

Strasser SI, McDonald GB (1999) Hepatitis viruses and hematopoietic cell transplantation: a guide to patient and donor management. Blood 93:1127–1136

Styczynski J, Balduzzi A, Gil L et al (2012) Risk of complications during hematopoietic stem cell collection in pediatric sibling donors: a prospective European Group for Blood and Marrow Transplantation Pediatric Diseases Working Party study. Blood 119:2935–2942

Suzuya H, Watanabe T, Nakagawa R et al (2005) Factors associated with granulocyte colony-stimulating factor-induced peripheral blood stem cell yield in healthy donors. Vox Sang 89:229–235

Switzer GE, Bruce J, Kiefer DM et al (2017) Health-related quality of life among older related hematopoietic stem cell donors (>60 Years) is equivalent to that of younger related donors (18 to 60 years): a related donor safety study. Biol Blood Marrow Transplant 23(1):165–171

The Foundation for the Accreditation of Cellular Therapy (FACT) (n.d.). International standards for cellular therapy product collection, processing and adminstration. 5th edition. http://www.factwebsite.org. Accessed 1 May 2017

Thomson JA, Wilson RM, Franklin IM (1995) Transmission of thyrotoxicosis of autoimmune type by sibling allogeneic bone marrow transplant. Eur J Endocrinol 133(5):564–566

Villalba R, Fornes G, Alvarez MA et al (1992) Acute Chagas' disease in a recipient of a bone marrow transplant in Spain: case report. Clin Infect Dis 14:594–595

Wendler D, Shah NN, Pulsipher MA et al (2016) Research involving pediatric stem cell donors: a way forward. Clin Trials 13(3):304–310

WHO statement on the first meeting of the International Health Regulations (2005) (IHR 2005) Emergency Committee on Zika virus and observed increase in neurological disorders and neonatal malformations 2016. http://www.who.int/mediacentre/news/statements/2016/1st-emergency-committee-zika/en/. Accessed 1 May 2017

Wiener LS, Steffen-Smith E, Fry T et al (2007) Hematopoietic stem cell donation in children: a review of the sibling donor experience. J Psychosoc Oncol 25:45–66

Worel N, Buser A, Greinix HT et al (2015) Suitability criteria for adult related donors: a consensus statement from the worldwide network for blood and marrow transplantation standing committee on donor issues. Biol Blood Marrow Transplant 21(12):2052–2060

5 Mobilization Strategies: HPC(A) Collections for Autologous Hematopoietic Cell Transplants

Nina Worel

5.1 Introduction

Autologous hematopoietic cell transplantation (auto-HCT) aims to restore bone marrow (BM) function after high-dose chemotherapy in patients with a variety of hemato-oncological diseases such as multiple myeloma (MM), non-Hodgkin's lymphoma (NHL), Hodgkin's lymphoma (HL), and other malignancies. For patients with MM and relapsed chemosensitive lymphomas, auto-HCT leads to improved progression-free survival (PFS) and overall survival (OS). Patients with MM achieve higher rates of complete remission with consolidative auto-HCT than with conventional induction therapy alone (Giralt et al. 2014; Passweg et al. 2016).

Under normal conditions, CD34⁺ cells circulate only in a very small number in the peripheral blood (PB) (Pusic and DiPersio 2008). Therefore, their mobilization from the BM into the PB is an essential part of apheresis collection process. Since the introduction of hematopoietic growth factors, mobilized PB CD34⁺ cells are the preferred source worldwide (Giralt et al. 2014; Mohty et al. 2014) as such growth factors allow enhanced CD34⁺ cell mobilization and improved collection results (Gianni et al. 1989). Auto-HCT from PB is favored because it leads to faster neutrophil and platelet engraftment and hematologic reconstitution compared to BM, resulting in potentially improved patient outcomes. In addition, some studies demonstrate that the use of PB grafts in auto-HCT is associated with better quality of life and reduced hospital stays, less need for transfusions and antibiotics, and reduced total costs (Mohty and Ho 2011; Vellenga et al. 2001; Vose et al. 2002). Granulocyte-macrophage colony-stimulating factor (GM-CSF) has been largely replaced by granulocyte colony-stimulating factor (G-CSF) for CD34⁺ cell mobilization.

N. Worel (✉)
Department of Blood Group Serology and Transfusion Medicine, Medical University of Vienna, Vienna, Austria
e-mail: nina.worel@meduniwien.ac.at

S. A. Abutalib et al. (eds.), *Best Practices of Apheresis in Hematopoietic Cell Transplantation*, Advances and Controversies in Hematopoietic Transplantation and Cell Therapy, https://doi.org/10.1007/978-3-319-55131-9_5

5.2 Mobilization Methods

Nowadays, there are two general approaches for autologous CD34$^+$ cell mobilization: steady-state mobilization using growth factors such as G-CSF alone and chemo-mobilization (i.e., chemotherapy and G-CSF) using chemotherapy either as part or apart of the disease-specific treatment protocol followed by growth factor application (Giralt et al. 2014; Mohty et al. 2014; Bensinger et al. 2009). The use of chemotherapy generally produces higher CD34$^+$ cell yields in a lower number of apheresis and, in theory, may reduce tumor contamination of the graft, although data to confirm this are still lacking (Mohty et al. 2014; Bensinger et al. 2009). Disadvantages of chemo-mobilization include increased toxicity and morbidity, the need for hospitalization, transfusion support, and anti-infectious treatment (Mohty et al. 2014; Bensinger et al. 2009).

Despite an established practice, current mobilization strategies vary between centers and differ in terms of feasibility and outcome (Mohty et al. 2014; Mohty and Ho 2011; Bensinger et al. 2009) (see Chap. 9). Although in the majority of patients sufficient CD34$^+$ cells for at least a single autologous transplantation can be collected, approximately 5–25% fail to mobilize an adequate number of cells (Pusic et al. 2008; Wuchter et al. 2010). If patients are scheduled for >1 transplant, even higher failure rates are reported. A more recent approach to improve mobilization and collection procedures includes the use of cell-binding inhibitors like plerixafor (Calandra et al. 2008; Chabannon et al. 2015; Worel et al. 2017). Nevertheless, it is necessary to optimize the current mobilization approaches and to identify upfront patients who are at risk of G-CSF mobilization failure (see Chap. 4).

5.3 Steady-State Cytokines Alone CD34$^+$ Cell Mobilization

5.3.1 Dose and Schedule

Administration of G-CSF (filgrastim and lenograstim) remains the only available treatment option for steady-state mobilization, as GM-CSF is no longer available in many countries and other growth factors (e.g., pegylated G-CSF) have no label for PB CD34$^+$ cell mobilization. G-CSF treatment leads to granulocyte activation and expansion and release of various proteases into the marrow, which then cleave adhesion molecules such as stromal-derived factor-1 (SDF-1), releasing hematopoietic stem and progenitor cells (specifically CD34$^+$ cells) into the PB (Giralt et al. 2014; Pusic and DiPersio 2008; Petit et al. 2002). Filgrastim and lenograstim are usually injected at a daily dose of 10 μg/kg of body weight subcutaneously. Doses can be divided in two applications of 5 μg/kg body weight and administered twice daily. The approved schedules of G-CSF are 5–7 consecutive days for filgrastim and 4–6 days for lenograstim (Fig. 5.1a). Leukapheresis normally is initiated if CD34$^+$ cells exceed a threshold of 20 μL or maybe lower (>10–15 CD34$^+$ cells/μL)

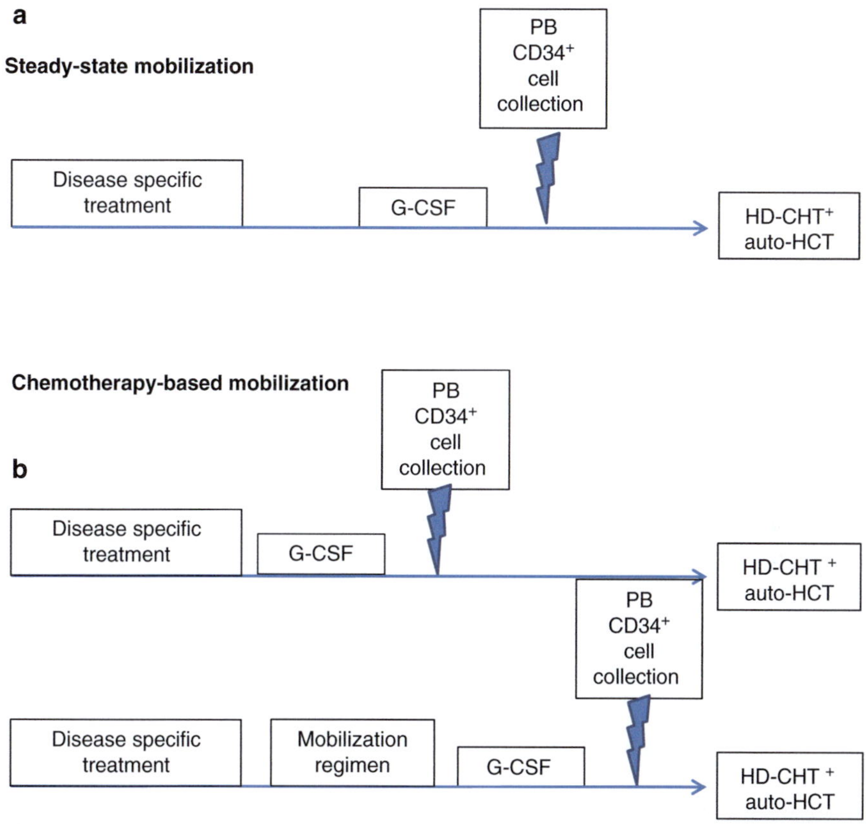

Fig. 5.1 Mobilization strategies for autologous PB CD34+ cell collection. *Auto-HCT* autologous hematopoietic cell transplantation, *CHT* chemotherapy, *HD* high dose, *G-CSF* granulocyte colony-stimulating factor, *PB* peripheral blood

according to institutional guidelines but should be started at least on days 5 or 6 after filgrastim and between days 5 and 7 after lenograstim. However, collection can also be started on day 4 of G-CSF if the institutional defined threshold of CD34+ is exceeded.

5.3.2 Adverse Events of Cytokine Administration

The most common adverse events of cytokine mobilization are bone pain in 52–84% of patients, which can be treated with common analgesics, such as acetaminophen, paracetamol, or ibuprofen (Anderlini et al. 1999; Tigue et al. 2007). Other associated symptoms include fatigue, headache, and fever. There have been reports of development or flare up of autoimmune events associated with G-CSF administration (e.g., autoimmune hyperthyroidism). A very rare but serious adverse event is splenic rupture which has been reported after G-CSF administration in healthy donors and patients and occurred in the majority of subjects at day 6 of G-CSF (Tigue et al. 2007). Several studies evaluated effects of short-term administration of G-CSF on the spleen. Spleen size was studied in healthy CD34$^+$ cell donors receiving G-CSF at a dose of 7.5 mg/kg b.w./day for 5 days. An average increase of 11 mm in spleen length and 10% increase in volume were noted, but baseline values normally are reached within 10 days after stop of G-CSF administration (Platzbecker et al. 2001; Stroncek et al. 2003). Until now, no increased risk for hematologic malignancies has been observed in healthy donors (Anderlini et al. 1999; Tigue et al. 2007) (see Chap. 6).

5.3.3 Practice Points

Mobilization with cytokines alone is generally well tolerated, needs less resources, and can be optimally timed. If the underlying disease does not necessarily need cytotoxic therapy and is treated with immunomodulatory drugs (i.e., MM with novel induction therapy) or antibodies, or patients are in remission, steady-state mobilization with cytokines alone would be the preferred option.

5.4 Chemotherapy-Based Mobilization

It is a matter of fact that chemotherapy decreases tumor burden and may increase PB CD34$^+$ cell yields in combination with growth factors (cytokines) (Mohty et al. 2014; Bensinger et al. 2009; Gertz 2010). However, compared to cytokine alone mobilization, chemotherapy-based regimens are associated with a higher incidence and severity of adverse events as neutropenic fever, sepsis, need for antibiotics and blood products, and hospital admission (Pusic et al. 2008; Gertz et al. 2009).

It is important to emphasize that DNA-topoisomerase II (i.e., etoposide) and alkylating agents (i.e., cyclophosphamide) are known to increase the risk of therapy-related myeloid neoplasms; hence, it is best to avoid them in a setting where such agents are solely being used to mobilize CD34$^+$ cells (Arber et al. 2016). Chemotherapy may be given as disease-specific treatment (e.g., R-CHOP; rituximab, cyclophosphamide, hydroxydaunorubicin, oncovin, and prednisone in NHL patients) or apart from the treatment protocol (e.g., cyclophosphamide in MM patients treated with new therapeutic agents). The choice of a chemotherapy-based mobilization regimen depends on the disease entity and institutional guidelines. After myelosuppressive chemotherapy, G-CSF is given at doses of 5–10 μg/kg b.w. per day starting between days 1 and 7 after initiation of chemotherapy and continues until the last day of apheresis (Fig. 5.1b).

There is doubt that especially in MM patients, in the era of novel induction therapy (e.g., proteasome inhibitors and immunomodulatory agents), chemotherapeutic drugs used for CD34$^+$ cell mobilization as cyclophosphamide or etoposide have an additional antitumor effect. In contrast in lymphoma patients, the myelosuppressive chemotherapy given as standard first-line or salvage therapy has a positive impact on CD34+ cell mobilization and eliminates the need for additional chemo- or steady-state mobilization in these heavily pretreated patients (Mohty et al. 2014; Pavone et al. 2002). In addition, disease-specific chemotherapy protocols using a combination of cytotoxic drugs (e.g., D-PACE for MM consisting of dexamethasone, platinum, doxorubicin, cyclophosphamide, etoposide or CHOP for NHL consisting of cyclophosphamide, doxorubicin, vincristine, prednisone) have been shown to be more effective than cyclophosphamide alone (Mohty et al. 2014; Pavone et al. 2002).

5.5 Binding Inhibitors: Plerixafor

5.5.1 Dose and Schedule

Plerixafor, a novel CD34+ cell-mobilizing agent, was launched in 2008 for use in the United States in combination with G-CSF for mobilization in patients with MM and lymphomas. In Europe, plerixafor was approved by the European Medicines Agency (EMA) with the restriction for patients whose CD34+ cells mobilize poorly (Genzyme Ltd: Suffolk U. Mozobil [Product information] 2009). Plerixafor is a reversible chemokine receptor 4 (CXCR4) antagonist that in combination with G-CSF augments the release of CD34+ cells from the BM by disrupting the binding site of CXCR4 with stromal cell-derived factor-1 (SDF-1). The recommended dose is 240 μg/kg b.w. subcutaneously approximately 6–11 h before initiation of leukapheresis following at least 4 days of G-CSF pretreatment. In patients with impaired renal function (creatinine clearance ≤50 mL/min), dose adjustment to 160 μg/kg b.w. is recommended (Genzyme Ltd: Suffolk U. Mozobil [Product information] 2009; DiPersio et al. 2009a, b). Until now, numerous studies have confirmed the efficacy of plerixafor in combination not only with G-CSF but also with G-CSF and chemotherapy, including poor mobilizing patients, with superior efficacy to other mobilization regimens (G-CSF alone or G-CSF and chemotherapy) without plerixafor (Calandra et al. 2008; Worel et al. 2017, 2011; DiPersio et al. 2009a, b; D'Addio et al. 2011). If plerixafor is given to improve or rescue chemotherapy-based mobilization, we prefer patients to have leukocyte counts of 5 G/L after at least 4 days of G-CSF pretreatment. Plerixafor can be used for remobilization in patents failing to collect a sufficient number of CD34+ cells, as immediate rescue in an ongoing mobilization attempt to prevent failure or preemptive in patients at risk for poor mobilization (Mohty et al. 2014; Chabannon et al. 2015; Worel et al. 2017, 2011; D'Addio et al. 2011).

5.5.2 Adverse Events of Plerixafor Administration

The most common adverse events observed are erythema at the injection site in 30% of patients and gastrointestinal disturbances (stomach discomfort, nausea, and diarrhea) in 30% of patients.

5.6 Suboptimal CD34⁺ Cell Mobilization: "Poor Mobilizers"

Factors adversely influencing PB CD34$^+$ mobilization and collection include older age, female gender, diagnosis (lymphomas more likely than MM), longer disease duration and therapy, more advanced disease, previous intensive radio- and/or chemotherapy (especially treatment with purine analogues, melphalan, and lenalidomide), and low platelet counts prior to collection (Mohty et al. 2014; Kumar et al. 2007) (Table 5.1). The definition of "poor" CD34$^+$ cell mobilization is heterogeneous. Parameters used to define poor mobilization range from the peak of CD34$^+$ cells in the PB to the cumulative apheresis yield or the percent of patients in whom CD34$^+$ cells

Table 5.1 Risk factors for suboptimal CD34$^+$ cell mobilization and mobilization failure

Risk factor	Proposed mechanism	Strategy for CD34$^+$ cell mobilization
Low platelet counts (Olivieri et al. 2012)	Reflects CD34$^+$ cell reserve	Regimens that support HSPC proliferation
Age (>60–65 years old) (Olivieri et al. 2012; Stiff 1999)	Reduced HSPC reserve: • HSPC senescence • Loss or dysfunction of the HSPC niche • Bone loss or altered bone metabolism	Regimens that support HSPC proliferation
Underlying disease (Pusic et al. 2008)	• Paraneoplastic dysfunction of the HSPC niche • Reduction of niches due to tumor mass	Reduce bone marrow infiltration before HSPC mobilization.
Extensive irradiation of marrow-bearing sites (Olivieri et al. 2012)	Direct HSPC toxicity, impairment of HSPC niche	Consider plerixafor.
Previous chemotherapy:		
• Melphalan (Olivieri et al. 2012)	Direct HSPC toxicity	Avoid melphalan before PB CD34$^+$ cell collection.
• Fludarabine (Olivieri et al. 2012; Berger et al. 2008)	Direct HSPC toxicity, impairment of HSPC niche	PB CD34$^+$ cell collection before 4 cycles of fludarabine
• Intensive CTH (Olivieri et al. 2012; Hill et al. 2011)	Impairment of HSPC niches, increased HSPC renewal with exhaustion	Consider plerixafor.
Previous prolong (>4 cycles) lenalidomide treatment (Kumar et al. 2007; Olivieri et al. 2012)	Possible effect on HSPC mobility (upregulation of CXCR4 expression), dysregulation of HSPC niche due to antiangiogenetic effects	PB CD34$^+$ cell collection before 4 cycles of lenalidomide. Stop lenalidomide during HSPC mobilization and collection, and consider plerixafor.
Diabetes (Fadini and Avogaro 2013)	Possible effect on BM microenvironment, impaired HSPC mobilization due to mobilopathy	Consider plerixafor.

BM bone marrow, *HSPC* hematopoietic stem and progenitor cell, *PB* peripheral blood, *CXCR4* CXC chemokine receptor 4

cannot be collected. Criteria to define a successful $CD34^+$ cell mobilization and an adequate apheresis yield have been proposed by several authors, but criteria vary between experts and centers. In a recent study of the Gruppo Italiano Trapianto di Midollo Osseo (GITMO), patients are defined as *proven poor mobilizers* when (1) after adequate mobilization (G-CSF 10 μg/kg body weight if used alone or ≥5 μg/kg body weight after chemotherapy), circulating $CD34^+$ cell peak is <20 cells/μL up to 6 days after mobilization with G-CSF alone or up to 20 days after chemotherapy and G-CSF, or (2) less than 2.0×10^6 $CD34^+$ cells per kg body weight in ≤3 apheresis are collected. Patients were defined as *predicted poor mobilizers* if (1) patients failed a previous collection attempt (not otherwise specified), (2) patients previously received extensive radiotherapy or full courses of chemotherapy affecting $CD34^+$ cell mobilization, and (3) patients met two of the following criteria: advanced disease (≥2 lines of chemotherapy), refractory disease, extensive BM involvement or cellularity <30% at the time of mobilization, and age ≥65 years (Olivieri et al. 2012). Besides these definitions, several other groups have developed algorithms to guide the use of the optimal mobilization regimen including "correct" timing of plerixafor application (Giralt et al. 2014; Olivieri et al. 2012; Chen et al. 2012; Costa et al. 2011). A very important finding is that the use of plerixafor as an immediate rescue approach also results in very high success rates (Worel et al. 2017; Costa et al. 2011). In one study, a decision-making algorithm based on the PB $CD34^+$ cell count on day 4 of G-CSF administration and the collection target of $CD34^+$ cells was developed to guide cost-effective use of plerixafor (continuing G-CSF only or adding plerixafor). The authors showed that patient-adapted plerixafor use based on this algorithm was superior to cyclophosphamide plus growth factor and successfully mobilized PB $CD34^+$ cells in MM patients previously treated with lenalidomide (Costa et al. 2011). Another study describes a risk-based approach to optimize PB $CD34^+$ cell collection with plerixafor by identifying potential poor mobilizers upfront. The algorithm takes into account the number of PB $CD34^+$ cells on day 5 of G-CSF mobilization, the desired amount of PB $CD34^+$ cells needed per transplant ($\geq 2.5 \times 10^6$/kg of recipient body weight for 1 transplant and $\geq 5 \times 10^6$/kg of recipient body weight for 2 transplants), and $CD34^+$ collection yield on the first apheresis day. The use of plerixafor was triggered by PB $CD34^+$ cells of ≤10/μL (for 1 transplant), or ≤20 cells per μL (for 2 transplants) on day 5 of G-CSF, or a $CD34^+$ collection yield of less than 50% of the total $CD34^+$ cell dose needed in the first leukapheresis (Abhyankar et al. 2012) (see Chap. 9).

5.7 What Is the Optimal $CD34^+$ Cell Dose/Kg for Successful Transplantation?

The infused $CD34^+$ cell dose influences the time to neutrophil and platelet engraftment, need for platelet and red blood cell transfusion, occurrence of febrile complications, need for antibiotics, and graft stability. Low $CD34^+$ cell doses (<2.0×10^6 $CD34^+$ cells/kg of recipient body weight) are associated with delayed engraftment and increased transfusion requirements, mostly for platelets (Table 5.2). However, a delay in platelet recovery also can be explained by other factors, such as intensive pretreatment, including irradiation to marrow-bearing sites, altering the matrix of the marrow, and the use of growth factors after transplantation, which could reflect

Table 5.2 Studies focusing on $CD34^+$ cell doses in autologous hematopoietic cell transplants

References	Cohort	Mobilization	Focus	Outcome
Weaver et al. (1995) *(Blood 1995)*	320 breast cancers 137 lymphomas 10 MM, 52 solid tumors	CHT ± HGF	Engraftment kinetics	<2.5 × 10^6/kg $CD34^+$ cells (2%) delayed PLT and ANC engraftment
Pérez-Simón et al. (1998) *(Transfusion 1998)*	38 breast cancers 23 lymphomas 6 MM, 4 solid tumors	Steady state, 5 μg/kg HGF	Collection, engraftment	0.75 × 10^6/kg $CD34^+$ cells/kg (13%) necessary to ensure engraftment
Pérez-Simón et al. (1999) *(BMT 1999)*	51 breast cancers 31 lymphomas 15 MM, 3 solid tumors	Not stated	Late engraftment Hospitalization, AB, transfusions, 1-year follow-up	>1.1 × 10^6/kg $CD34^+$ cells/kg stable engraftment >2.2 × 10^6/kg $CD34^+$ cells/kg reduced transfusions
Siena S. (2000) *(JCO 2000)*	MEDLINE search was conducted to identify relevant publications.	Different	Clinical outcomes	≥8 × 10^6 $CD34^+$ cells/kg associated with better clinical outcome

AB antibiotic treatment, *ANC* absolute neutrophil count, *CHT* chemotherapy, *FU* follow-up, *HGF* hematopoietic growth factor, *MM* multiple myeloma, *PLT* platelets

the ability of cytokines to influence cells of intermediate lineage that have the potential to become either neutrophils or platelets, leading to an accelerated neutrophil maturation and later platelets recovery (Jillella and Ustun 2004).

Clinical studies investigating the optimal $CD34^+$ cell dose to be reinfused in patients undergoing autologous transplantation showed that using high $CD34^+$ cell doses (>5 to >10 × 10^6/kg) is associated with faster neutrophil and platelet recovery, but, apart from a reduced need for platelet transfusions, the full effect and real clinical benefit of this strategy is unknown (Table 5.2). Indeed, studies investigating the effect of the $CD34^+$ cell dose on engraftment have yielded contrary results. More recent studies have found a correlation between $CD34^+$ cell dose, progression-free survival (PFS), and overall survival (OS) in patients with MM and non-Hodgkin's lymphoma (NHL). Possible reasons for better PFS and OS in this good or "super"-mobilizers are a sustained and more rapid hematopoietic reconstitution that leads to a lower non-relapse mortality (NRM) and the fact that higher numbers of $CD34^+$ cells in the graft coincide with an increased number of T cells, which may accelerate immune reconstitution after auto-HCT and, therefore, induce tumor-specific T cells (Bolwell et al. 2007). In contrast, another study in NHL patients demonstrated that higher $CD3^+$ T-cell doses infused with the graft, and not $CD34^+$ numbers, have an effect on absolute lymphocyte and natural killer (NK) cell count at day +15, thereby positively influencing PFS and OS. Patients with lymphocytes of at least 500 cells/μL and NK cells greater than 80 cells/μL on day 15 after auto-HCT had significantly better PFS and OS in this study (Porrata et al. 2008).

5.8 Practice Points

Until now, there is no golden standard for the kind of mobilization regimen for autologous $CD34^+$ cell collection. Both steady-state and chemotherapy-based regimens have their advantages and disadvantages. PB $CD34^+$ cell mobilization can be optimized with an appropriate strategy adapted to each patient, based on the patient's disease, existing risk factors for poor mobilization, and the individual collection aim. A low PB $CD34^+$ cell count before apheresis is a predictor for poor collection results. Therefore, $CD34^+$ cell counts are an important factor helping to estimate the patient's risk for poor mobilization and collection and may allow immediate intervention to rescue mobilization failure. A possible algorithm of $CD34^+$ cell mobilization in daily routine is given in Fig. 5.2.

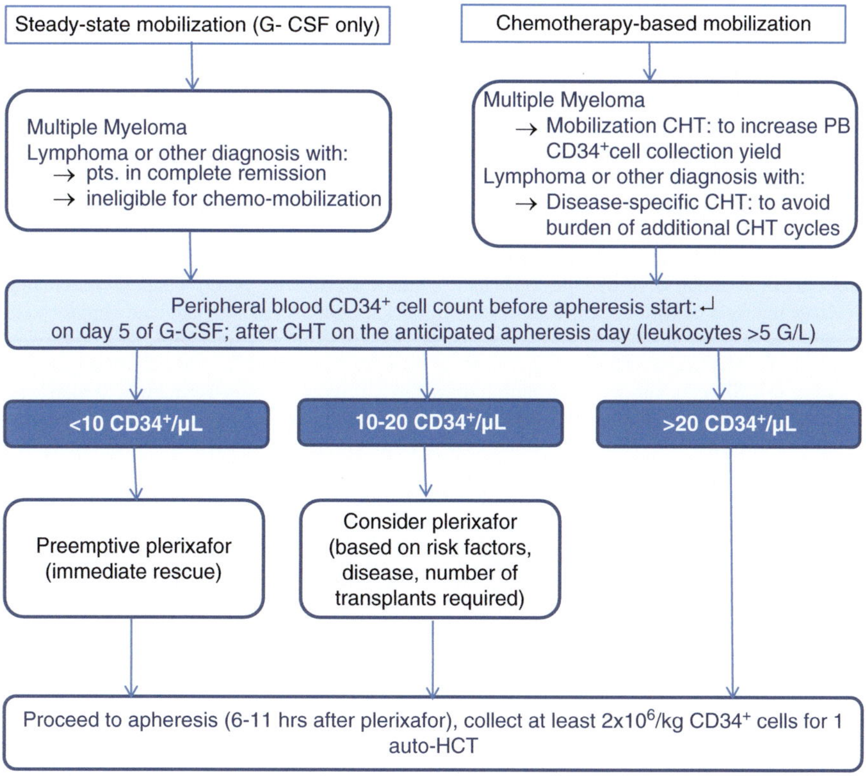

Fig. 5.2 Possible algorithm of $CD34^+$ cell mobilization in daily routine. *PB* peripheral blood, *auto-HCT* autologous hematopoietic cell transplantation, *CHT* chemotherapy, *hrs* hours, *G-CSF* granulocyte colony-stimulating factor, *pts* patients

The minimum recommended dose of 2.0×10^6 $CD34^+$ cells/kg b.w. is associated with regular and timely engraftment. Although doses less than 2.0×10^6 $CD34^+$ cells/kg b.w. result in hematopoietic engraftment, they are associated with a delay in neutrophil and platelet recovery and a risk for graft failure or transitory loss of engraftment. To determine the optimum dose of $CD34^+$ cells/kg of b.w. and possibly other cells, not only for regular and stable engraftment but also for improved PFS and OS, randomized studies with sufficient numbers of patients need to be conducted.

References

Abhyankar S, DeJarnette S, Aljitawi O, Ganguly S, Merkel D, McGuirk J (2012) A risk-based approach to optimize autologous hematopoietic stem cell (HSC) collection with the use of plerixafor. Bone Marrow Transplant 47(4):483–487

Anderlini P, Donato M, Chan KW, Huh YO, Gee AP, Lauppe MJ et al (1999) Allogeneic blood progenitor cell collection in normal donors after mobilization with filgrastim: the M.D. Anderson Cancer Center experience. Transfusion 39(6):555–560

Arber DA, Orazi A, Hasserjian R, Thiele J, Borowitz MJ, Le Beau MM et al (2016) The 2016 revision to the World Health Organization classification of myeloid neoplasms and acute leukemia. Blood 127(20):2391–2405

Bensinger W, DiPersio JF, McCarty JM (2009) Improving stem cell mobilization strategies: future directions. Bone Marrow Transplant 43(3):181–195

Berger MG, Berger J, Richard C, Jeanpierre S, Nicolini FE, Tournilhac O et al (2008) Preferential sensitivity of hematopoietic (HPs) and mesenchymal (MPs) progenitors to fludarabine suggests impaired bone marrow niche and HP mobilization. Leukemia 22(11):2131–2134

Bolwell BJ, Pohlman B, Rybicki L, Sobecks R, Dean R, Curtis J et al (2007) Patients mobilizing large numbers of CD34+ cells ('super mobilizers') have improved survival in autologous stem cell transplantation for lymphoid malignancies. Bone Marrow Transplant 40(5):437–441

Calandra G, McCarty J, McGuirk J, Tricot G, Crocker SA, Badel K et al (2008) AMD3100 plus G-CSF can successfully mobilize CD34+ cells from non-Hodgkin's lymphoma, Hodgkin's disease and multiple myeloma patients previously failing mobilization with chemotherapy and/or cytokine treatment: compassionate use data. Bone Marrow Transplant 41(4):331–338

Chabannon C, Bijou F, Miclea JM, Milpied N, Grouin JM, Mohty M (2015) A nationwide survey of the use of plerixafor in patients with lymphoid malignancies who mobilize poorly demonstrates the predominant use of the "on-demand" scheme of administration at French autologous hematopoietic stem cell transplant programs. Transfusion 55(9):2149–2157

Chen AI, Bains T, Murray S, Knight R, Shoop K, Bubalo J et al (2012) Clinical experience with a simple algorithm for plerixafor utilization in autologous stem cell mobilization. Bone Marrow Transplant 47(12):1526–1529

Costa LJ, Alexander ET, Hogan KR, Schaub C, Fouts TV, Stuart RK (2011) Development and validation of a decision-making algorithm to guide the use of plerixafor for autologous hematopoietic stem cell mobilization. Bone Marrow Transplant 46(1):64–69

D'Addio A, Curti A, Worel N, Douglas K, Motta MR, Rizzi S et al (2011) The addition of plerixafor is safe and allows adequate PBSC collection in multiple myeloma and lymphoma patients poor mobilizers after chemotherapy and G-CSF. Bone Marrow Transplant 46(3):356–363

DiPersio JF, Micallef IN, Stiff PJ, Bolwell BJ, Maziarz RT, Jacobsen E et al (2009a) Phase III prospective randomized double-blind placebo-controlled trial of plerixafor plus granulocyte colony-stimulating factor compared with placebo plus granulocyte colony-stimulating factor for autologous stem-cell mobilization and transplantation for patients with non-Hodgkin's lymphoma. J Clin Oncol Off J Am Soc Clin Oncol 27(28):4767–4773

DiPersio JF, Stadtmauer EA, Nademanee A, Micallef IN, Stiff PJ, Kaufman JL et al (2009b) Plerixafor and G-CSF versus placebo and G-CSF to mobilize hematopoietic stem cells for autologous stem cell transplantation in patients with multiple myeloma. Blood 113(23):5720–5726

Fadini GP, Avogaro A (2013) Diabetes impairs mobilization of stem cells for the treatment of cardiovascular disease: a meta-regression analysis. Int J Cardiol 168(2):892–897

Genzyme Ltd: Suffolk U. Mozobil [Product information] (2009). http://www.ema.europa.eu/docs/en_GB/document_library/EPAR_-_Product_Information/human/001030/WC500030686.pdf. Accessed 28 Aug 2013

Gertz MA (2010) Current status of stem cell mobilization. Br J Haematol 150(6):647–662

Gertz MA, Kumar SK, Lacy MQ, Dispenzieri A, Hayman SR, Buadi FK et al (2009) Comparison of high-dose CY and growth factor with growth factor alone for mobilization of stem cells for transplantation in patients with multiple myeloma. Bone Marrow Transplant 43(8):619–625

Gianni AM, Siena S, Bregni M, Tarella C, Stern AC, Pileri A et al (1989) Granulocyte-macrophage colony-stimulating factor to harvest circulating haemopoietic stem cells for autotransplantation. Lancet 2(8663):580–585

Giralt S, Costa L, Schriber J, DiPersio J, Maziarz R, McCarty J et al (2014) Optimizing autologous stem cell mobilization strategies to improve patient outcomes: consensus guidelines and recommendations. Biol Blood Marrow Tr 20(3):295–308. English

Hill BT, Rybicki L, Smith S, Dean R, Kalaycio M, Pohlman B et al (2011) Treatment with hyperfractionated cyclophosphamide, vincristine, doxorubicin, and dexamethasone combined with cytarabine and methotrexate results in poor mobilization of peripheral blood stem cells in patients with mantle cell lymphoma. Leuk Lymphoma 52(6):986–993

Jillella AP, Ustun C (2004) What is the optimum number of CD34+ peripheral blood stem cells for an autologous transplant? Stem Cells Dev 13(6):598–606

Kumar S, Dispenzieri A, Lacy MQ, Hayman SR, Buadi FK, Gastineau DA et al (2007) Impact of lenalidomide therapy on stem cell mobilization and engraftment post-peripheral blood stem cell transplantation in patients with newly diagnosed myeloma. Leukemia 21(9):2035–2042

Mohty M, Ho AD (2011) In and out of the niche: perspectives in mobilization of hematopoietic stem cells. Exp Hematol 39(7):723–729

Mohty M, Hubel K, Kroger N, Aljurf M, Apperley J, Basak GW et al (2014) Autologous haematopoietic stem cell mobilisation in multiple myeloma and lymphoma patients: a position statement from the European Group for Blood and Marrow Transplantation. Bone Marrow Transplant 49(7):865–872. English

Olivieri A, Marchetti M, Lemoli R, Tarella C, Iacone A, Lanza F et al (2012) Proposed definition of 'poor mobilizer' in lymphoma and multiple myeloma: an analytic hierarchy process by ad hoc working group Gruppo Italiano Trapianto di Midollo Osseo. Bone Marrow Transplant 47(3):342–351

Passweg JR, Baldomero H, Bader P, Bonini C, Cesaro S, Dreger P et al (2016) Hematopoietic stem cell transplantation in Europe 2014: more than 40000 transplants annually. Bone Marrow Transplant 51(6):786–792. English

Pavone V, Gaudio F, Guarini A, Perrone T, Zonno A, Curci P et al (2002) Mobilization of peripheral blood stem cells with high-dose cyclophosphamide or the DHAP regimen plus G-CSF in non-Hodgkin's lymphoma. Bone Marrow Transplant 29(4):285–290

Perez-Simon JA, Caballero MD, Corral M, Nieto MJ, Orfao A, Vazquez L et al (1998) Minimal number of circulating CD34+ cells to ensure successful leukapheresis and engraftment in autologous peripheral blood progenitor cell transplantation. Transfusion 38(4):385–391

Perez-Simon JA, Martin A, Caballero D, Corral M, Nieto MJ, Gonzalez M et al (1999) Clinical significance of CD34+ cell dose in long-term engraftment following autologous peripheral blood stem cell transplantation. Bone Marrow Transplant 24(12):1279–1283

Petit I, Szyper-Kravitz M, Nagler A, Lahav M, Peled A, Habler L et al (2002) G-CSF induces stem cell mobilization by decreasing bone marrow SDF-1 and up-regulating CXCR4. Nat Immunol 3(7):687–694

Platzbecker U, Prange-Krex G, Bornhauser M, Koch R, Soucek S, Aikele P et al (2001) Spleen enlargement in healthy donors during G-CSF mobilization of PBPCs. Transfusion 41(2):184–189

Porrata LF, Inwards DJ, Ansell SM, Micallef IN, Johnston PB, Gastineau DA et al (2008) Early lymphocyte recovery predicts superior survival after autologous stem cell transplantation in non-Hodgkin lymphoma: a prospective study. Biol Blood Marrow Transplant 14(7):807–816

Pusic I, DiPersio JF (2008) The use of growth factors in hematopoietic stem cell transplantation. Curr Pharm Des 14(20):1950–1961

Pusic I, Jiang SY, Landua S, Uy GL, Rettig MP, Cashen AF et al (2008) Impact of mobilization and remobilization strategies on achieving sufficient stem cell yields for autologous transplantation. Biol Blood Marrow Transplant 14(9):1045–1056

Siena S, Schiavo R, Pedrazzoli P, Carlo-Stella C (2000) Therapeutic relevance of CD34 cell dose in blood cell transplantation for cancer therapy. J Clin Oncol Off J Am Soc Clin Oncol 18(6):1360–1377

Stiff PJ (1999) Management strategies for the hard-to-mobilize patient. Bone Marrow Transplant 23(Suppl 2):S29–S33

Stroncek D, Shawker T, Follmann D, Leitman SF (2003) G-CSF-induced spleen size changes in peripheral blood progenitor cell donors. Transfusion 43(5):609–613

Tigue CC, McKoy JM, Evens AM, Trifilio SM, Tallman MS, Bennett CL (2007) Granulocyte-colony stimulating factor administration to healthy individuals and persons with chronic neutropenia or cancer: an overview of safety considerations from the Research on Adverse Drug Events and Reports project. Bone Marrow Transplant 40(3):185–192

Vellenga E, van Agthoven M, Croockewit AJ, Verdonck LF, Wijermans PJ, van Oers MH et al (2001) Autologous peripheral blood stem cell transplantation in patients with relapsed lymphoma results in accelerated haematopoietic reconstitution, improved quality of life and cost reduction compared with bone marrow transplantation: the Hovon 22 study. Br J Haematol 114(2):319–326

Vose JM, Sharp G, Chan WC, Nichols C, Loh K, Inwards D et al (2002) Autologous transplantation for aggressive non-Hodgkin's lymphoma: results of a randomized trial evaluating graft source and minimal residual disease. J Clin Oncol Off J Am Soc Clin Oncol 20(9):2344–2352

Weaver CH, Hazelton B, Birch R, Palmer P, Allen C, Schwartzberg L et al (1995) An analysis of engraftment kinetics as a function of the CD34 content of peripheral blood progenitor cell collections in 692 patients after the administration of myeloablative chemotherapy. Blood 86(10):3961–3969

Worel N, Rosskopf K, Neumeister P, Kasparu H, Nachbaur D, Russ G et al (2011) Plerixafor and granulocyte-colony-stimulating factor (G-CSF) in patients with lymphoma and multiple myeloma previously failing mobilization with G-CSF with or without chemotherapy for autologous hematopoietic stem cell mobilization: the Austrian experience on a named patient program. Transfusion 51(5):968–975

Worel N, Fritsch G, Agis H, Bohm A, Engelich G, Leitner GC et al (2017) Plerixafor as preemptive strategy results in high success rates in autologous stem cell mobilization failure. J Clin Apher 32:224–234

Wuchter P, Ran D, Bruckner T, Schmitt T, Witzens-Harig M, Neben K et al (2010) Poor mobilization of hematopoietic stem cells-definitions, incidence, risk factors, and impact on outcome of autologous transplantation. Biol Blood Marrow Transplant 16(4):490–499

Mobilization Strategies: HPC(A) Collections for Allogeneic Hematopoietic Cell Transplants

6

Pavan Kumar Bhamidipati, Mark A. Fiala, and John F. DiPersio

6.1 Introduction

Historically, CD34⁺ cells were harvested from donors by repeated aspiration of the bone marrow (BM), a procedure that is associated with a great deal of discomfort and requires general or regional anesthesia. Over the last 20 years, peripheral blood (PB) has become the preferred graft source for allo-HCT. Hematopoietic progenitor cells (HPCs) mobilized by hematopoietic cytokines and/or chemokine receptor antagonists are pluripotent hematopoietic stem cells that have the capability of self-renewal and multi-lineage reconstitution after HCT. HPCs can be identified by their surface expression of numerous stem cell markers including CD34, CD90, CD117, and CD133.

There are advantages and disadvantages of utilizing PB-mobilized HPCs compared to BM. These include the relative ease of mobilization and collection of HPCs and larger number of CD34⁺ hematopoietic progenitor cells (HPC) that can be obtained. According to National Marrow Donor Program (NMDP) guidelines, no more than 20 mL of marrow/kg is collected in one bone marrow harvest which may limit the number of CD34⁺ HPCs that can be collected. Conversely, donors can undergo multiple days of apheresis, and any restrictions on volumes are for logistical concerns rather than safety.

Although HPCs circulate in the PB, they do so in small numbers in the normal resting state. Stress factors such as infection, trauma, or chemotherapy will increase HPC circulation (Baldridge et al. 2011). A higher number of HPCs are needed for successful allo-HCT than it is possible to collect under normal conditions; thus, donors must undergo HPC mobilization prior to collection.

P. K. Bhamidipati · M. A. Fiala · J. F. DiPersio (✉)
Division of Oncology, Washington University School of Medicine, Saint Louis, MO, USA
e-mail: pbhamidipati@wustl.edu; mfiala@wustl.edu; jdipersi@wustl.edu

S. A. Abutalib et al. (eds.), *Best Practices of Apheresis in Hematopoietic Cell Transplantation*, Advances and Controversies in Hematopoietic Transplantation and Cell Therapy, https://doi.org/10.1007/978-3-319-55131-9_6

6.2 Mobilization Methods in Healthy Donors

HPC mobilization in healthy donors is performed utilizing cytokines exclusively. Typically, granulocyte colony-stimulating factor (G-CSF) or less commonly granulocyte-macrophage colony-stimulating factor (GM-CSF) are utilized, although CXCR4 antagonists such as plerixafor and BL-8040 and balixafortide (previously POL6326) have been tested in clinical trials (Abraham et al. 2017; Karpova et al. 2017).

6.2.1 G-CSF/GM-CSF

The mobilization of HPCs with cytokines was first introduced in 1989 when Gianni et al. utilized GM-CSF to mobilize patients with non-Hodgkin lymphoma undergoing autologous HCT (auto-HCT) (Gianni et al. 1989). Since that time, HPC mobilization and collection from PB has developed into an alternative and pragmatic approach (Baumann et al. 1993; Bensinger et al. 1995; Dreger et al. 1994).

Standard-dose G-CSF (10 μg/kg/day) is a highly effective regimen for HPC mobilization yielding adequate HPC collection in up to 95% of healthy donors (Ings et al. 2006). Studies testing higher-dose G-CSF (either once daily or split dosing schedules) have shown slightly improved HPC yields and mobilization success rates but were associated with more toxicity and increased costs (Engelhardt et al. 1999).

G-CSF (10 μg/kg/day) is given subcutaneously over 4.5 consecutive days with apheresis occurring on the fifth day. If a sufficient HPC yield, typically $>2 \times 10^6$ (up to maximum $8–10 \times 10^6$ based on institution preference) $CD34^+$ cells/kg recipient body weight, is not collected after the first day of 3–4 total blood volume aphereses, the donor can undergo additional days of G-CSF and apheresis. Most centers typically perform 1–2 days for normal allogeneic donors and 3–4 days for patients undergoing auto-HCT as the daily collection yield generally declines each day.

The patent on filgrastim, the first FDA-approved G-CSF, expired in 2006 in Europe and in 2013 in the United States. Since that time, several biosimilars have come to market. Biosimilars are biochemically identical molecules of the parent biologics (Abraham et al. 2013). Due to complexity of manufacturing of many biologics, biosimilars usually not referred to as "generics" (which usually are the exact copies of small-molecule drugs) but instead as "biosimilars."

Filgrastim-Sndz (Novartis), lenograstim (Chugai Pharmaceuticals), and tevagrastim (Teva Pharmaceutical Industries) are all currently available G-CSF biosimilars. There are additional biosimilar agents available in Europe. In general, all have similar safety and efficacy profiles with no significant differences to filgrastim (Abraham et al. 2013). However, much of this data has been generated in the auto-HCT setting. The National Comprehensive Cancer Network (NCCN) recently assigned G-CSF biosimilars category 2A (based upon lower-level evidence, there is uniform NCCN consensus that the intervention is appropriate) recommendation in the auto-HCT setting and category 2B (based upon lower-level evidence, there is

NCCN consensus that the intervention is appropriate) in the allogeneic setting (Zelenetz and Becker 2016). While the evidence supporting their use in the allogeneic setting is not yet overwhelming, biosimilars often result in cost-saving benefits and thus their clinical utilization is increasing.

In the limited number of studies where it has been tested, polyethylene glycol-conjugated (Peg)-G-CSF has shown similar kinetics of mobilization, but data on recipient outcomes is lacking (Kroschinsky et al. 2005). Peg-G-CSF has not been widely accepted by transplant centers, probably because of ease and experience in usage of G-CSF and cost-related issues. Among patients undergoing auto-HCT, a higher dose of Peg-G-CSF was required and was shown to be not cost-effective compared to G-CSF (Hill et al. 2006; Martino et al. 2014).

GM-CSF can be administered alternatively to G-CSF, but at standard doses (5–10 μg/kg), it mobilizes fewer CD34$^+$ cells than G-CSF. And, thus, additional days of apheresis and/or higher apheresis volumes are required to collect a similar number of HPCs (Lane et al. 1999; Sohn et al. 2002). Interestingly, in a study of 230 donors at our center, we noted slightly lower rates of grade II–IV graft-versus-host disease (GvHD) among GM-CSF-mobilized grafts compared to G-CSF. The graft composition was different in the GM-CSF cohorts, suggesting that GM-CSF mobilizes a different subset of both CD34$^+$ HPC and non-CD34$^+$-mobilized peripheral blood cells compared to G-CSF (Devine et al. 2005).

GM-CSF has also been used to augment G-CSF mobilization in clinical trials. In a randomized clinical trial of GM-CSF with G-CSF compared to G-CSF alone, combination treatment resulted in higher CD34$^+$ HSC yields. It was also noted that the grafts from donors receiving combination treatment contained fewer plasmacytoid dendritic cells and had enhanced donor T-cell engraftment with Th1 polarization; however, this did not result in any differences in recipient outcomes (Lonial et al. 2013).

6.2.2 Adverse Reactions

Side effects of G-CSF/GM-CSF are mostly mild and serious complications are rare (Pulsipher et al. 2013). Common side effects of G-CSF are bone pain, headache, and flu-like symptoms such as malaise, nausea, myalgias, bone pain, and night sweats (Holig 2013; Rhodes and Anderlini 2008; Holig et al. 2009). Allergic reactions including anaphylaxis may occur on initial exposure. G-CSF/GM-CSF should be given cautiously to donors with a history of allergic reactions. Acute respiratory distress syndrome (ARDS) is a rare but serious toxicity primarily in donors receiving high or intravenous doses of GM-CSF. Patients who develop fevers, shortness of breath, and chills should be evaluated for lung infiltrates or respiratory distress.

Although rare, precipitation of sickle cell crisis can occur in donors with sickle cell trait; however, several studies have been conducted in this population, and toxicity is similar to that of the general population (Rosenbaum et al. 2008; Horowitz and Confer 2005). In spite of these studies, most transplant physicians try to avoid G-CSF for mobilization in SS patients and sickle trait patients. The risk of precipitation of acute chest syndrome and splenic infarction/rupture is higher in SS patients, resulting in some groups looking at alternative mobilizing regimens (CXCR4 inhibitors) in this patient population. Most transplant physicians feel that G-CSF-/GM-CSF-based mobilization should be considered in sickle trait patients and not in SS patients.

The spleen is commonly enlarged following extended administration of G-CSF/GM-CSF, but this generally normalizes after few days. The increase of splenic volume after G-CSF ranges between 10 and 20% in various studies (Stroncek et al. 2003; Platzbecker et al. 2001). Life-threatening complications, such as spontaneous splenic rupture, are extremely rare with only a few cases reported mainly in patients that have received a higher dose or longer duration of G-CSF than normally administered (Nuamah et al. 2006). In donors who develop severe, sudden-onset upper abdominal pain or shoulder pain during the administration phase, G-CSF/GM-CSF should be discontinued and should be evaluated for this rare complication.

There was once a concern for increased incidence of hematological malignancies due to growth factor stimulation/exposure. There are only sporadic reports suggesting higher occurrences of acute leukemia and lymphoma in normal donors exposed to G-CSF. Of note is that G-CSF does induce changes in gene and microRNA expression in CD34$^+$ HPCs that can persist for at least 1 year after exposure to the drug (Baez et al. 2014). The consequence of this remains unclear. In a large retrospective survey of 15,445 individuals who donated peripheral blood progenitor cells (PBPCs) or bone marrow (BM) between 1992 and 2009, there was no evidence that either PBPC or BM donation was associated with increased risks of hematological malignancies (Schmidt et al. 2017; Shaw et al. 2015). The standardized incidence ratio (SIR) for a diagnosis of leukemia was essentially 0 (95% CI, 0 to 1.88).

The World Marrow Donor Association (WMDA) released a statement in 2015 that the risk of developing cancer within several years after the use of G-CSF is not increased compared with donors not receiving G-CSF (Shaw et al. 2015; Anderlini et al. 1999; Tigue et al. 2007). However, due to the concern for underreporting and heterogeneity of the retrospective registry analyses, a caution is often advised by NMDP and EBMT (Shaw et al. 2015). To evaluate this, long-term follow-up of HPC donors is desirable once every 1–2 years for at least 10 years (Halter et al. 2013; Stroncek and McCullough 2012).

6.2.3 CXCR4 Antagonists/Inhibitors

CXCR4 antagonists/inhibitors reduce the binding and chemotaxis of HSCs to the stromal factor 1-a (SDF-1) expressing BM stroma and osteoblasts, thus increasing the number in circulation (Uy et al. 2008). Plerixafor is the most studied CXCR4 antagonist for CD34$^+$ cell mobilization to date. It is FDA approved when administered in combination with G-CSF for autologous mobilization in patients with multiple myeloma and non-Hodgkin lymphoma but not in healthy donors.

In the auto-HCT setting, the recommended dose of plerixafor is 240 μg/kg/day by SC injection, applied on fourth day of G-CSF. Plerixafor has generally been dosed in the evening before the scheduled apheresis prior to beginning stem cell apheresis because the maximum increase in circulating CD34+ cells occurs approximately 4–10 h after SC injection (Stewart et al. 2009). Plerixafor is often used with risk-adapted algorithms in three ways: preemptive usage in expected poor mobilizers, immediate rescue for patients with suboptimal mobilization, and planned remobilization in failed mobilizers.

In the allo-HCT mobilization setting, plerixafor alone has had modest success. Up to a third (33%) of the donors fail to mobilize the minimal CD34+ yield needed for allogeneic transplantation after conventional dose plerixafor (240 μg/kg) is administered subcutaneous the morning of apheresis (Devine et al. 2008). At 480 μg/kg, HPC yield and success rates improve slightly but are still inferior to that of standard-dose G-CSF (Pantin et al. 2017).

In attempt to improve mobilization success, intravenous (IV) administration of plerixafor has been tested; the optimal dose was determined to be 320 μg/kg (Schroeder et al. 2017). IV plerixafor was found to be safe and effective similar to subcutaneous, but mobilization failure was still common and identical to that seen by the same group testing subcutaneous plerixafor in normal allogeneic donors (Devine et al. 2008). It's notable that recipients had lower rates of GvHD and CMV viremia compared to historical data with G-CSF. The favorable outcomes were attributed to a graft composition that is rich in plasmacytoid dendritic cell progenitors (pre-pDCs) and mature plasmacytoid dendritic cells.

When combined with G-CSF, plerixafor augments mobilization much like what is observed in the auto-HCT setting. Again, graft composition is significantly different with enhanced CD4 and CD8 mobilization and skewing CD34+ cells to an increased population of dendritic cell precursors and mature plasmacytoid dendritic cells, but with low numbers of pro-inflammatory dendritic cells. However, this has not been shown to translate to lower rates of acute GVHD or the reactivation of viral infections perhaps due to the addition of G-CSF (Schroeder et al. 2017; Rutella et al. 2014). Based on the limited efficacy of plerixafor in the allo-HCT setting, its use should be limited to clinical trials and as a salvage strategy in the case of mobilization failures following G-CSF (see below) (Nadeau et al. 2015).

Additional agents targeting the hematopoietic niche are currently undergoing evaluation in the clinic for normal allo-HCT mobilization including CXCR4 antagonists TG-0054 (TaiGen Biotechnology), balixafortide (POL6326; Polyphor Ltd) (clinicaltrials.gov # NCT01841476), and BL-8040 (BioLineRx) (clinicaltrials.gov # NCT02639559), a high-affinity, long-acting inhibitor of CXCR4.

6.2.4 Novel Targets

We have shown in a murine preclinical HCT mobilization model that bortezomib, a proteasome inhibitor used in patients with myeloma, induced rapid (12–18 h) mobilization of mouse HPCs via modulation of the VCAM-1/VLA-4 axis (Ghobadi et al. 2014). We have also shown that another small-molecule inhibitor of VLA-4 (BIO5192), when used alone, induced rapid mobilization of HSC with kinetics even faster than plerixafor (~30 min). When administered in combination with G-CSF or

AMD3100, it induced rapid and additive/synergistic HSPC mobilization (Ramirez et al. 2009). A dual small-molecule integrin inhibitor of α9β1 and α4β1 (R-BC154), similarly to BIO5192, induced rapid mobilization of murine HPC (Cao et al. 2016). Of note, bortezomib, BIO5192, and R-BC154 are all relatively weak mobilizing agents compared to G-CSF or even plerixafor and will likely require the addition of other mobilizing agents to be effective in the clinic.

Two recent reports suggest that the combination of the chemokine receptor CXCR2 agonist, Gro-beta (Gro-β), with either plerixafor or several novel VLA-4 inhibitors results in dramatic, synergistic, and rapid HSC mobilization in mouse preclinical models. The combination of these agents (Gro-β and either plerixafor or VLA-4 inhibitors) dramatically is more potent and superior to G-CSF, plerixafor, and VLA4 inhibitors but is extremely rapid (approximately 15–20 min) compared to 30–60 min with VLA-4 inhibitors, 2–3 h with plerixafor, and 12–18 h with bortezomib. The combination of Gro-β and both plerixafor and VLA4 inhibitors will be tested in the clinic in the next 12–18 months (Karpova et al. 2016; Hoggatt et al. 2018). TXA127 (angiotensin 1–7 agonist), thioridazine, NOX-A12 (novel CXCL12 inhibitor), SB-751689 (ronacaleret, a calcium-sensing receptor antagonist), α4β7 integrin blocker (natalizumab), and others are also being actively investigated in various preclinical models.

6.3 Healthy Donors as Poor Mobilizers

Unlike auto-HCT, otherwise healthy allo-HCT donors do not have prior chemotherapy/radiation exposure and have no marrow infiltration that would impair $CD34^+$ HPC collection. However, even among healthy donors, approximately 2–6% are unable to collect a minimum of 2×10^6 $CD34^+$ cells/kg body weight ("minimal goal") after two apheresis procedures and constitute "poor mobilizers" (Ings et al. 2006; Rinaldi et al. 2012).

Poor mobilization is often due to defective bone marrow reserves or a damaged niche. Impaired mobilization is often seen in donors with preexistent diabetes (diabetic stem cell "mobilopathy (DSCM)") (DiPersio 2011; Fadini et al. 2013; Fadini and Avogaro 2013). It is postulated that DSCM may be due to impaired β3 adrenergic nerve innervation of the bone marrow resulting in altered BM niche function (Ferraro et al. 2011), to enhanced integrin α4β1-mediated adhesion (Abplanalp et al. 2016), or possibly to maladaptive CD26/DPP-4 regulation (Fadini et al. 2013) that contributes to a mobilization defect of endothelial progenitor cells and HSCs in diabetes. Plerixafor, in contrast to G-CSF, was shown to overcome this limitation in patients with diabetes (Fadini et al. 2015). Diabetes is also associated with a deficit of circulating endothelial progenitor cells (EPCs), which has been attributed to their defective mobilization from the bone marrow. Enhanced integrin α4β1-mediated adhesion-related mobilization defect was shown in a streptozotocin diabetic mouse model, and the mobilization defect was reversed by α4-integrin modulating mutations and agents (Abplanalp et al. 2016). α4β1 inhibitors could therefore be used to improve mobilization in these patients in the future (Cao et al. 2016).

Even among donors with successful collection, there is great heterogeneity in HPC yield and in the apheresis volume and number of procedures needed for successful collection. Several factors are associated with $CD34^+$ cell mobilization. Among these, donor factors that have been associated with poorer stem cell yield include advancing age, sex, lower BMI, and resting total white blood cell or $CD34^+$ count (Rinaldi et al. 2012; Wang et al. 2008; Vasu et al. 2008; Martino et al. 2017, 2006; Brown et al. 1997; de la Rubia et al. 2004). As collection yields are measured in cells per kg of recipient weight, having a donor-to-recipient weight ratio below one increases the likelihood of mobilization failure (Fiala et al. 2014). On contrary, factors associated with an improved mobilization success include male sex, higher body mass index, higher G-CSF dosage, higher premobilization WBC, and the use of lenograstim rather than filgrastim (Chen et al. 2014; Bertani et al. 2014). Non-donor factors noted in various studies that can affect mobilization include G-CSF dose and timing of the apheresis procedure (see text later) (Martino et al. 2017; Martinez et al. 1999; Demirer et al. 2002; Krejci et al. 2015).

6.4 Second/Subsequent HPC Collections from Same Donor: What Are the Data?

Repeat HPC mobilization is uncommon in the allo-HCT setting, and most data regarding this come from small retrospective studies. Of interest, $CD34^+$ cell yield does seem to be reduced in second/subsequent collections in healthy donors. Guo et al. evaluated the $CD34^+$ yield in 100 donors undergoing second collection and noticed a reduction in apheresis yields compared to the initial collections. Further, lymphocyte counts of $>2.0 \times 10^9$/L prior to their first collections predicted a better $CD34^+$ HPC collected after a second cycle. Male sex and an inter-transplantation interval >9 months between collections were associated with better yield (Guo et al. 2016). Similar findings were seen in previous studies that showed a reduced $CD34^+$ yield with second PBPC mobilization (De la Rubia et al. 2002). A retrospective study from our institution included 62 healthy donors that underwent mobilization with G-CSF followed by remobilization with G-CSF and showed reduced $CD34^+$ HPC yield after remobilization compared to those normal allogeneic donors initially mobilized with plerixafor followed by remobilization with G-CSF (Fiala et al. 2016). This data suggests that donors undergoing repeat mobilization when initially mobilized with G-CSF may benefit from the addition of CXCR4 antagonists/inhibitors.

6.5 Apheresis Procedure

Hematopoietic progenitor ("$CD34^+$") cell harvesting is a two-part procedure. During the initial phase of administration of mobilization agents, donors receive cytokines or other mobilizing agents. In the second phase of HPC collection, the apheresis procedure is initiated using conventional apheresis equipment via peripheral or central venous access (see Chaps. 5 and 7).

Based on the circulating $CD34^+$ cells in the peripheral blood on day 4, an empirical algorithm can be used to estimate the mean volume of blood that needs to be processed to achieve the collection goal (see Chap. 9). Due to logistical issues, most centers limit apheresis to 12–24 L or 3–4 blood volumes per day. If the collection goal is not achieved after one apheresis procedure, additional procedures can be performed on subsequent days. In a retrospective analysis of >1400 donors registered with the International Bone Marrow Transplant Registry (IBMTR) and the European Blood and Marrow Transplant Group (EBMT), 60% of donors required more than one leukapheresis procedure to collect the target number of CD34⁺ cells, and 15% required three or more (Anderlini et al. 2001) (Fig. 6.1).

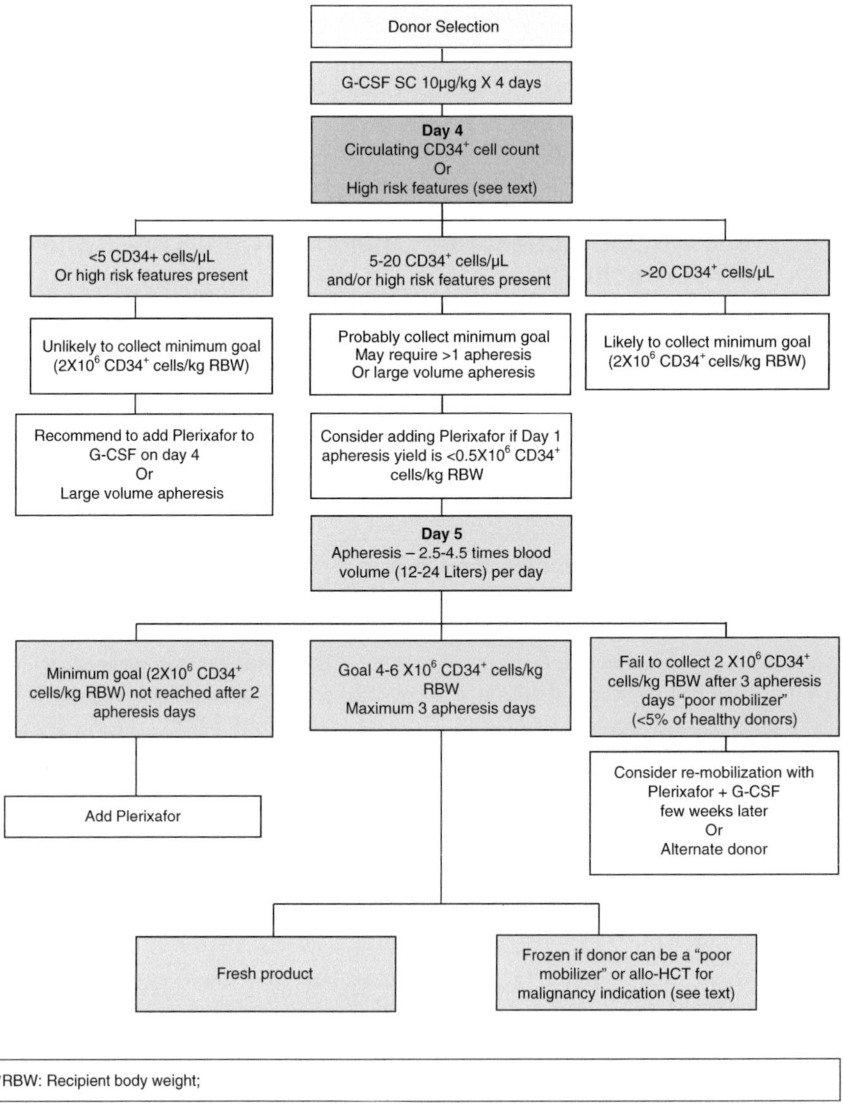

Fig. 6.1 Standard algorithm for CD34⁺ cell mobilization in healthy donors

Even though relatively safe, the apheresis procedure is not without complications. The rate of serious complications from G-CSF mobilization and PBPC collection was reported to be 1.1%, as compared with 0.5% following bone marrow collection in one retrospective study (Anderlini et al. 2001). Apart from the risks associated with central line placement (i.e., bleeding, infection, and thrombosis risk) and shift in blood volumes (hypotension), the apheresis procedure can be associated with hypocalcemia (Pulsipher et al. 2009a). This is predominantly due to citrate that is used as anticoagulant during procedure. Citrate toxicity leads to hypocalcemia through increased calcium ion binding that often requires correction during the procedure. Further toxicities of citrate include hypomagnesemia, hypokalemia, and metabolic alkalosis. Thrombocytopenia develops either due to contemporary collection with leukocytes or due to the adherence of platelets to the apheresis machine. Decreased platelet counts can be seen particularly after 2 days of apheresis, although only 2% of donors drop their platelet counts to $<50 \times 10^9$/L, and this drop is often transient in nature and does not require platelet transfusions with few exceptions (Pulsipher et al. 2013). Thrombocytopenia compounds the bleeding risk already inherent in large-volume apheresis that often requires anticoagulation (see Chaps. 8 and 14).

6.5.1 Collection Goal: Do We Know the Answer?

For a successful allo-HCT, mobilization and collection of adequate HSCs are essential. Sufficient numbers of HPCs provide a faster and more consistent and sustained multi-lineage hematopoietic recovery resulting in reduced hospitalization, blood product usage, infections, and other associated hospital costs. In general, the aim is to collect the "optimal" $CD34^+$ dose in minimal number of apheresis procedures. An optimal dose is the $CD34^+$ dose per kilogram body weight of recipient that results in successful multi-lineage hematopoietic recovery and decreased transfusion requirements after allo-HCT (Siena et al. 2000). As such, careful donor selection and improving the apheresis procedure are essential (Kollman et al. 2001; Flomenberg et al. 2004; De la Rubia et al. 2001).

What constitutes an optimal $CD34^+$ dose varies across institutions. Based on recent studies, consensus is that 5×10^6 cells/kg is the optimal dose as it results in more rapid, consistent, and sustained engraftment (Duong et al. 2014; Pulsipher et al. 2009b). With myeloablative conditioning, the $CD34^+$ dose is important in hematopoietic reconstitution and an optimal dose of 5×10^6 cells/kg is shown to be associated with enhanced survival, decreased graft rejection, and decreased incidence of infections and relapse (Ringden et al. 2003; Sierra et al. 1997; Przepiorka et al. 1999; Rocha et al. 2002; Schulman et al. 1999; Heimfeld 2002) However, with reduced intensity/non-myeloablative conditioning, a $CD34^+$ dose of $<4 \times 10^6$ cells/kg from sibling donors and a dose $<6 \times 10^6$ cells/kg from unrelated donor were associated with higher NRM, poor OS, and lower neutrophil and platelet recovery after allo-HCT (Torlen et al. 2014).

The accepted minimal CD34$^+$ HPC number is 2 × 10^6 CD34$^+$ cells/kg recipient body weight. Even though successful engraftment can occur at doses as low as 0.75 × 10^6 CD34$^+$cells/kg recipient body weight, neutrophil and platelet engraftment are often delayed and can increase the morbidity associated with allo-HCT (Torlen et al. 2014; Pérez-Simón et al. 2003). Although the ideal number of CD34$^+$ required for multi-lineage engraftment is controversial, a minimum of 2 × 10^6 or an ideal 4–5 × 10^6 CD34$^+$/kg recipient body weight are accepted norms. CD34$^+$ doses <5 × 10^6 CD34$^+$/kg are associated with successful neutrophil but impaired platelet engraftment and are associated with increased number of hospital days.

Administration of a higher CD34$^+$ dose (>5 × 10^6 cells/kg recipient weight), although was shown to be associated with faster neutrophil and platelet recovery, higher lymphocyte recovery at day 30, and reduced relapse, was not associated with improved OS (Nakamura et al. 2008). Several studies have shown similar findings and that higher doses of CD34$^+$ (ranging from 8 to 10 × 10^6 cells/kg recipient weight) result in an increased risk of GvHD and most notably extensive chronic GvHD (Przepiorka et al. 1999; Torlen et al. 2014; Barrett et al. 2000; Remberger et al. 2008; Mohty et al. 2003; Urbano-Ispizua et al. 2001; Zaucha et al. 2001). Even higher CD34$^+$ doses (>10 × 10^6 CD34$^+$/kg recipient body weight) are associated with rapid and improved engraftment rates (neutrophil and platelet recovery), decreased transfusion dependency, and shorter hospitalization but were associated with increased risk of both acute and chronic GvHD and with a modest decreased survival (Przepiorka et al. 1999; Mohty et al. 2003; Zaucha et al. 2001; Remberger et al. 2015).

In HLA-haploidentical HCT (haplo-HCT) and prior to the use of posttransplant cyclophosphamide (PT-Cy), T-cell depletion was extensively used to reduce GvHD. To minimize graft rejection, "megadose" CD34$^+$-selected HPC was used resulting in rapid engraftment and reduced GvHD but with increased non-relapse mortality secondary to infections and relapse rates (Aversa et al. 1994, 1998). CD34$^+$ doses of ≥10 × 10^6 CD34$^+$ cells/kg body weight were often used in these studies (Aversa et al. 2007). However, with the advent of in vivo depletion using PT-Cy, a CD34$^+$ dose of 4–6 × 10^6 cells/kg recipient body weight is considered acceptable for successful haplo-HCT (Stiehl et al. 2014). As such, many transplant centers now accept a minimum CD34$^+$ dose of 2 × 10^6 cells/kg and an optimum dose of 4–6 × 10^6 cells/kg for a successful allo-HCT (Pulsipher et al. 2009b). Recent (2017) literature analysis by Mohammadi et al. suggests that >8 × 10^6 CD34$^+$/kg for sibling donors and >9 × 10^6 CD34$^+$/kg from unrelated donors are considered not beneficial (Mohammadi et al. 2017).

6.5.2 Timing

For donors receiving cytokines for mobilization, apheresis is often performed on day 5 after starting G-CSF. Peak HPC mobilization generally occurs on day 4–6 (Dreger et al. 1994; Tjonnfjord et al. 1994). However, collection of HPCs on day 4 has been shown to be feasible and effective while reducing G-CSF exposure to healthy donors but is associated with inferior yields (Flommersfeld et al. 2015; van

Oostrum et al. 2017). In one study, the mobilization success rate on day 4 of standard G-CSF mobilization was only 22.6% (van Oostrum et al. 2017). In addition, optimal $CD34^+$ cell yields after GM-CSF-induced mobilization occurs on day 6 and not day 5 (Devine et al. 2005). If institutional restrictions allow, optimal timing can be varied for each donor. The peripheral blood (PB) $CD34^+$ cell count is the best predictor of apheresis harvest, and using it to time apheresis has been shown to reduce costs (Armitage et al. 1997; Gutensohn et al. 2010). In a retrospective study of 95 patients by Armitage et al., 94% of donors with ≥20/μL $CD34^+$ cell on day 4 yielded $>2 \times 10^6$ $CD34^+$ cells/kg in one apheresis (Armitage et al. 1997).

There is no agreement on the minimum threshold of PB $CD34^+$ cell count required for apheresis; institutional practices vary from 5 to 20 μL. Adequate yield is not expected in patients with <5/μL $CD34^+$ (Armitage et al. 1997; Coluccia et al. 2012). If the count is between 5 and 20/μL, sufficient HPCs may be collected, but frequently more than one apheresis procedure is required (Pérez-Simón et al. 1998; Elliott et al. 1996). An alternative prediction algorithm has been proposed based on age, sex, lactate dehydrogenase (LDH) on day 4, and RBC count at the baseline that has been shown to predict collection of at least 2×10^6 $CD34^+$ cells/donor body weight in one apheresis procedure (Yoshizato et al. 2013).

6.6 Fresh Versus Frozen Cell Product in Allo-HCT: What Is Preferred?

Apheresis can be planned to coincide with conditioning regimen in the case of related donor allo-HCT, and as such, apheresis product can be transfused without cryopreserving ("fresh"). However, apheresis product can be collected in advance and cryopreserved. Cryopreservation facilitates the assurance of quality of the product and assures against unforeseen "poor mobilization issues." Further, the unused cryopreserved cells can be utilized at a later date for $CD34^+$-selected boost or for $CD3^+$-selected donor lymphocyte infusion (DLI) in the post-allo-HCT period. Most centers favor infusion of fresh apheresis products due to the theoretical concern that cryopreservation and thawing may lead to loss of viability of HPCs, T cells, and other mononuclear cells (Frey et al. 2006). Additional hypothetical concerns of frozen products include the possibility of transfusion reactions associated with dimethyl sulfoxide (DMSO), concern for bacterial contamination with increased handling, increased risk of GvHD, and reduced engraftment and higher non-relapse mortality. However, multiple studies suggest that no differences in outcomes exist between fresh and cryopreserved products (Frey et al. 2006; Parody et al. 2013; Kim et al. 2007; Ghobadi et al. 2017).

6.7 Expert Point of View

Mobilization of HPCs has evolved over the past 30 years to primarily utilize cytokines and peripheral blood as mobilizing agents and stem cell sources for allo-HCT. Multiple studies have identified various donor and non-donor risk factors that may impact both outcome of allo-HCT mobilization and engraftment and survival of recipients. A goal of 4–6 × 10^6 $CD34^+$ cells/kg recipient body weight is the optimal goal to be collected in up to 2–3 days of apheresis procedures. G-CSF-based mobilization is the current standard and is relatively safe with long-term data suggesting no untoward effects to the donors. Other cytokines (GM-CSF/PEG-filgrastim) and chemokine antagonists (plerixafor) have not currently replaced G-CSF. New mobilizing agents and combinations of agents are making their way through preclinical and early clinical trials and may eventually provide more rapid, robust, and safe alternatives to mobilizing normal donors for allo-HCT. Although adding plerixafor to G-CSF has made significant impact on improving the mobilization yields and overcoming "poor mobilization (collecting <2 × 10^6 $CD34^+$ cells/kg recipient body weight) in auto-HCT, it is a relatively weak mobilizing agent when used in mice and man by itself and has not been tested in combination with G-CSF in normal allogeneic donors. The impact of adding plerixafor (and other agents) to G-CSF in healthy donors may not be great since the likelihood of mobilization failure is very low with G-CSF alone. However, plerixafor can still be utilized in either preemptive or "just-in-time" approach to overcome the poor mobilization risk based on pre-apheresis circulating $CD34^+$ numbers or based on the yields of $CD34^+$/kg or circulating $CD34^+$ cells/ml after G-CSF-only mobilization. Further, novel molecules such as GroB, VLA4 inhibitors, and novel CXCR4 antagonists may help overcome the slow mobilization and occasional poor mobilization seen with G-CSF in allogeneic donors in the future.

References

Abplanalp WT, Conklin DJ, Cantor JM, Ginsberg MH, Wysoczynski M, Bhatnagar A et al (2016) Enhanced Integrin alpha4beta1-mediated adhesion contributes to a mobilization defect of endothelial progenitor cells in diabetes. Diabetes 65(11):3505–3515

Abraham I, Tharmarajah S, MacDonald K (2013) Clinical safety of biosimilar recombinant human granulocyte colony-stimulating factors. Expert Opin Drug Saf 12(2):235–246

Abraham M, Pereg Y, Bulvik B, Klein S, Mishalian I, Wald H et al (2017) Single dose of the CXCR4 antagonist BL-8040 induces rapid mobilization for the collection of human CD34+ cells in healthy volunteers. Clin Cancer Res 23(22):6790–6801

Anderlini P, Donato M, Chan KW, Huh YO, Gee AP, Lauppe MJ et al (1999) Allogeneic blood progenitor cell collection in normal donors after mobilization with filgrastim: the M.D. Anderson Cancer Center experience. Transfusion 39(6):555–560

Anderlini P, Rizzo JD, Nugent ML, Schmitz N, Champlin RE, Horowitz MM et al (2001) Peripheral blood stem cell donation: an analysis from the International Bone Marrow Transplant Registry (IBMTR) and European Group for Blood and Marrow Transplant (EBMT) databases. Bone Marrow Transplant 27(7):689–692

Armitage S, Hargreaves R, Samson D, Brennan M, Kanfer E, Navarrete C (1997) CD34 counts to predict the adequate collection of peripheral blood progenitor cells. Bone Marrow Transplant 20(7):587–591

Aversa F, Tabilio A, Terenzi A, Velardi A, Falzetti F, Giannoni C et al (1994) Successful engraftment of T-cell-depleted haploidentical "three-loci" incompatible transplants in leukemia patients by addition of recombinant human granulocyte colony-stimulating factor-mobilized peripheral blood progenitor cells to bone marrow inoculum. Blood 84(11):3948–3955

Aversa F, Tabilio A, Velardi A, Cunningham I, Terenzi A, Falzetti F et al (1998) Treatment of high-risk acute leukemia with T-cell-depleted stem cells from related donors with one fully mismatched HLA haplotype. N Engl J Med 339(17):1186–1193

Aversa F, Tabilio A, Velardi A, Terenzi A, Falzetti F, Carotti A et al (2007) Hematopoietic stem cell transplantation from alternative donors for high-risk acute leukemia: the haploidentical option. Curr Stem Cell Res Ther 2(1):105–112

Baez A, Martin-Antonio B, Piruat JI, Prats C, Alvarez-Laderas I, Barbado MV et al (2014) Granulocyte colony-stimulating factor produces long-term changes in gene and microRNA expression profiles in CD34+ cells from healthy donors. Haematologica 99(2):243–251

Baldridge MT, King KY, Goodell MA (2011) Inflammatory signals regulate hematopoietic stem cells. Trends Immunol 32(2):57–65

Barrett AJ, Ringden O, Zhang MJ, Bashey A, Cahn JY, Cairo MS et al (2000) Effect of nucleated marrow cell dose on relapse and survival in identical twin bone marrow transplants for leukemia. Blood 95(11):3323–3327

Baumann I, Testa NG, Lange C, de Wynter E, Luft T, Dexter TM et al (1993) Haemopoietic cells mobilised into the circulation by lenograstim as alternative to bone marrow for allogeneic transplants. Lancet 341(8841):369

Bensinger WI, Weaver CH, Appelbaum FR, Rowley S, Demirer T, Sanders J et al (1995) Transplantation of allogeneic peripheral blood stem cells mobilized by recombinant human granulocyte colony-stimulating factor. Blood 85(6):1655–1658

Bertani G, Santoleri L, Martino M, Fedele R, Moscato T, Marenco P et al (2014) Identification of hematopoietic progenitor cell donor characteristics predicting successful mobilization: results of an Italian multicenter study. Transfusion 54(8):2028–2033

Brown RA, Adkins D, Goodnough LT, Haug JS, Todd G, Wehde M et al (1997) Factors that influence the collection and engraftment of allogeneic peripheral-blood stem cells in patients with hematologic malignancies. J Clin Oncol 15(9):3067–3074

Cao B, Zhang Z, Grassinger J, Williams B, Heazlewood CK, Churches QI et al (2016) Therapeutic targeting and rapid mobilization of endosteal HSC using a small molecule integrin antagonist. Nat Commun 7:11007

Chen J, Burns KM, Babic A, Carrum G, Kennedy M, Segura FJ et al (2014) Donor body mass index is an important factor that affects peripheral blood progenitor cell yield in healthy donors after mobilization with granulocyte-colony-stimulating factor. Transfusion 54(1):203–210

Coluccia P, Crovetti G, Del Fante C, Dallavalle FM, Laszlò D, Ferremi P et al (2012) Screening of related donors and peripheral blood stem cell collection practices at different Italian apheresis centres. J Geophys Res Space Physics 10(4):440–447

De la Rubia J, Díaz MA, Verdeguer A, Pascual Maria J, Arbona C, Arrieta R et al (2001) Donor age-related differences in PBPC mobilization with rHuG-CSF. Transfusion 41(2):201–205

De la Rubia J, Arbona C, Del Canizo C, Arrieta R, De Arriba F, Pascual MJ et al (2002) Second mobilization and collection of peripheral blood progenitor cells in healthy donors is associated with lower CD34(+) cell yields. J Hematother Stem Cell Res 11(4):705–709

de la Rubia J, Lorenzo JI, Torrabadella M, Marin P, Insunza A, Sanz MA (2004) Basal CD34(+) cell count predicts peripheral blood progenitor cell mobilization and collection in healthy donors after administration of granulocyte colony-stimulating factor. Haematologica 89(12):1530–1532

Demirer T, Ayli M, Ozcan M, Gunel N, Haznedar R, Dagli M et al (2002) Mobilization of peripheral blood stem cells with chemotherapy and recombinant human granulocyte colony-stimulating factor (rhG-CSF): a randomized evaluation of different doses of rhG-CSF. Br J Haematol 116(2):468–474

Devine SM, Brown RA, Mathews V, Trinkaus K, Khoury H, Adkins D et al (2005) Reduced risk of acute GVHD following mobilization of HLA-identical sibling donors with GM-CSF alone. Bone Marrow Transplant 36(6):531–538

Devine SM, Vij R, Rettig M, Todt L, McGlauchlen K, Fisher N et al (2008) Rapid mobilization of functional donor hematopoietic cells without G-CSF using AMD3100, an antagonist of the CXCR4/SDF-1 interaction. Blood 112(4):990

DiPersio JF (2011) Diabetic stem-cell "mobilopathy". N Engl J Med 365(26):2536–2538

Dreger P, Haferlach T, Eckstein V, Jacobs S, Suttorp M, Loffler H et al (1994) G-CSF-mobilized peripheral blood progenitor cells for allogeneic transplantation: safety, kinetics of mobilization, and composition of the graft. Br J Haematol 87(3):609–613

Duong HK, Savani BN, Copelan E, Devine S, Costa LJ, Wingard JR et al (2014) Peripheral blood progenitor cell mobilization for autologous and allogeneic hematopoietic cell transplantation: guidelines from the American Society for Blood and Marrow Transplantation. Biol Blood Marrow Transplant 20(9):1262–1273

Elliott C, Samson DM, Armitage S, Lyttelton MP, McGuigan D, Hargreaves R et al (1996) When to harvest peripheral-blood stem cells after mobilization therapy: prediction of CD34-positive cell yield by preceding day CD34-positive concentration in peripheral blood. J Clin Oncol 14(3):970–973

Engelhardt M, Bertz H, Afting M, Waller CF, Finke J (1999) High-versus standard-dose filgrastim (rhG-CSF) for mobilization of peripheral-blood progenitor cells from allogeneic donors and CD34(+) immunoselection. J Clin Oncol 17(7):2160–2172

Fadini GP, Avogaro A (2013) Diabetes impairs mobilization of stem cells for the treatment of cardiovascular disease: a meta-regression analysis. Int J Cardiol 168(2):892–897

Fadini GP, Albiero M, Vigili de Kreutzenberg S, Boscaro E, Cappellari R, Marescotti M et al (2013) Diabetes impairs stem cell and proangiogenic cell mobilization in humans. Diabetes Care 36(4):943–949

Fadini GP, Fiala M, Cappellari R, Danna M, Park S, Poncina N et al (2015) Diabetes limits stem cell mobilization following G-CSF but not plerixafor. Diabetes 64(8):2969–2977

Ferraro F, Lymperi S, Mendez-Ferrer S, Saez B, Spencer JA, Yeap BY et al (2011) Diabetes impairs hematopoietic stem cell mobilization by altering niche function. Sci Transl Med 3(104):104ra1

Fiala MA, Park S, Abboud CN, Cashen AF, Jacoby M, Pusic I et al (2014) Donor-to-recipient weight ratio is independently associated with $CD34^+$ yield in healthy donors undergoing peripheral blood stem cell collection for allogeneic transplantation. Blood 124(21):2456

Fiala MA, Park S, Slade M, DiPersio JF, Stockerl-Goldstein KE (2016) Remobilization of hematopoietic stem cells in healthy donors for allogeneic transplantation. Transfusion 56(9):2331–2335

Flomenberg N, Baxter-Lowe LA, Confer D, Fernandez-Vina M, Filipovich A, Horowitz M et al (2004) Impact of HLA class I and class II high-resolution matching on outcomes of unrelated donor bone marrow transplantation: HLA-C mismatching is associated with a strong adverse effect on transplantation outcome. Blood 104(7):1923

Flommersfeld S, Sohlbach K, Jaques G, Bein G, Hoffmann J, Kostrewa P et al (2015) Collection of peripheral blood progenitor cells on day 4 is feasible and effective while reducing granulocyte-colony-stimulating factor exposure to healthy donors. Transfusion 55(6):1269–1274

Frey NV, Lazarus HM, Goldstein SC (2006) Has allogeneic stem cell cryopreservation been given the 'cold shoulder'? An analysis of the pros and cons of using frozen versus fresh stem cell products in allogeneic stem cell transplantation. Bone Marrow Transplant 38(6):399–405

Ghobadi A, Rettig MP, Cooper ML, Holt MS, Ritchey JK, Eissenberg L et al (2014) Bortezomib is a rapid mobilizer of hematopoietic stem cells in mice via modulation of the VCAM-1/VLA-4 axis. Blood 124(17):2752–2754

Ghobadi A, Fiala MA, Ramsingh G, Gao F, Abboud CN, Stockerl-Goldstein K et al (2017) Fresh or cryopreserved CD34+-selected mobilized peripheral blood stem and progenitor cells for the treatment of poor graft function after allogeneic hematopoietic cell transplantation. Biol Blood Marrow Transplant 23(7):1072–1077

Gianni AM, Siena S, Bregni M, Tarella C, Stern AC, Pileri A et al (1989) Granulocyte-macrophage colony-stimulating factor to harvest circulating haemopoietic stem cells for autotransplantation. Lancet 2(8663):580–585

Guo Z-P, Wang T, Xu L-P, Zhang X-H, Wang Y, Huang X-J et al (2016) Factors affecting the $CD34^+$ cell yields from the second donations of healthy donors: the steady-state lymphocyte count is a good predictive factor. Transfus Apheres Sci 55(3):311–317

Gutensohn K, Magens MM, Kuehnl P, Zeller W (2010) Increasing the economic efficacy of peripheral blood progenitor cell collections by monitoring peripheral blood CD34+ concentrations. Transfusion 50(3):656–662

Halter J, Van Walraven S, Worel N, Bengtsson M, Hägglund H, De Faveri GN et al (2013) Allogeneic hematopoietic stem cell donation--standardized assessment of donor outcome data: a consensus statement from the Worldwide Network for Blood and Marrow Transplantation (WBMT). Bone Marrow Transplant 48(2):220

Heimfeld S (2002) Bone marrow transplantation: how important is CD34 cell dose in HLA-identical stem cell transplantation? Leukemia 17(5):856–858

Hill GR, Morris ES, Fuery M, Hutchins C, Butler J, Grigg A et al (2006) Allogeneic stem cell transplantation with peripheral blood stem cells mobilized by pegylated G-CSF. Biol Blood Marrow Transplant 12(6):603–607

Hoggatt J, Singh P, Tate TA, Chou B-K, Datari SR, Fukuda S et al (2018) Rapid mobilization reveals a highly engraftable hematopoietic stem cell. Cell 172(1):191–204.e10

Holig K (2013) G-CSF in healthy allogeneic stem cell donors. Transfus Med Hemother 40(4):225–235

Holig K, Kramer M, Kroschinsky F, Bornhauser M, Mengling T, Schmidt AH et al (2009) Safety and efficacy of hematopoietic stem cell collection from mobilized peripheral blood in unrelated volunteers: 12 years of single-center experience in 3928 donors. Blood 114(18):3757–3763

Horowitz MM, Confer DL (2005) Evaluation of hematopoietic stem cell donors. Hematology Am Soc Hematol Educ Program:469–475

Ings SJ, Balsa C, Leverett D, Mackinnon S, Linch DC, Watts MJ (2006) Peripheral blood stem cell yield in 400 normal donors mobilised with granulocyte colony-stimulating factor (G-CSF): impact of age, sex, donor weight and type of G-CSF used. Br J Haematol 134(5):517–525

Karpova D, Rettig MP, Eissenberg L, Ritchey J, Holt M, Heier R et al (2016) Combined targeting of CXCR2 and VLA4 results in rapid and synergistic mobilization of hematopoietic stem and progenitor cells in mice. Blood 128(22):659

Karpova D, Bräuninger S, Wiercinska E, Krämer A, Stock B, Graff J et al (2017) Mobilization of hematopoietic stem cells with the novel CXCR4 antagonist POL6326 (balixafortide) in healthy volunteers—results of a dose escalation trial. J Transl Med 15:2

Kim DH, Jamal N, Saragosa R, Loach D, Wright J, Gupta V et al (2007) Similar outcomes of cryopreserved allogeneic peripheral stem cell transplants (PBSCT) compared to fresh allografts. Biol Blood Marrow Transplant 13(10):1233–1243

Kollman C, Howe CWS, Anasetti C, Antin JH, Davies SM, Filipovich AH et al (2001) Donor characteristics as risk factors in recipients after transplantation of bone marrow from unrelated donors: the effect of donor age. Blood 98(7):2043

Krejci M, Janikova A, Folber F, Kral Z, Mayer J (2015) Outcomes of 167 healthy sibling donors after peripheral blood stem cell mobilization with G-CSF 16mug/kg/day: efficacy and safety. Neoplasma 62(5):787–792

Kroschinsky F, Holig K, Poppe-Thiede K, Zimmer K, Ordemann R, Blechschmidt M et al (2005) Single-dose pegfilgrastim for the mobilization of allogeneic CD34+ peripheral blood progenitor cells in healthy family and unrelated donors. Haematologica 90(12):1665–1671

Lane TA, Ho AD, Bashey A, Peterson S, Young D, Law P (1999) Mobilization of blood-derived stem and progenitor cells in normal subjects by granulocyte-macrophage- and granulocyte-colony-stimulating factors. Transfusion 39(1):39–47

Lonial S, Akhtari M, Kaufman J, Torre C, Lechowicz MJ, Flowers C et al (2013) Mobilization of hematopoietic progenitors from normal donors using the combination of granulocyte-macrophage colony-stimulating factor and granulocyte colony-stimulating factor results in fewer plasmacytoid dendritic cells in the graft and enhanced donor T cell engraftment with Th1 polarization: results from a randomized clinical trial. Biol Blood Marrow Transplant 19(3):460–467

Martinez C, Urbano-Ispizua A, Marin P, Merino A, Rovira M, Carreras E et al (1999) Efficacy and toxicity of a high-dose G-CSF schedule for peripheral blood progenitor cell mobilization in healthy donors. Bone Marrow Transplant 24(12):1273–1278

Martino M, Callea I, Condemi A, Dattola A, Irrera G, Marcuccio D et al (2006) Predictive factors that affect the mobilization of CD34+cells in healthy donors treated with recombinant granulocyte colony-stimulating factor (G-CSF). J Clin Apher 21(3):169–175

Martino M, Laszlo D, Lanza F (2014) Long-active granulocyte colony-stimulating factor for peripheral blood hematopoietic progenitor cell mobilization. Expert Opin Biol Ther 14(6):757–772

Martino M, Gori M, Pitino A, Gentile M, Dattola A, Pontari A et al (2017) Basal $CD34^+$ cell count predicts peripheral blood stem cell mobilization in healthy donors after administration of granulocyte colony; stimulating factor: a longitudinal, prospective, observational, single-center, cohort study. Biol Blood Marrow Transplant 23(7):1215–1220

Mohammadi S, Malek Mohammadi A, Nikbakht M, Norooznezhad AH, Alimoghaddam K, Ghavamzadeh A (2017) Optimizing stem cells mobilization strategies to ameliorate patient outcomes: a review of guide- lines and recommendations. Int J Hematol Oncol Stem Cell Res 11(1):78–88

Mohty M, Bilger K, Jourdan E, Kuentz M, Michallet M, Bourhis JH et al (2003) Higher doses of CD34+ peripheral blood stem cells are associated with increased mortality from chronic graft-versus-host disease after allogeneic HLA-identical sibling transplantation. Leukemia 17(5):869–875

Nadeau M, George L, Yeager AM, Anwer F, McBride A (2015) Plerixafor as a salvage mobilization strategy for haploidentical peripheral blood allogeneic stem cell transplantation. Clinical Case Rep 3(9):728–730

Nakamura R, Auayporn N, Smith DD, Palmer J, Sun JY, Schriber J et al (2008) Impact of graft cell dose on transplant outcomes following unrelated donor allogeneic peripheral blood stem cell transplantation: higher CD34+ cell doses are associated with decreased relapse rates. Biol Blood Marrow Transplant 14(4):449–457

Nuamah NM, Goker H, Kilic YA, Dagmoura H, Cakmak A (2006) Spontaneous splenic rupture in a healthy allogeneic donor of peripheral-blood stem cell following the administration of granulocyte colony-stimulating factor (g-csf). A case report and review of the literature. Haematologica 91(5 Suppl):ECR08

Pantin J, Purev E, Tian X, Cook L, Donohue-Jerussi T, Cho E et al (2017) Effect of high-dose plerixafor on CD34+ cell mobilization in healthy stem cell donors: results of a randomized crossover trial. Haematologica 102(3):600–609

Parody R, Caballero D, Marquez-Malaver FJ, Vazquez L, Saldana R, Madrigal MD et al (2013) To freeze or not to freeze peripheral blood stem cells prior to allogeneic transplantation from matched related donors. Eur J Haematol 91(5):448–455

Pérez-Simón JA, Caballero MD, Corral M, Nieto MJ, Orfao A, Vazquez L et al (1998) Minimal number of circulating CD34+ cells to ensure successful leukapheresis and engraftment in autologous peripheral blood progenitor cell transplantation. Transfusion 38(4):385–391

Pérez-Simón JA, Díez-Campelo M, Martino R, Sureda A, Caballero D, Cañizo C et al (2003) Impact of $CD34^+$ cell dose on the outcome of patients undergoing reduced-intensity-conditioning allogeneic peripheral blood stem cell transplantation. Blood 102(3):1108–1113

Platzbecker U, Prange-Krex G, Bornhauser M, Koch R, Soucek S, Aikele P et al (2001) Spleen enlargement in healthy donors during G-CSF mobilization of PBPCs. Transfusion 41(2):184–189

Przepiorka D, Smith TL, Folloder J, Khouri I, Ueno NT, Mehra R et al (1999) Risk factors for acute graft-versus-host disease after allogeneic blood stem cell transplantation. Blood 94(4):1465–1470

Pulsipher MA, Chitphakdithai P, Miller JP, Logan BR, King RJ, Rizzo JD et al (2009a) Adverse events among 2408 unrelated donors of peripheral blood stem cells: results of a prospective trial from the National Marrow Donor Program. Blood 113(15):3604–3611

Pulsipher MA, Chitphakdithai P, Logan BR, Leitman SF, Anderlini P, Klein JP et al (2009b) Donor, recipient, and transplant characteristics as risk factors after unrelated donor PBSC transplantation: beneficial effects of higher CD34+ cell dose. Blood 114(13):2606–2616

Pulsipher MA, Chitphakdithai P, Logan BR, Shaw BE, Wingard JR, Lazarus HM et al (2013) Acute toxicities of unrelated bone marrow versus peripheral blood stem cell donation: results of a prospective trial from the National Marrow Donor Program. Blood 121(1):197

Ramirez P, Rettig MP, Uy GL, Deych E, Holt MS, Ritchey JK et al (2009) BIO5192, a small molecule inhibitor of VLA-4, mobilizes hematopoietic stem and progenitor cells. Blood 114(7):1340–1343

Remberger M, Mattsson J, Hassan Z, Karlsson N, LeBlanc K, Omazic B et al (2008) Risk factors for acute graft-versus-host disease grades II-IV after reduced intensity conditioning allogeneic stem cell transplantation with unrelated donors: a single centre study. Bone Marrow Transplant 41(4):399–405

Remberger M, Torlen J, Ringden O, Engstrom M, Watz E, Uhlin M et al (2015) Effect of total nucleated and CD34(+) cell dose on outcome after allogeneic hematopoietic stem cell transplantation. Biol Blood Marrow Transplant 21(5):889–893

Rhodes B, Anderlini P (2008) Allogeneic peripheral blood stem cell collection as of 2008. Transfus Apher Sci 38(3):219–227

Rinaldi C, Savignano C, Pasca S, Sperotto A, Patriarca F, Isola M et al (2012) Efficacy and safety of peripheral blood stem cell mobilization and collection: a single-center experience in 190 allogeneic donors. Transfusion 52(11):2387–2394

Ringden O, Barrett AJ, Zhang MJ, Loberiza FR, Bolwell BJ, Cairo MS et al (2003) Decreased treatment failure in recipients of HLA-identical bone marrow or peripheral blood stem cell transplants with high CD34 cell doses. Br J Haematol 121(6):874–885

Rocha V, Labopin M, Gluckman E, Powles R, Arcese W, Bacigalupo A et al (2002) Relevance of bone marrow cell dose on allogeneic transplantation outcomes for patients with acute myeloid leukemia in first complete remission: results of a European survey. J Clin Oncol 20(21):4324–4330

Rosenbaum C, Peace D, Rich E, Van Besien K (2008) Granulocyte colony-stimulating factor-based stem cell mobilization in patients with sickle cell disease. Biol Blood Marrow Transplant 14(6):719–723

Rutella S, Filippini P, Bertaina V, Li Pira G, Altomare L, Ceccarelli S et al (2014) Mobilization of healthy donors with plerixafor affects the cellular composition of T-cell receptor (TCR)-αβ/CD19-depleted haploidentical stem cell grafts. J Transl Med 12(1):240

Schmidt AH, Mengling T, Hernández-Frederick CJ, Rall G, Pingel J, Schetelig J et al (2017) Retrospective analysis of 37,287 observation years after peripheral blood stem cell donation. Biol Blood Marrow Transplant 23(6):1011–1020

Schroeder MA, Rettig MP, Lopez S, Christ S, Fiala M, Eades W et al (2017) Mobilization of allogeneic peripheral blood stem cell donors with intravenous plerixafor mobilizes a unique graft. Blood 129(19):2680–2692

Schulman KA, Birch R, Zhen B, Pania N, Weaver CH (1999) Effect of CD34+ cell dose on resource utilization in patients after high-dose chemotherapy with peripheral-blood stem-cell support. J Clin Oncol 17(4):1227

Shaw BE, Confer DL, Hwang W, Pulsipher MA (2015) A review of the genetic and long-term effects of G-CSF injections in healthy donors: a reassuring lack of evidence for the development of haematological malignancies. Bone Marrow Transplant 50(3):334–340

Siena S, Schiavo R, Pedrazzoli P, Carlo-Stella C (2000) Therapeutic relevance of CD34 cell dose in blood cell transplantation for cancer therapy. J Clin Oncol 18(6):1360–1377

Sierra J, Storer B, Hansen JA, Bjerke JW, Martin PJ, Petersdorf EW et al (1997) Transplantation of marrow cells from unrelated donors for treatment of high-risk acute leukemia: the effect of leukemic burden, donor HLA-matching, and marrow cell dose. Blood 89(11):4226–4235

Sohn S, Kim J, Seo K, Chae Y, Jung J, Suh J et al (2002) GM-CSF-based mobilization effect in normal healthy donors for allogeneic peripheral blood stem cell transplantation. Bone Marrow Transplant 30(2):81

Stewart DA, Smith C, MacFarland R, Calandra G (2009) Pharmacokinetics and pharmacodynamics of plerixafor in patients with non-Hodgkin lymphoma and multiple myeloma. Biol Blood Marrow Transplant 15(1):39–46

Stiehl T, Ho AD, Marciniak-Czochra A (2014) The impact of CD34+ cell dose on engraftment after SCTs: personalized estimates based on mathematical modeling. Bone Marrow Transplant 49(1):30–37

Stroncek D, McCullough J (2012) Safeguarding the long-term health of hematopoietic stem cell donors: a continuous and evolving process to maintain donor safety and trust. Expert Rev Hematol 5(1):1–3

Stroncek D, Shawker T, Follmann D, Leitman SF (2003) G-CSF-induced spleen size changes in peripheral blood progenitor cell donors. Transfusion 43(5):609–613

Tigue CC, McKoy JM, Evens AM, Trifilio SM, Tallman MS, Bennett CL (2007) Granulocyte-colony stimulating factor administration to healthy individuals and persons with chronic neutropenia or cancer: an overview of safety considerations from the Research on Adverse Drug Events and Reports project. Bone Marrow Transplant 40(3):185–192

Tjonnfjord GE, Steen R, Evensen SA, Thorsby E, Egeland T (1994) Characterization of CD34+ peripheral blood cells from healthy adults mobilized by recombinant human granulocyte colony-stimulating factor. Blood 84(8):2795–2801

Torlen J, Ringden O, Le Rademacher J, Batiwalla M, Chen J, Erkers T et al (2014) Low CD34 dose is associated with poor survival after reduced-intensity conditioning allogeneic transplantation for acute myeloid leukemia and myelodysplastic syndrome. Biol Blood Marrow Transplant 20(9):1418–1425

Urbano-Ispizua A, Carreras E, Marin P, Rovira M, Martinez C, Fernandez-Aviles F et al (2001) Allogeneic transplantation of CD34(+) selected cells from peripheral blood from human leukocyte antigen-identical siblings: detrimental effect of a high number of donor CD34(+) cells? Blood 98(8):2352–2357

Uy GL, Rettig MP, Cashen AF (2008) Plerixafor, a CXCR4 antagonist for the mobilization of hematopoietic stem cells. Expert Opin Biol Ther 8(11):1797–1804

van Oostrum A, Zwaginga JJ, Croockewit S, Overdevest J, Fechter M, Ruiterkamp B et al (2017) Predictors for successful PBSC collection on the fourth day of G-CSF-induced mobilization in allogeneic stem cell donors. J Clin Apher 32(6):397–404

Vasu S, Leitman SF, Tisdale JF, Hsieh MM, Childs RW, Barrett AJ et al (2008) Donor demographic and laboratory predictors of allogeneic peripheral blood stem cell mobilization in an ethnically diverse population. Blood 112(5):2092–2100

Wang TF, Wen SH, Chen RL, Lu CJ, Zheng YJ, Yang SH et al (2008) Factors associated with peripheral blood stem cell yield in volunteer donors mobilized with granulocyte colony-stimulating factors: the impact of donor characteristics and procedural settings. Biol Blood Marrow Transplant 14(11):1305–1311

Yoshizato T, Watanabe-Okochi N, Nannya Y, Ichikawa M, Takahashi T, Sato T et al (2013) Prediction model for CD34 positive cell yield in peripheral blood stem cell collection on the fourth day after G-CSF administration in healthy donors. Int J Hematol 98(1):56–65

Zaucha JM, Gooley T, Bensinger WI, Heimfeld S, Chauncey TR, Zaucha R et al (2001) CD34 cell dose in granulocyte colony-stimulating factor-mobilized peripheral blood mononuclear cell grafts affects engraftment kinetics and development of extensive chronic graft-versus-host disease after human leukocyte antigen-identical sibling transplantation. Blood 98(12):3221–3227

Zelenetz AD, Becker PS (2016) The role of biosimilars. J Natl Compr Cancer Netw 14(5 Suppl):626–629

7 Hematopoietic Progenitor Cells, Apheresis and Therapeutic Cells, T-Cells Collection: Instrumentation, Operating Parameters, and Troubleshooting

Edwin A. Burgstaler and Jeffrey L. Winters

7.1 Introduction

The focus of this chapter will be to discuss the current instrumentation used for the collection of cellular therapy products from the peripheral blood by apheresis methods, specifically hematopoietic progenitor cells, apheresis (HPC[A]), and therapeutic cells, T cells (TC-T). The chapter will not include a discussion of legacy apheresis instruments, such as the *Fenwal CS3000 Plus* or *COBE Spectra*, as these devices are or will soon no longer be supported by their manufacturers, even though still widely used in some parts of the world. Instead, discussion will focus on the *Fenwal Amicus* and *Terumo BCT Spectra Optia*, including both the MNC and continuous MNC (CMNC) protocols for the latter, with the goals of describing (1) the methods of cell separation and collection for each device/protocol; (2) the advantages, disadvantages, and operating parameters; and (3) troubleshooting for both devices. The content of this chapter is derived from information made available by the instruments' manufacturers, publications in the peer-reviewed medical literature, and the authors' personal experiences in using these devices, including both *Spectra Optia protocols*, in a busy therapeutic apheresis service which collects more than 1000 HPC(A) and TC-T products, annually.

E. A. Burgstaler
Development Technologist, Therapeutic Apheresis Treatment Unit, Division of Transfusion Medicine, Department of Laboratory Medicine and Pathology, Mayo Clinic, Rochester, MN, USA
e-mail: Burgstaler.edwin@mayo.edu

J. L. Winters (✉)
Therapeutic Apheresis Treatment Unit, Division of Transfusion Medicine, Department of Laboratory Medicine and Pathology, Mayo Clinic, Rochester, MN, USA
e-mail: Winters.Jeffrey@mayo.edu

S. A. Abutalib et al. (eds.), *Best Practices of Apheresis in Hematopoietic Cell Transplantation*, Advances and Controversies in Hematopoietic Transplantation and Cell Therapy, https://doi.org/10.1007/978-3-319-55131-9_7

7.2 Hematopoietic Progenitor Cells, Apheresis

HPC(A) products are collected from autologous or allogeneic donors in order to restore hematopoiesis following myeloablative (all cases of autologous and select cases of allogeneic transplants) and reduced intensity/nonmyeloablative (select cases of allogeneic transplant) conditioning regimens of chemotherapy with or without concurrent radiation therapy. In the context of allogeneic transplantation, the goal is to replace the recipient's immune system with that of the donor's in the hope of producing an immune response to the recipient's tumor, i.e., graft-versus-tumor (GvT) effect. In the autologous setting, the goal of the graft is to "rescue hematopoiesis" of the patient following high-dose chemotherapy, i.e., myeloablative condition regimen (MAC). Evidence does, however, suggest that there is an immune component to autologous transplants similar to that observed in allogeneic transplant recipients. When collecting $CD34^+$ cells via HPC(A), the goal is to collect sufficient $CD34^+$cells that would result in timely restoration of hematopoiesis. A variety of targets have been used to define an adequate product, but most commonly, it is a dose, on a per kilogram of recipient weight, of $CD34^+$ cells. Stem and progenitor cells represent a subset of $CD34^+$ cells. The usual collection targets in the autologous setting are anywhere in the ranges of $2–5 \times 10^6$ $CD34^+$ cells/kg while that for allogeneic transplants is usually in the range of $4–8 \times 10^6$ $CD34^+$ cells/kg of recipient weight. These doses may be achieved by processing a fixed volume of blood per collection (e.g., 2–3 blood volumes), measuring $CD34^+$ cells within the product during the collection and adjusting the duration of the collection accordingly or by processing blood for a fixed length of time (e.g., 4–6 h). Significant variability in clinical practice means that there is no standard in this regard (see Chaps. 4 and 5).

7.3 Therapeutic Cells, T Cells

TC-T are lymphocytes collected either for subsequent genetic modification (e.g., chimeric antigen receptor T cells [CAR-T cells]) or other manipulations or for infusion into patients after allogeneic hematopoietic cell transplantation (allo-HCT) in order to induce a GvT effect. The $CD3^+$ T-cells targets vary depending upon the medical use. The number collected for subsequent modification will vary depending upon the protocols and methods used to modify, and potentially expand, the T cells. When used without modification such as for conventional donor lymphocyte infusion (DLI), typically doses of $1–2 \times 10^8$ $CD3^+$ cells are collected and divided in specific aliquots for cryopreservation; this is usually done after administration of initial first fresh dose of DLI to the transplant recipient. In order to achieve these doses, collections may be performed using a blood volume target (e.g., 2–3 total blood volumes) or procedure length target (e.g., 4-h collection); again, there is no standard but institutional practices vary on the length of procedure.

7.4 Instrumentation

7.4.1 Fenwal Amicus (Fresenius Kabi, Lake Zurich, IL)

The *Fenwal Amicus* has been capable of TC and HPC(A) collections since clearance by the Food and Drug Administration (FDA) for these procedures in 2002. The separation kit is a disposable flexible plastic belt-shaped chamber that is wrapped around and secured to a rigid spool (Fig. 7.1). There are two chambers in the belt *(separation and collection chambers)*; however, only the *separation chamber* is used for TC and HPC(A) collection. A ramp is molded into the spool which directs flow within the separation chamber (Fig. 7.1).

As whole blood enters the *separation chamber*, the blood separates into the cell and plasma layers. Blood enters at a lower hematocrit (approximately 35%) and flows to the far end of the *separation chamber*. Platelets quickly separate and are returned by the platelet-rich plasma pump (Fig. 7.2). The granulocytes drop down into the RBC layer and flow to the outlet. As the whole blood flows through the chamber, the hematocrit increases to about 80%. As the mononuclear cells (MNCs) enter, they are heavier than platelets and drop to the cellular layer and move toward the outlet. However, as the hematocrit increases, the MNCs separate from the granulocytes and RBC and flow back to the inlet (Fig. 7.2). When they encounter the lower hematocrit, they drop down to the cellular layer resulting in the MNC recirculation in the center of the *separation chamber* (Fig. 7.2). Set volumes of whole blood are processed (usually 1000 mL or 1400 mL, depending on peripheral white blood cell (WBC) count) to allow buildup of the MNC layer prior to MNC harvesting. When the programmed volume has been processed, the *Amicus machine*

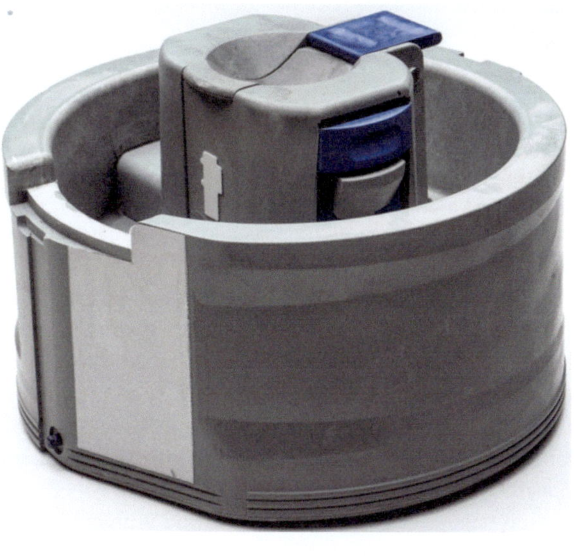

Fig. 7.1 Amicus mononuclear cell (MNC) spool. From left to right, note the slope of the ramp for the separation chamber (see text)

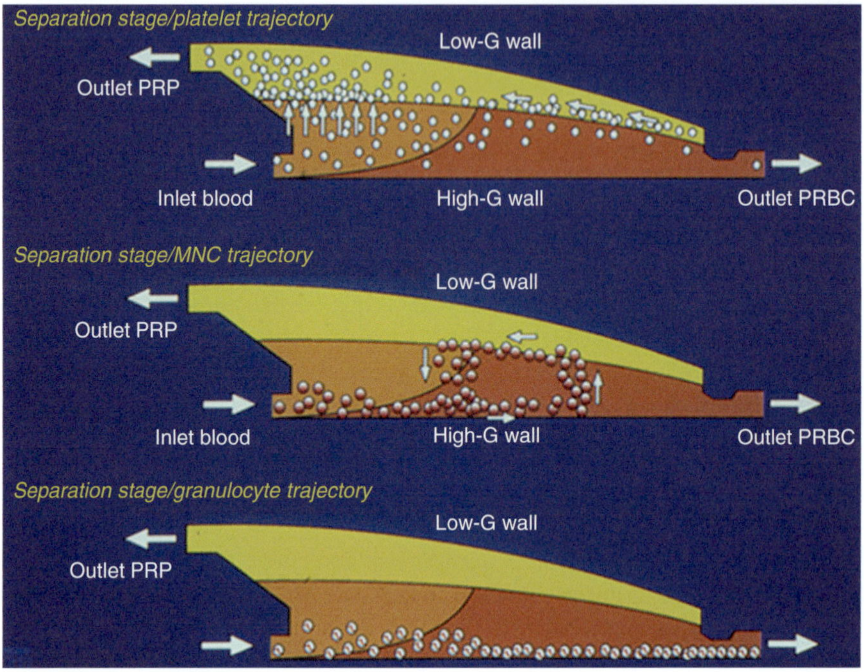

Fig. 7.2 Amicus blood separation in the centrifuge. Circulation of the various cells during separation and harvest of mononuclear cells (MNC). Platelet-rich plasma is returned to the patient/donor through the platelet-rich port (left). MNCs recirculate in the center of the chamber until harvest, and then they exit out the platelet-rich port (left) with the addition of packed RBC. Packed RBCs and granulocytes are returned to the patient/donor through the RBC port (right). (Used with permission from Fresenius Kabi)

automatically diverts about 30 mL of the high-hematocrit RBC to a small collection bag outside the *separation chamber* to be used to push the MNC out of the centrifuge. The MNC transfer then ensues. The inlet speed is dropped, and the cell/plasma interface that has been maintained on the ramp at about 60% is allowed to rise on the ramp and exit the *separation chamber*. The MNCs then pass through an optical sensor outside the centrifuge. When a designated amount of light is blocked (sense level), a whole blood pumped counter is activated. There are two settings used to open and close the valves to the collection bag: (1) the MNC and (2) the RBC offsets. The *MNC offset* is used to open the valve. It allows the platelet-rich plasma to be diverted back to the donor/patient. When the *MNC offset* is reached, the valve to the collection bag is opened and the MNCs continue to flow into the collection bag until the *RBC offset* setting is reached. When the collection valve closes, a small amount of platelet-rich plasma is flushed back to the donor, and the platelet-poor plasma (about 8–10 mL) is used to flush the MNC in the collection line to the collection bag. A new cycle is then started with cycles continuing until the end of the HPC(A) procedure.

During most of the procedure, plasma leaving the centrifuge is platelet rich. Platelet-poor plasma is usually collected at the very beginning or at end of the procedure that can be added to the product/graft or as a separate collection, if desired.

The settings for the *MNC offset*, *RBC offset*, ramp position, and light blockage (sense level) in the optical sensor can be adjusted by the operator (Burgstaler et al. 2010; Burgstaler and Winters 2014). Various cycle volumes have also been used and are operator programmable (Burgstaler and Winters 2011a).

7.4.2 Spectra Optia (Terumo BCT, Lakewood, CO, USA)

The *Spectra Optia* has two HPC(A)/TC collection protocols, each of which has different disposable supplies. The *Spectra Optia* was cleared by the FDA for the collection of TC and HPC(A) in 2012 using the MNC protocol and 2015 using the CMNC protocol. The MNC protocol works in cycles and uses an additional *separation chamber* to separate the MNC from the platelets (Fig. 7.3). The CMNC protocol continually collects MNC, similar to the *COBE Spectra* MNC procedure, and does not utilize the separate *separation chamber* (Fig. 7.4).

7.4.2.1 Spectra Optia MNC

The *Spectra Optia MNC protocol* uses a flexible circular centrifuge chamber that fits in a rigid insert (Fig. 7.5). The centrifuge chamber is the same diameter throughout. Whole blood enters the chamber and flows counterclockwise to the collection ports. There are three ports in the collector area: (1) the plasma port which is closest

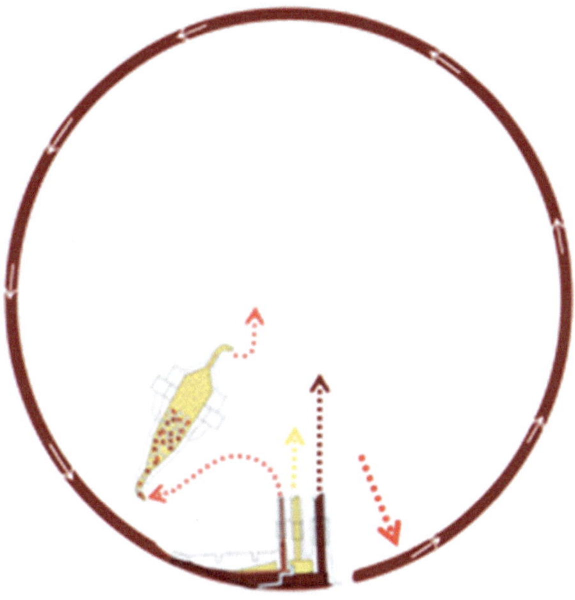

Fig. 7.3 Spectra Optia blood separation in the centrifuge using the MNC protocol. Whole blood flows counterclockwise with separation of the MNC and platelets that are drawn into the conical chamber (left) and then into the collection bag, during the harvest cycles. Platelet-poor plasma is drawn from the plasma port (center) to be returned to the patient/donor. Packed RBCs (right port) are returned to the patient/donor. (Used with permission from Terumo BCT)

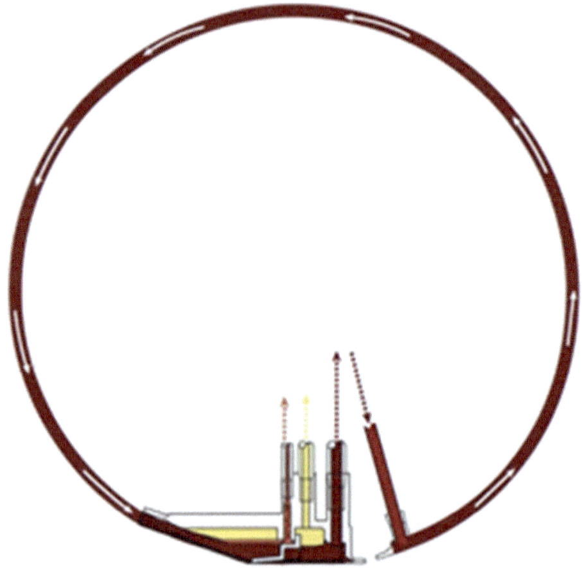

Fig. 7.4 Spectra Optia blood separation in the centrifuge using the CMNC protocol. Whole blood flows counterclockwise with separation of the MNCs that are drawn from the left port and into the collection bag, continuously. Platelet-rich plasma is drawn from the plasma port (center) to be returned to the patient/donor. Packed RBCs (right port) are returned to the patient/donor. (Used with permission from Terumo BCT)

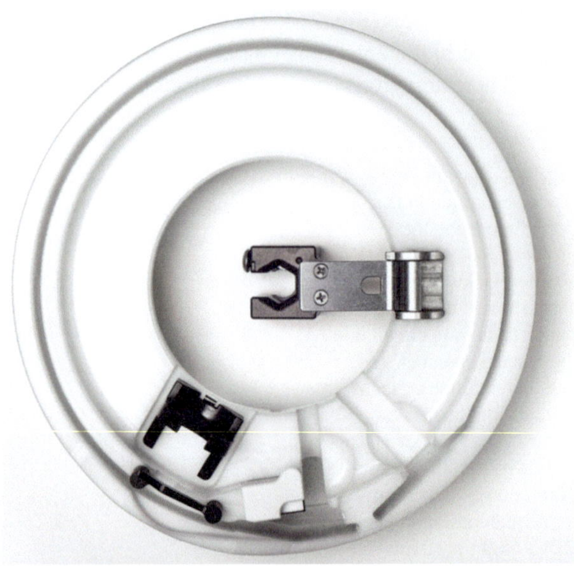

Fig. 7.5 Spectra Optia MNC insert. Circular channel with vertical walls and the secondary conical chamber holder

to the center, (2) the packed cell (RBC) line which is closest to the outside, and (3) the collection port is the first port (Fig. 7.3). The collection port is connected to the collection pump, while the plasma port is connected to the plasma pump. The remaining blood components are pushed out of the centrifuge chamber by the inlet pump. The *Spectra Optia* has an optical system, the automated interface management (AIM) system, which monitors and controls the cell/plasma interface. With the MNC program, the centrifuge packing factor is high, driving platelets into the buffy coat layer. The buffy coat is drawn off in a small collect line that is connected to a conical chamber located in the centrifuge (Fig. 7.3). The first stage of separation uses cell density to separate red blood cells from the buffy coat in the flexible circular *separation chamber*. The conical chamber located near the axis of rotation for the centrifuge then separates the platelets and MNC according to cell size using two forces: (1) centrifuge g-force and (2) fluid flow from the collect pump. The centrifuge g-force pushes components away from the axis of rotation, while the collect pump pulls components toward the center of the centrifuge, toward the axis of rotation, causing separation of the cells. First, the chamber fills with platelets. Then as RBC and MNC enter the chamber, based on their sizes, the MNC stays on the inlet side of the chamber while RBC percolates through the MNC and layer on top toward the outlet and the axis of rotation. As the chamber fills with MNC, the RBC eventually reaches the outlet and exits the chamber. An optical sensor detects the RBC-blocking light and triggers a chamber flush. The collect valve opens, and the MNCs are harvested into the collect bag (set volume is collected). A plasma flush then clears the line of MNC, flushing them into the collection bag. This is then followed by the start of a new cycle. The collect volume and plasma flush volume can be adjusted by the operator. The operator can also change the optical sensor control to use either the cycle volume or operator interaction (manual initiation) to trigger the MNC harvest. The operator can also determine the amount of RBC entering the chamber by adjusting the Collection Preference which controls the plasma pump speed. Donors with very high WBC counts will have many cycles because the chamber fills quickly resulting in frequent MNC harvests. This, in turn, results in larger collection volumes due to both the number of cells collected and the plasma flush used to clear the chamber and lines.

7.4.2.2 Spectra Optia CMNC

The *Spectra Optia CMNC* uses a different insert, the Intermediate Density Layer (IDL), for collections (Fig. 7.6). As with the MNC *separation chamber*, the CMNC chamber has the same diameter throughout, but it does not have a chamber bracket or the conical separation chamber present in the MNC kit (Fig. 7.6). The slot that the flexible chamber fits into is pear-shaped rather than rectangular which increases the extracorporeal volume of the device by approximately 100 mL compared to the MNC disposable kit. As with the *Spectra Optia MNC*, whole blood is pumped counterclockwise to the collection area. A lower packing factor is used to prevent platelets from being forced into the buffy coat. The same collection ports present in the MNC disposables are used; however, the collect line does not have a separate chamber attached, as with the *Spectra Optia MNC* kit (Fig. 7.4). The AIM system monitors and adjusts the position of the buffy coat interface. The collect pump continuously draws the MNC off and pumps them into the collection bag. The color of the collection is monitored by the operator, similar to what was done with the *COBE Spectra*, and adjusted by changing the Collection Preference, which adjusts

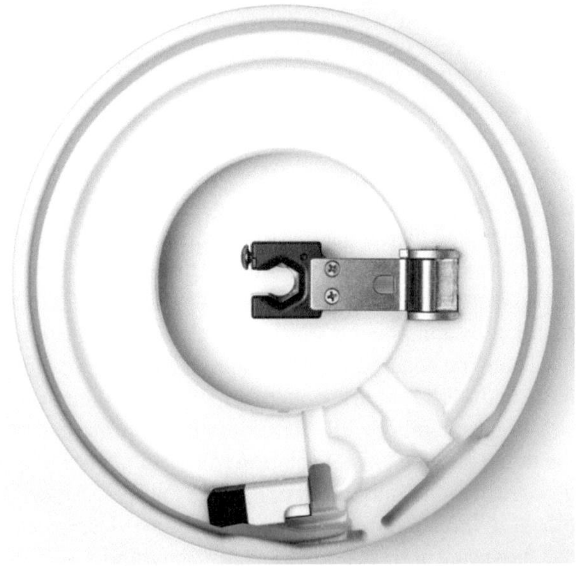

Fig. 7.6 Spectra Optia CMNC (IDL) insert. Circular channel with pear-shaped walls and no secondary conical chamber holder

the plasma pump. The plasma is platelet rich and is returned to the donor/patient. For that reason, there are only certain times that platelet-poor plasma can be collected. Separate plasma can be collected for addition to the collection or separate plasma collection. The *Spectra Optia* has a monitoring screen that can indicate if the AIM system is correctly adjusting the cell/plasma interface. The collect pump speed can be adjusted, and the collect volume is more predictable, compared to the MNC protocol, because of the continual collection.

7.5 Advantages and Disadvantages

Both of the instruments (described above), as well as the different protocols available for the *Spectra Optia*, offer advantages and disadvantages depending upon the characteristics of the patient/donor undergoing collection, experience of the operators, the processes and workflow of the apheresis collection center, and laboratory responsible for processing the cellular therapy product. Table 7.1 represents the authors' opinions of the advantages and disadvantages of the *Amicus* and the *Spectra Optia* protocols. It is important to acknowledge that one person's advantage may be another's disadvantage and vice versa. It should be noted that the authors utilize both devices in their practice with success, tailoring their use to the characteristics of those undergoing collection in order to maximize the safety and efficacy of the collection procedures. Table 7.2 provides how the authors utilize both devices in tailoring collections based upon patient/donor characteristics.

Table 7.1 Advantages and disadvantages

Advantages	Disadvantages
Fresenius Kabi Fenwal Amicus • Automated with manual adjustments possible • Low extracorporeal volume (ECV)—163 mL • Platelet sparing • Good MNC differentials, low granulocyte content • Low RBC content • Heparin/ACD-A anticoagulant solutions can be used. • CD34$^+$ cell and MNC collection efficiencies (CE) are as expected. • With AC ratios to 26:1 when using heparin/ACD-A anticoagulant: Less citrate toxicity Less volume to patient Higher inlet rates • Can collect separate plasma • Custom prime for low blood volumes	*Fresenius Kabi Fenwal Amicus* • Does not have sterile addition of AC to product bag • Cannot see into centrifuge • Works in cycles, which prolongs procedures due to transfers • Product size can vary slightly. • Slightly harder to control RBC and granulocyte content
Terumo BCT Spectra Optia—CMNC • Automated with manual adjustments possible • Simple to adjust, provides continuous collection • Very predictable product size • Sterile addition of AC to product bag • Tracking monitor on interface position • Can observe action in centrifuge • Can collect separate plasma • Very good MNC differentials, very low granulocyte content • Very low RBC content • Custom prime for low blood volumes • CD34$^+$ cell and MNC (CE) are as expected.	*Terumo BCT Spectra Optia—CMNC* • Poorly compatible with heparin/ACD-A anticoagulant solutions due to platelet clumping • Without 26:1 AC ratios: More citrate given More fluid to patient Slower inlet rates • Larger ECV—297 mL • Platelet loss is moderate to high.
Terumo BCT Spectra Optia—MNC • Automated with manual adjustments possible • Low ECV—191 mL • Low RBC content • Good MNC differential; low granulocyte content, but more than CMNC • Custom prime for low blood volumes • Sterile addition of AC to collection bag • CD34$^+$ cell and MNC (CE) are as expected.	*Terumo BCT Spectra Optia—MNC* • Poorly compatible with heparin/ACD-A anticoagulant solutions due to platelet clumping • Without 26:1 AC ratios: More citrate given More fluid to patient Slower inlet rates • Product volume variable due to WBC count • Large products with high WBC counts • Works in cycles, which prolongs procedures due to transfers • Platelet loss is moderate to high. • Requires more manipulation and observation of interface and platelets in chamber

Table 7.2 Patient/donor characteristics and optimal apheresis instrument

Characteristic	Optimal instrument	Rationale
Concerns about/ sensitivity to excessive fluid	Amicus	Heparin/ACD-A AC and 26:1 ratio will infuse half as much fluid per collection with Amicus, while heparin AC is associated with platelet clumping in the Spectra Optia. Due to the cycles, less blood and AC are processed compared to Spectra Optia CMNC with no cycles.
Very lipemic plasma	Spectra Optia CMNC or MNC	Interface detector is more tolerant of high lipids than Amicus.
Low platelet count	Amicus	Amicus demonstrates greater platelet sparing.
High granulocyte count	Spectra Optia CMNC	CMNC collects the least granulocytes.
Small patient with small blood volume	1st choice: Amicus 2nd choice: Spectra Optia MNC	Amicus has the lowest ECV of 163 mL Spectra Optia MNC ECV: 191 mLs Spectra Optia CMNC ECV: 297 mLs Amicus is also more compatible with heparin/ ACD-A AC and less citrate can be given.

AC anticoagulant, *CMNC* continuous mononuclear cell, *ECV* extracorporeal volume

7.6 Product Content and Characteristics

Both instruments and protocols can collect HPC(A) and TC products which are pure, potent, and efficacious. There are, however, differences in product content which may influence which device or protocol is used in certain circumstances or patients/donors. Table 7.3 provides a summary of the HPC(A) product content reported in the medical literature for each of the instruments and protocols, while Table 7.4 provides a summary of characteristics reported for TC collections.

7.7 Troubleshooting

As indicated above, both devices can collect an appropriate HPC(A) or TC product. However, at times, the content of the product may not be what is expected or desired. When this occurs, it is necessary to examine the collection procedure and the product content to be able to effectively troubleshoot. Etiology of unexpected hematopoietic graft yields and product content can result from patient/donor characteristics, operator errors, and equipment malfunction.

Troubleshooting for poor TC and HPC(A) collection yields can be very complex, especially in patients who have been mobilized with chemotherapy and/or cytokines. Usually, the problem is not the machine or the operator; the biggest variables in suboptimal collections are the donors/patients and the number of $CD34^+$ cells mobilized in the PB or the number of circulating lymphocytes. Factors such as the

Table 7.3 HPC(A) product content and collection procedure parameters reported in the medical literature

Source	Proc. N	Pt. N	Pre CD34+ cells/μL	Pre WBC ×10^9/L	CD34+ cell CE1 %	CD34+ cell CE2 %	CD34+ cell ×10^6/kg or ×10^6	PLT CE %	PLT loss % or ×10^11	RBC mL	Product volume mL	WB processed mL/TBV	Time min	Gran %	Gran ×10^9
AMICUS															
Tarik et al. (2013)	17				44.4 ± 14.8		6.3 ± 11.0		11.4 ± 11.0%				295 ± 42		
Sputtek et al. (2013)	36	15			64.6 ± 14.6		386 ± 413 × 10^6		0.7 ± 0.3 × 10^{11}			10,900 ± 1900	250 ± 15		
Burgstaler and Winters (2014)	20	20	49	56.5	55.0		3.28		2.2 × 10^{11}	25		15,800	300		15.7
Burgstaler and Winters (2014)	20	20	51	58.0	59.6		3.74		1.9 × 10^{11}	28		15,800	300		15.3
Burgstaler et al. (2012)		30		50.2			234.2 × 10^6		1.3 × 10^{11}	30			300	20	13.5
Burgstaler et al. (2012)		30		44.1			346.7 × 10^6		1.3 × 10^{11}	28			300	30	14.6
Burgstaler et al. (2010)	120	156		3.0–118.0			0.89–2.91		1.1–2.3 × 10^{11}	16–33		13,000–22,000	300	13–36	4.8–18.8
Burgstaler and Winters (2011b)	200	63		45.2			1.5		1.3 × 10^{11}	21			300	24	9.8
Burgstaler and Winters (2011b)	200	66		53.6			0.89		1.2 × 10^{11}	17			300	23	7.2
Burgstaler and Winters (2011c)	50	20		51.6			3.07		23%, 2.3 × 10^{11}	26		15,800	300	28	15.1
Burgstaler and Winters (2011a)	24	12	63 77	50.4 52.4	37.0 46.7		3.48 4.04		2.4 × 10^{11} 3.2 × 10^{11}	30 36	305 340	15,700 14,900	300 300	33 41	21.9 27.8
Gumogda et al. (2015)		20				37.04 ± 14.8						2.5 (TBV)			
Burgstaler et al. (2004)	80	65		33.3 36.8			2.1 1.5		1.1 × 10^{11} 1.1 × 10^{11}	14 15		13,400 20,300	300	25–40	5.3–15.1
Burgstaler and Pineda (2002)	40			12.3–43.3	37.0 46.7		60.5 × 10^6 285 × 10^6		2.4 × 10^{11} 3.2 × 10^{11}	30 36		10,000–29,000	300	33 41	21.9 27.8

(continued)

Table 7.3 (continued)

Source	Proc. N	Pt. N	Pre CD34⁺ cells/μL	Pre WBC ×10⁹/L	CD34⁺ cell CE1 %	CD34⁺ cell CE2 %	CD34⁺ cell ×10⁶/kg or ×10⁶	PLT CE %	PLT loss % or ×10¹¹	RBC mL	Product volume mL	WB processed mL/TBV	Time min	Gran %	Gran ×10⁹
SPECTRA OPTIA MNC															
Sputtek et al. (2013)	36	15			71.1 ± 12.0		$378 + 404 \times 10^6$		$2.6 \pm 1.5 \times 10^{11}$			9800 ± 1600	244 ± 15		
Burgstaler and Winters (2015)	80		32–55	48–51		50.3–59.2	$265–379 \times 10^6$	17.3–21.2	32.2–40.6%	8–11		12,500–20,700	300	18–28	10.5–19.3
Burgstaler and Winters (2016)	20		41.0	49.9		49.0	379.3×10^6	14.5 (CE2)	4.1×10^{11}	11	382	20,700	300	28	19.1
Brauninger et al. (2012)	50		103.6 ± 7.4		68 ± 0.02	51 ± 0.01	9.4 ± 0.6		Approx. 5.4%	388 ± 9				38	
Brauninger et al. (2011)	30		100.2 ± 8.9		41.1 ± 0.7		8.0 ± 0.7		37.2 ± 1.4%		270.8	14,100		39.2	
Karafin et al. (2014)	30				77 (43–111)	65 (12–173)								15 (0–48)	
Reinhardt et al. (2011)	35				47 ± 1.9				36.9 ± 1.5%		233.6± 13.3	2.8			
Lisenko et al. (2017)	98	78	6–433	3–80		7–116	0.5–40.4		1–63%			≤4 TBV	≤300		
SPECTRA OPTIA CMNC															
Lisenko et al. (2017)	94	72	4–531	5–113		8–87	0.3–237		0.57%			≤4 TBV	≤300		
Lozano et al. (2014)	10	9	40.2 12.0–252.9		60.7 40.5–90.1						191 146–257	3.3 1.7–4.7 (TBV)	210 111–293		
Gumogda et al. (2015)	20	20				50.2 ± 11.2						2.5 (TBV)			
Lamb and Stevens (2015)	40	25	39.2 7–446	35.9 4.0–69.6		52 29–114	2.5 0.45–27.4				268 114–389				
Watts et al. (2015)	50	41				54 50–62 44 41–47 43 38–52					192 191–194 156 152–157 112 111–113		200		

Marculescu et al. (2015)	10	10				47.4 34.4–56.5	7 2.8–8.1	12.8 (CE1)		3.7 1.4–6.5	9256–18,052				
Toney et al. (2015)		11	30 ± 5 or 421 ± 94	38.6 ± 4.9		47.5 ± 4.6 36.2 ± 5.6	8.75 ± 2.11	(CE1)	16.7 ± 3.4%		164.4 ± 0.02	8090 ± 900			
Sanderson et al. (2017)	39	23					2.92		27.3%	4.4% HCT	220		239		
Burgstaler and Winters (2017)	34 63			41.8 51.6			4.79 3.38	14.6 (CE2) 13.4 (CE2)		7 6	340 339	23,300 22,300	300 300	13 8.9	11.1 5.9
Burgstaler and Winters (2016)	20			45.5		57.1	363.0 × 10^6	14.5 (CE2)	31%	13	340	23,900	300	12	9.4
Schmidt et al. (2015)	17		86.2 ± 47.6	43.1 ± 11.2					110 ± 27 × 10^9/L		277 ± 30				

Empty cells no data reported, *Proc* number of procedures, *Pt* number of patients, *WBC* white blood cell count, *CE* collection efficiency, *PLT* platelet, *RBC* red blood cell, *WB* whole blood, *Gran* granulocyte

$$\mathrm{CE1} = \frac{\mathrm{CD34+cell/\mu L\,product \times PV}}{\frac{\mathrm{CD34+cell/\mu L\,pre + CD34+cell/\mu L\,post}}{2} \times \mathrm{TVP}}$$

$$\mathrm{CE2} = \frac{\mathrm{CD34+cell/\mu L\,product \times PV}}{\mathrm{CD34+cell/\mu L\,pre \times TVP}}$$

where *PV* product volume, *pre* pre-apheresis, *post* post-apheresis, and *TVP* total volume processed

Table 7.4 Therapeutic cell product content and collection procedure parameters reported in the medical literature

Source	Device (# Procedures)	Lymphocyte CE1 % or ×10^9	Monocyte CE1	MNC CE1 % or ×10^9	MNC Purity %	Platelet CE1 %	Volume mL	Throughput MNC × 10^6/mL
Robitzsch et al. (2015)	AM (40)	57 ± 19	39 ± 16	52 ± 16	96 ± 3			53 ± 25
Robitzsch et al. (2015)	SP CMNC (20)	56 ± 17	65 ± 15	64 ± 11	90 ± 7			69 ± 34
Robitzsch et al. (2015)	SP MNC (31)	54 ± 19	61 ± 21	55 ± 17	92 ± 7			57 ± 22
Steininger et al. (2014)	AM (12)	1.20 ± 0.37 2.80 ± 1.1 ×10^9						
Steininger et al. (2014)	SP MNC (20)	1.64 ± 0.70 2.36 ± 0.96 ×10^9						
Punzel et al. (2015)	SP CMNC (17)	60 ± 13			85 ± 10		176 ± 54	
Punzel et al. (2015)	SP MNC (18)	64 ± 15			87 ± 4		238 ± 47	
Fischer et al. (2013)	AM (40)	57	18%	51		7		
Fischer et al. (2013)	SP MNC (10)	64	33			24		
Burgstaler et al. (2005)	AM (20)	9.6 × 10^9	3.3 × 10^9	13 × 10^9	98		155	

Empty cells no data reported, *AM* amicus, *SP* Spectra Optia, *CMNC* continuous mononuclear cell, *MNC* mononuclear cell

$$\text{CE1} = \frac{\text{Cell count}/\mu\text{L product} \times \text{PV}}{\dfrac{\text{Cell count}/\mu\text{L pre} + \text{Cell count}/\mu\text{L post}}{2} \times \text{TVP}}$$

where *PV* product volume, *pre* pre-apheresis, *post* post-apheresis, and *TVP* total volume processed

type and extent of previous chemotherapy and radiation treatments, the marrow's ability to mobilize CD34$^+$ cells, the number of cells present in the circulation, the number of unwanted cells such as granulocytes, patient vascular access, the presence of high concentrations of plasma proteins such as seen in some plasma cell disorders, and other patient-specific issues can produce poor collection yields. The influence of these factors is unpredictable and fluctuates, changing over the course of the collections frequently in less than 24 h.

When investigating a suboptimal or poor collection, it is best to consider all of the components of collection rather than just CD34$^+$ cell or MNC yield. The MNC content should indicate if the collection was drawn from the proper layer. A product with a high percentage of MNC with a low percentage of granulocytes would indicate that the collection was appropriate. High granulocyte and RBC contents indicate the collection was too deep and that the buffy coat containing the desired cells was not harvested. A high platelet content and low total WBC and RBC contents would indicate the collection was too high, missing the portion of the buffy coat containing the desired cells.

If a product collected on the *Amicus* has a low WBC content, this can occur due to either a thick layer of platelets or a blush of RBCs triggering the optical sensor in the *Amicus* which opens and closes the valves during the harvest (see previous description). The *Amicus* uses the amount of light detected by the optical sensor (sense level) to open *(MNC offset)* and close *(RBC offset)* the valve to the collection bag. When the amount of light blocked reaches the programed level (sense level), the harvest is initiated with a volume of blood pumped *(MNC offset)* until the valves to the collection bag open. This is then followed by a volume of blood *(RBC offset)* pumped into the collect bag and then the valve closes. Once triggered, further changes in the amount of blocked light during the harvest are ignored by the device. If a thick layer of platelets or an RBC blush passes through the collect line, it can trigger the optical sensor by blocking sufficient light to reach the *sense level* with the valve opening and closing too early resulting in a failure to harvest the desired cells. This will occur even if the platelets or RBC blush clears as once the *sense level* is reached, the offsets are triggered. Using the default MNC (2.3 mL) and RBC (6.8 mL) offsets on *Amicus* without observing the actual color of the collection can result in some very poor collections. The operator monitoring the first cycle (manual monitoring) and making adjustments in the *RBC offset* can produce more consistent yields and lower cross cellular content (Burgstaler and Winters 2011b). This relatively simple procedure requires the operator to observe the upper right pump cassette to ensure that the RBCs make it to the top of the cassette (Fig. 7.7). If this does not occur, then the *RBC offset* can be adjusted by the operator for subsequent cycles (Burgstaler and Winters 2011b).

7.7.1 Poor CD34$^+$ Cell Yields

Obviously, high PB CD34$^+$ cell counts are required for high CD34$^+$ cell yields, but many patients do not mobilize well and therefore poor yields are not related to the actual collection procedure. It is thought that the CD34$^+$ cells have a specific gravity similar to that of lymphocytes and monocytes; therefore, the goal during collection would be to target that layer of the buffy coat between the platelets and the granulocytes. The only real indication of the layer being harvested is the red color of the collected cells as they are being harvested. Some RBCs are needed in the product in order to collect an appropriate product, but too many or too few indicate that the buffy coat has not been appropriately collected. If the collection contains primarily platelets and lymphocytes, attempts should be made to go deeper (darker red) for the next collection. If the collection contains large numbers of granulocytes and RBC, going lighter in the RBC color should harvest the buffy coat. Unfortunately, at times there are collections with appropriate RBC, granulocytes, and good MNC yield, but poor CD34$^+$ cell yields despite adequate numbers of circulating CD34$^+$ cells. With the *Amicus machine*, if there are good yields of WBC, but poor yields of CD34$^+$ cells, the operator should inspect the window on the spool holder for cracks. Cracks can affect CD34$^+$ cell yields by interfering with the interface detector.

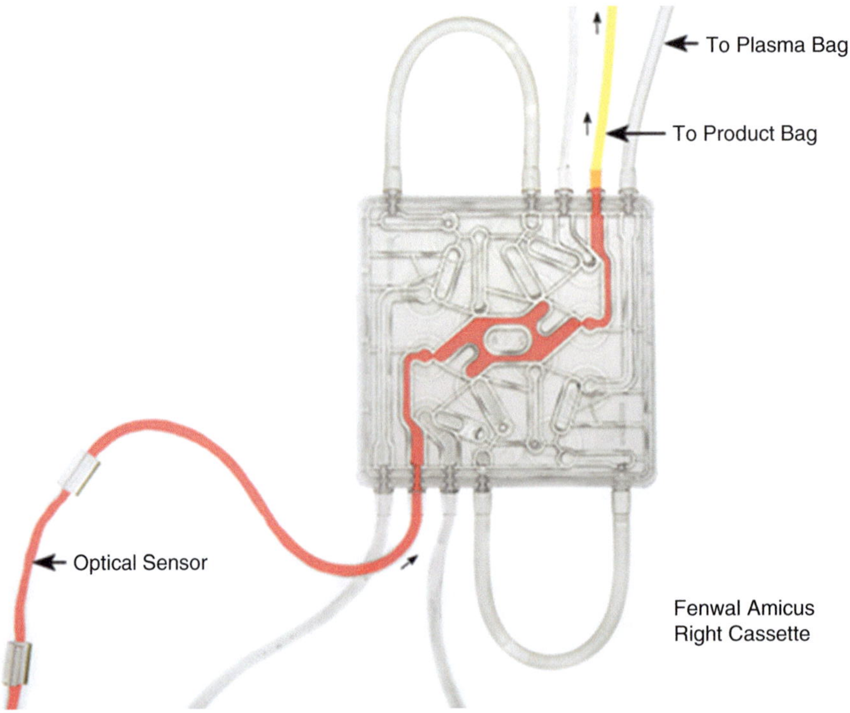

Fig. 7.7 Amicus right cassette during MNC transfer. Red blood cells should be present to the top of the cassette, prior to plasma flush. (Used with permission of Wiley-Blackwell)

Another factor that can affect CD34$^+$ cell yield is the mean corpuscular volume (MCV) of the RBC. Small RBCs, such as those present in patients/donors with iron-deficient anemia (IDA), can migrate up into the buffy coat layer and be harvested with the MNC. If the operator uses the normal color indicator for these (with low MCV) collections, the product will appear to be sufficiently red, but when cell content is measured, they will have small numbers of CD34$^+$ cells and MNC. In order to correct this problem, the operator must target a darker than normal red color in the product in patients with concomitant IDA with low MCV.

Very lipemic plasma can also adversely affect the performance of the instrument optical sensors and operator's perception of red color. A darker red color should be sought to overcome the white color of the lipemic plasma.

7.7.2 Excessive Platelet Loss

The platelets have a specific gravity (1.040) close to that of MNC (lymphocytes 1.050–1.061 and monocytes 1.065–1.066). As a result, there will be platelets in the collection; however, the amount of platelets can be modified. The *Amicus* is more platelet sparing than the *Spectra Optia* as seen in Table 7.3 (Sputtek et al. 2013). On the *Amicus*, a larger MNC offset will direct more of the platelets back to the donor. Using a high *MNC offset*, >2.3 mL, could, however, reduce the number of CD34$^+$ cells. It has been reported that using an *MNC offset* of 1.5 mL rather than the default setting of 2.3 mL can still achieve similar platelet loss and CD34$^+$ cell yields (Burgstaler et al. 2010). An unexpected finding from this study was that going too deep into the RBC layer also increased platelet loss on the *Amicus* (Burgstaler et al. 2010). Using a very light red color on the *Spectra Optia* can increase platelet loss.

High circulating WBC counts, as well as the combination of high WBC counts and high inlet flow rates, can adversely affect CD34$^+$ cell collection (Burgstaler et al. 2004; Burgstaler and Pineda 2002; Cooling et al. 2010). Therefore, in the presence of high WBC, inlet flow rates should be limited to increase centrifuge dwell time to allow for adequate separation and subsequent collection of the CD34$^+$ cells.

7.7.3 Excessive Granulocyte Content

Excessive granulocyte content is usually a result of harvesting too deep into the RBC layer (darker red color). When this occurs, using a lighter red color will decrease granulocyte content. However, even with the correct amount of RBC in the product, high granulocyte content may occur. This can be due to the high content of neutrophil precursors in the products due to the patient's/donor's response to mobilization. Immature, neutrophil precursors such as myelocytes (1.070) and promyelocytes (1.058–1.066) have a similar specific gravity as MNC (lymphocytes 1.050–1.061 and monocytes 1.065–1.066) and will be harvested with the MNC. Since the red color is the operator's only indication of the types of cells being collected, they are not able to prevent the collection of these immature/precursor neutrophils and a higher percent of granulocytes may be present in the collection in this setting.

7.7.4 Excessive RBC Content

Excessive RBC content usually indicates that the collect color was too dark. RBCs hemolyze during the freezing process, and usually large numbers of granulocytes in high RBC products are also collected due to the similar densities of granulocytes and RBC. Low red cell MCV is associated with poor CD34$^+$ cell and MNC yields (Cantilena et al. 2017; Panch et al. 2015; Wang et al. 2013; Leitman et al. 2010). If the red cell MCV is low, it may be necessary to go deeper into the RBC layer to get MNC and HPC (discussed above), but the collection will also contain increased numbers of RBC and granulocytes. For the *Terumo Optia*, an increase in the packing factor may help (seek the advice of the manufacturer). If graft appears to contain large volumes of RBCs, then one must consider evaluation of hematology analyzer used to determine the RBC content of the product. Some analyzers, such as the *Beckman-Coulter ACT 10* (Beckman-Coulter Corp., Miami, FL), are adversely affected by large numbers of WBC when determining the MCV and hematocrit (Seigneurin and Passe 1983). These devices were, after all, designed to measure PB cell counts and not cell counts on highly concentrated cellular therapy products. We have found that by using the donor's peripheral MCV and the collection RBC count, we were able to correct the RBC volume with similar results reported by others for the same apheresis equipment when utilizing the *Beckman-Coulter ACT 10* to measure RBC content.

7.8 Conclusion

Both the *Amicus* and *Spectra Optia* are flexible, highly automated apheresis systems capable of collecting high-quality HPC(A) and TC products. Each device, and in the case of the *Spectra Optia* each protocol, collects cells in a slightly different manner resulting in differences in product content, and each is influenced in slightly different ways by patient/donor characteristics such as lipemia and WBC count. These differences can be utilized to tailor the collection to specific patient characteristics. In the absence of both devices being available, either device can be used to effectively collect cellular therapy products as long as procedures are adjusted for variables related to individual patient.

When troubleshooting poor collections, it is important not to focus solely on the $CD34^+$ cell or lymphocyte yields but also to consider the content of other cells including granulocytes, platelets, and red blood cells as their presence, or absence, provides important clues in optimizing subsequent collections (Table 7.5).

Table 7.5 Clinical pearls

- *Amicus* and *Spectra Optia* are flexible, highly automated apheresis systems capable of collecting high-quality HPC(A) and TC products.
- The *Spectra Optia* was cleared by the FDA for the collection of TC and HPC(A) in 2012 using the MNC protocol and 2015 using the CMNC protocol.
- Etiology of unexpected hematopoietic graft yields and product content can result from patient/donor characteristics, operator errors, and equipment malfunction.
- The MNC content should indicate if the collection was drawn from the proper layer.
- High granulocyte and RBC contents indicate the collection was too deep and that the buffy coat containing the desired cells was not harvested.
- A high platelet content and low total WBC and RBC contents would indicate the collection was too high, missing the portion of the buffy coat containing the desired cells.
- The only real indication of the layer being harvested is the *red color* of the collected cells as they are being harvested.
- If graft appears to contain large volumes of RBCs, then one must consider evaluation of hematology analyzer used to determine the RBC content of the product. Hyperleukocytosis leads to an overestimation of the determination by Coulter Counter Model S of RBC count, hemoglobin, MCV, and packed cell volume.

References

Brauninger S et al (2011) Mobilized allogeneic peripheral stem/progenitor cell apheresis with spectra Optia v. 5.0. a novel automatic interface controlled apheresis system: results from the first feasibility trial. Vox Sang 101:217–246

Brauninger S et al (2012) Allogeneic donor peripheral blood "stem cell" apheresis: prospective comparison of two apheresis systems. Transfusion 52:1137–1145

Burgstaler EA, Pineda AA (2002) The negative effect of high peripheral white blood cell count on CD34+ cell recovery. J Clin Apher 17:148

Burgstaler EA, Winters JL (2011a) The effects of shorter cycles to improve CD34+ cell yields in patients with elevated circulating CD34+ cell levels using the Fenwal amicus. Transfusion 51(Suppl):226A

Burgstaler EA, Winters JL (2011b) Manual color monitoring to optimize hematopoietic progenitor cell collection on the Fenwal amicus. J Clin Apher 26:123–130

Burgstaler EA, Winters JL (2011c) Comparison of hematopoietic progenitor cell (HPC) collections using the COBE spectra version 7 and amicus version 3.1 for patients with AL amyloidosis. J Clin Apher 26:186–194

Burgstaler EA, Winters JL (2014) The effects of adjusting the mononuclear cell sense level to improve automation of Fenwal amicus hematopoietic progenitor cell collections. J Clin Apher 29:1

Burgstaler EA, Winters JL (2015) Comparison of 3 anticoagulant techniques used during hematopoietic progenitor cell collection using the TerumoBCT spectra Optia. J Clin Apher 30:64

Burgstaler EA, Winters JL (2016) Comparison of hematopoietic progenitor cell (HPC) collection using the new spectra Optia continuous mononuclear cell (CMNC) collection program vs. the spectra Optia mononuclear cell (MNC) program. J Clin Apher 31:23

Burgstaler EA, Winters JL. Comparison of hematopoietic progenitor cell (HPC) collection using the spectra optia continuous mononuclear cell (CMNC) collections with a 26:1 anticoagulant ratio versus an anticoagulant ratio ramping technique. J Clin Apher 2017; publication pending

Burgstaler EA, Pineda AA, Winters JL (2004) Hematopoietic progenitor cell large volume leukapheresis (LVL) on the Fenwal amicus blood separator. J Clin Apher 19:103–111

Burgstaler EA, Winters JL, Pineda AA (2005) Mononuclear cell collection with the Fenwal amicus versus Fenwal CS3000 plus. J Clin Apher 20:57

Burgstaler EA, Porrata LF, Markovic SN, Winters JL (2010) Use of various offset settings in the fenwal amicus during hematopoietic progenitor cell collection to increase lymphocyte yield and reduce cross-cellular contamination. J Clin Apher 25:301–309

Burgstaler EA, Kreuter JD, Winters JL (2012) Plerixafor plus G-CSF mobilization results in similar CD34+ cells to total nucleated cells ratio and number of freezer bags as G-CSF only. J Clin Apher 27:1

Cantilena CC, Yau YY, West K, Klein HG (2017) Red cell mean corpuscular volume predicts mononuclear cell apheresis collection efficiency and yield #47. Special Issue Abstracts From the American Society for Apheresis 38th Annual Meeting May 3–6, 2017 Fort Lauderdale, Florida. J Clin Apher 32:71–142. https://doi.org/10.1002/jca.21537

Cooling L, Hoffman S, Herrst M, Muck C, Armelagos H, Davenport R (2010) A prospective randomized trial of two popular mononuclear cell collection sets for autologous peripheral blood stem cell collection in multiple myeloma. Transfusion 50:100–119

Fischer JC, Wenzel F, Rox JM (2013) Comparison of the apheresis devices amicus, spectra Optia, and COBE spectra in non-stimulated mononuclear cell collections. Transfus Med Hemother 40:75

Gumogda M et al (2015) Comparative study of the collection efficiency of continuous mononuclear cell collection (CMNC) spectra Optia apheresis system device versus amicus cell separator device in mononuclear cell collection (AMNC). Bone Marrow Transplant 50(Suppl 1):5349

Karafin RM et al (2014) Evaluation of the spectra Optia apheresis system for mononuclear cell (MNC) collection in G-CSF mobilized and nonmobilized healthy donors: results of a multicenter study. J Clin Apher 29(5):273–280

Lamb R, Stevens J (2015) Single center experience with the continuous mononuclear cell collection (CMNC) protocol on the spectra optia apheresis system. Bone Marrow Transplant 50(Suppl 1):S349

Leitman SF, Yau Y, Matthews CL, Hopkins JA, Min K (2010) Optimization of unstimulated mononuclear cell collection using the amicus continuous-flow apheresis device. Transfusion 50:15A

Lisenko K, Pavel P, Bruckner T, Puthenparambi J, Hundemer M, Schmitt A, Witzens-Harig M, Ho A, Wuchter P (2017) Comparison between intermittent and continuous spectra Optia leukapheresis systems for autologous peripheral blood stem cell collection. J Clin Apher 32:27–34

Lozano M et al (2014) Evaluation of white blood cell depletion kit in the spectra optia separator for CD34+ collection in mobilized patients. Bone Marrow Transplant 49(Suppl 1):5529

Marculescu A et al (2015) Stem cell apheresis using the spectra optia CMNC protocol-experience of Fundeni Clinical Institute, Bucharest, Romania. Bone Marrow Transplant 50(Suppl 1):S336–S337

Panch SR, Yau YY, Kang EM, DeRavin SS, Malech HL, Leitman SF (2015) Mobilization characteristics and strategies to improve hematopoietic progenitor cell mobilization and collection in patients with chronic granulomatous disease and severe combined immunodeficiency. Transfusion 55:265–274

Punzel M et al (2015) Feasibility and advantages of a novel continuous spectra optia apheresis system (CMNC system) to collect non-stimulated mononuclear cells (MNC) for cellular therapy. Bone Marrow Transplant 50(Suppl 1):S348

Reinhardt P et al (2011) Automatic interface-controlled apheresis collection of stem/progenitor cells: results from an autologous donor validation trial of a novel stem cell apheresis device. Transfusion 51:1321–1330

Robitzsch JT, Rox JM, Fischer JC (2015) Comparison of four apheresis systems (COBE spectra, spectra optia, spectra optia CMNC and amicus) for non-stimulated mononuclear cell collections. Bone Marrow Transplant 50:S344

Sanderson F, Poullin P, Smith R, Nicolino-Brunet C, Philip P, Chaib A, Costello R (2017) Peripheral blood stem cells collection on spectra optia apheresis system using the continuous mononuclear cell collection protocol: a single center report of 39 procedures. J Clin Apher 32(3):182–190. https://doi.org/10.1002/jca.21485

Schmidt JP, Grabowski C, Winterfeld S, Kroll H (2015) Comparison of three different cell separators for the collection of peripheral blood stem cells. Transfus Med Hemother 42:24

Seigneurin D, Passe D (1983) Interference of hyperleukocytosis on coulter model S blood counts: methods for correction. Biomed Pharmacother 37:401–404

Sputtek A, Schubert C, Peine S, Rowe AW (2013) Safe collection of peripheral blood stem cells in patients and donors using the amicus separator and the spectra Optia apheresis system. Vox Sang 105:294–295

Steininger PA, Strasser EF, Weiss D, Achenbach S, Zimmerman R, Eckstein R (2014) First comparative evaluation of a new leukapheresis technology in non-cytokine-stimulated donors. Vox Sang 106(3):248–255

Tarik K, Pascal L, Bouhya S (2013) Evaluation of the amicus separator for mononuclear cell collection. J Clin Apher 28:118–119

Toney I et al (2015) Stem cell apheresis using the new spectra Optia CMNC platform. Bone Marrow Transplant 50(Suppl 1):S343

Wang TF, Chen SH, Yang SH, Su YC, Chu SC, Li DK (2013) Poor harvest of peripheral blood stem cells in donors with microcytic red blood cells. Transfusion 53:91–95

Watts M et al (2015) Predetermined small volume HPC-A harvests for cryopreservation using the continuous mononuclear cell (CMNC) procedure of the Terumo Optia apheresis machine. Cytotherapy 17(6):S59

Anticoagulation and Other Periprocedural Considerations for Apheresis

8

Matthew S. Karafin and Mehraboon S. Irani

8.1 Introduction

Hematopoietic progenitor cell (HPC) collection by apheresis is an increasingly common procedure for autologous and allogeneic hematopoietic cell transplantation. Successful apheresis collection procedures cannot be performed without the establishment and maintenance of adequate venous access and appropriate anticoagulation of the extracorporeal circuit to sustain flow rates of 50–100 mL/min. This chapter discusses these practical considerations regarding apheresis HPC collections and how one might maximize procedure efficacy and safety.

8.1.1 Anticoagulation

Anticoagulation of the extracorporeal circuit is required for all apheresis procedures, and peripheral blood HPC collections are no exception. The selection of the anticoagulant used is often based on institutional policy or donor registry standards but, in selected situations, can also be made on a patient-to-patient basis. The options commonly used for HPC collections are citrate only (ACD-A, acid citrate dextrose formula A) or a combination of unfractionated heparin and ACD-A (e.g., 10 units heparin/mL and ACD-A). Currently, the anticoagulant selected does not appear to influence collection efficacy or yield, and thus these two options can be used interchangeably, keeping risk and benefits in mind (Dettke et al. 2012).

M. S. Karafin (✉) · M. S. Irani
Medical Sciences Institute, Blood Center of Wisconsin, Milwaukee, WI, USA
e-mail: matthew.karafin@bcw.edu; mehraboon.irani@bcw.edu

S. A. Abutalib et al. (eds.), *Best Practices of Apheresis in Hematopoietic Cell Transplantation*, Advances and Controversies in Hematopoietic Transplantation and Cell Therapy, https://doi.org/10.1007/978-3-319-55131-9_8

The usual choice for many is ACD-A, especially in adult (age >18 years) donors. ACD-A for HPC collections can be used at an inlet ratio (anticoagulant: whole blood) of 1:12 to 1:15 (Pulsipher et al. 2009; Bolan et al. 2003; Ings et al. 2006). The benefit of this anticoagulant is that it is well established in the apheresis literature and has a known risk/safety profile. ACD-A does not act as an in vivo anticoagulant and therefore is not known to cause a bleeding diathesis as opposed to heparin. However, it does lower ionized calcium, and symptoms of hypocalcemia can be common in these procedures. An estimated 51% of all HPC adverse events are calcium-related complications from citrate administration (tingling, numbness, and rarely carpal-pedal spasm) (Pulsipher et al. 2009) (see Chap. 14). Fortunately, these complications are predominantly minor with appropriate preventive measures and can be easily managed with calcium administration or briefly slowing or pausing the collection (Gašova et al. 2010). Due to the slower inlet ratio, ACD-A-only HPC collections also generally result in higher fluid gains for the patient. Consequently, while most patients can tolerate procedures with only ACD-A, patients who are significantly volume sensitive, such as those with severe heart or renal disease (low glomerular filtration rate), should be considered for partial heparin anticoagulation if no contraindications to heparin is noted.

Unlike ACD-A only, ACD-A and heparin in combination can be run at a 1:15 to 1:35 inlet ratio and thus has the benefit of being a faster procedure with reduced volume returned to the patient at the end of the collection (Rowley et al. 2001a; Sevilla et al. 2004, 2009; Holig et al. 2009). The use of heparin also reduces, but does not eliminate, the risk of hypocalcemia and associated side effects and the need for calcium replacement. Unlike ACD-only collections, however, heparin from the HPC collection does act as an in vivo anticoagulant and increases the bleeding risk for the patient/donor. This may be significant in patients already predisposed to bleeding events, such as those who are already on oral anticoagulants, are already thrombocytopenic, or have baseline coagulopathy. Patients with such comorbidities should avoid receiving HPC collections with heparin in addition to those with history of heparin-induced thrombocytopenia (HIT). It should be noted, the use of heparin carries the risk of a new diagnosis of heparin-induced thrombocytopenia (HIT) and the associated thrombotic complications from exposure (Schwartz et al. 2010).

8.1.2 Vascular Access

Successful collection procedures cannot be performed without the establishment of adequate venous access. Although the majority of healthy allogeneic donors have adequate peripheral venous access, up to 10–30% may require placement of a central venous catheter (CVC) (Pulsipher et al. 2009; Favre et al. 2003; Anderlini et al. 2001; Murata et al. 1999; Lysak et al. 2005). Recently, ultrasound-guided peripheral vein placement has been used in lieu of a CVC for therapeutic apheresis applications and could be used for collections of HPCs (Salazar et al. 2017). This advancement could be particularly useful in allogeneic donors with apparently poor peripheral venous access. In either case, for adequate flow rates, most HPC collections for adults require either two 16–20 gauge or larger catheters peripherally or a 10–11 Fr dual-lumen temporary CVC.

Temporary CVC lines are used when needed for adult and pediatric allogeneic HPC donors. Dual-lumen apheresis/dialysis-type CVCs are most commonly inserted into the jugular vein, but other insertion sites are possible as described in the next paragraph. Patients who undergo autologous HPC collection may be best managed with a semipermanent, tunneled apheresis/dialysis-type CVC that will be adequate for both the apheresis procedure itself and for their future posttransplant infusion needs. Like the choice of anticoagulant, current policies and practices regarding the assessment, placement, and management of venous access for HPC collections are based on institutional preferences or nationally mandated policies.

The pros and cons of different anatomic sites for catheterization have been well established (Hamilton and Foxcroft 2007). Jugular and subclavian access minimize bacterial contamination and maintain patient or donor mobility (Hamilton and Foxcroft 2007). Major disadvantages of these two sites are the risk of pneumothorax or hemothorax during cannulation and the difficulty of applying compression if bleeding occurs (Hamilton and Foxcroft 2007). Another risk is air embolism due to inadequate insertion, disconnection, or removal of the catheter, which can be fatal in rare cases (Heckmann et al. 2000). Lastly, placement of a CVC in the femoral vein is often discouraged because it has a higher incidence of bacterial infection and thrombosis. The need to stay supine during the whole time the catheter is in use also makes femoral catheters less convenient for HPC collection patients/donors (Hölig et al. 2012). One large retrospective evaluation of severe adverse events in marrow and HPC donors reported a single local hemorrhage and a maximum of five catheter-related infections, which corresponds to a maximum incidence of only 2.6 access complications in 10,000 donations (Halter et al. 2009). Ultrasound-guided peripheral vein access as referred to above (Salazar et al. 2017) could potentially obviate the need for such catheters in allogeneic HPC donors.

O'Leary and colleagues performed a recent international survey of current practices of autologous and allogeneic HPC collections (O'Leary et al. 2016). In this survey, they established that donor vein assessment is most often performed by apheresis staff prior to collection, suggesting that peripheral veins are the preferred access site for most HPC collection services. Other studies support this survey finding, as patients who receive HPC collections using peripheral veins report significantly less pain and a greater willingness to donate again in comparison to those who get a CVC (Hölig et al. 2012). When CVC catheter placement is medically necessary, temporary lines are most frequently placed in the jugular vein by interventional radiology, and verification of adequate central line placement is confirmed before its use in both autologous and allogeneic donors (O'Leary et al. 2016).

Evidence supporting best practice recommendations for HPC collection vascular access locking and occlusion management is limited. Locking can be done using saline, low-dose heparin (i.e., 10 IU/mL), or high-dose heparin (100 IU/mL). One advantage of saline or low-dose heparin is the decreased risk for systemic anticoagulation if injected into the bloodstream by accident. In contrast, while there does not appear to be a statistically significant difference in the maintenance of catheter patency when using low-dose heparin compared with normal saline (Rabe et al. 2002), there does appear to be an increased risk for clotting when normal saline is compared with higher-dose heparin (Schallom et al. 2012). Evidence is also limited surrounding the best use of alteplase in the setting of an established catheter occlusion. One small study in 60 patients with occluded catheters found no difference in the rate of established patency at the next procedure when randomly assigned to a short alteplase dwell time (<1 h) or a long dwell time (48–72 h) (Macrae et al. 2005).

Catheter removal usually takes place at the end of the collection procedure and differs between autologous and allogeneic donors. For autologous donors, line removal generally takes place after laboratory confirmation of an adequate HPC collection yield (O'Leary et al. 2016). In contrast, most centers do not base the line removal for healthy allogeneic donors on donor laboratory values, although some centers require a minimum platelet count; a platelet count greater than 50,000/μL is considered a reasonable threshold for line removal (O'Leary et al. 2016).

8.1.3 Hematologic and Electrolyte Parameters

Many autologous HPC donors and some allogeneic donors present with abnormal laboratory values, and these values can be altered further by HPC collections. Schlenke and colleagues (Schlenke et al. 2000) found that potassium concentrations can fall by 11.3% mmol/L post-apheresis, and the mean citrate-induced reduction of total calcium can be up to 11% in some patients (mean 5.5%). Cellular blood components also fall with HPC collections, as Schlenke and colleagues also found a relative loss of hemoglobin and platelet counts to be 10.7% and 24.2%, respectively, per apheresis collection (Schlenke et al. 2000). Other investigators have documented even greater cellular losses during HPC collection, including a 33–41% reduction in platelet count after a single allogeneic collection with 13 L of blood processed (Schreiner et al. 1998), and a 50% or greater reduction when 30 L of blood is processed (Rowley et al. 2001b). Moreover, >50% of healthy allogeneic donors in a separate study demonstrated platelet counts <100/μL after two consecutive HPC collections (Miflin et al. 1996). Lastly, ionized calcium levels can decrease by 31% or more with HPC collections, supporting the observation that citrate toxicity is the most common adverse event with HPC collections (Olson et al. 1977). The variability noted in these studies is likely due to differences in volumes processed, patient gender, techniques used, operator variability, and the apheresis collection machines used. Regardless of the cause, however, these changes can become clinically significant with longer collection procedures or increased numbers of consecutive collection days, and consequently, regular monitoring of these values is recommended. Replacement therapy beyond standard calcium replacement protocols may become necessary based on laboratory values or clinical symptoms (see Chap. 14).

8.1.4 Pediatric Considerations

HPC collection can be performed safely in pediatric populations, but some additional considerations are necessary. While anticoagulant choice is similar to adults, and citrate-only procedures are preferred, the exposure to citrate and heparin can be more pronounced and require closer monitoring. Like adults, ACD-A for HPC collections can be used at an inlet ratio (anticoagulant: whole blood) of 1:12 to 1:15, but the inlet flow rate will be slower (between 10 and 30 mL/min) due to smaller patient size. Rapid changes in blood volume are also not well tolerated in this donor population due to smaller patient total blood volume (TBV). Symptoms of hypovolemia with HPC collections are thus more of a concern than for adults (Orbach et al. 2003). To prevent adverse events associated with these expected volume changes, using an irradiated red cell blood (RBC) prime is recommended when 10%–15% of the TBV of the donor will be in the extracorporeal circuit during the HPC collection (Alegre et al. 1996). The total amount of blood needed to prime the system varies based on the apheresis machine used for the collection.

Vascular access in pediatric populations can also be more challenging than adults. Like adults, vascular access that allows for a sufficient blood flow rate is a prerequisite for successful apheresis and HPC collections (Kim 2000). Establishing peripheral access is much more challenging in small-size children and infants, as their peripheral veins often do not have the diameter needed to accommodate the required large-bore needles (see text above), and their veins may collapse against the negative pressures applied during the collection, requiring staff to either reduce the inlet blood flow rate and extend the time of apheresis or halt the collection altogether (Kim 2000). A 7–8 Fr rigid dual-lumen temporary CVC is often needed in these cases (Kim 2000).

Lastly, managing patient anxiety and fear can play a larger role in the success of a collection, as patients can pull their apheresis access or move during the collection, leading to procedure delays or patient harm. Depending on age and cognitive ability, some children cannot understand what is happening to them, and procedure length may increase this anxiety further (Kim 2000). Noninvasive management strategies for anxiety include a warm environment in the apheresis room, having the donor's parents at the bedside, and the presence of distractions such as books, art projects, television programs or movies, and video games (Kim 2000). In more severe cases of procedure-related anxiety, low doses of intravenous anxiolytic drugs (i.e. midazolam) can be also used under the appropriate supervision for sedation (Salazar-Riojas et al. 2015).

8.2 Expert Point of View

HPC collection by apheresis is already a common procedure for autologous and allogeneic hematopoietic cell transplantation in both children and adult populations. For standard adult donors, peripheral access and use of citrate (ACD-A) as the sole anticoagulant for collections are preferable due to its maximized safety profile and overall convenience. Use of partial heparin anticoagulation can be made on a case-by-case basis and should be dependent on the severity of patient cardiac and renal function. Use of central venous catheters are also generally well-tolerated in adults but carry additional, albeit rare, risks to the donor, such as air embolus (see text above) and should be reserved for those who cannot tolerate or maintain peripheral intravenous access. For pediatric populations, central access is preferable to peripheral access to maximize flow rates for HPC collections. Like adults, the use of citrate anticoagulation is also preferred when possible.

References

Alegre A, Diaz MA, Madero L, Granda A, de la Vega A, Villa M et al (1996) Large-volume leukapheresis for peripheral blood stem cell collection in children: a simplified single-apheresis approach. Bone Marrow Transplant 17:923–927

Anderlini P, Rizzo JD, Nugent ML, Schmitz N, Champlin RE, Horowitz MM (2001) Peripheral blood stem cell donation: an analysis from the International Bone Marrow Transplant Registry (IBMTR) and European Group for Blood and Marrow Transplant (EBMT) databases. Bone Marrow Transplant 27:689–692

Bolan CD, Carter CS, Wesley RA et al (2003) Prospective evaluation of cell kinetics, yields and donor experiences during a single large-volume apheresis versus two smaller volume consecutive day collections of allogeneic peripheral blood stem cells. Br J Haematol 120(5):801–807

Dettke M, Buchta C, Wiesinger H et al (2012) Anticoagulation in large-volume leukapheresis: comparison between citrate- versus heparin-based anticoagulation on safety and CD34 (+) cell collection efficiency. a 14(3):350–358

Favre G, Beksac¸ M, Bacigalupo A, Ruutu T, Nagler A, Gluckman E, Russell N, Apperley J, Szer J, Bradstock K, Buzyn A, Matcham J, Gratwohl A, Schmitz N (2003) Differences between graft product and donor side effects following bone marrow or stem cell donation. Bone Marrow Transplant 32:873–880

Gašova Z, Bhuiyan-Ludvikova Z, Bohmova M et al (2010) PBPC collections: management, techniques and risks. Transfus Apher Sci 43:237–243

Halter J, Kodera Y, Ispizua AU et al (2009) Severe events in donors after allogeneic hematopoietic stem cell donation. Haematologica 94:94–101

Hamilton HC, Foxcroft D (2007) Central venous access sites for the prevention of venous thrombosis, stenosis and infection in patients requiring long-term intravenous therapy (review). Cochrane Database Syst Rev 3:1–18

Heckmann JG, Lang CJ, Kindler K, Huk W, Erbguth FJ, Neundörfer B (2000) Neurologic manifestations of cerebral air embolism as a complication of central venous catheterization. Crit Care Med 28:1621–1625

Holig K, Kramer M, Krochinsky F et al (2009) Safety and efficacy of hematopoietic stem cell collection from mobilized peripheral blood in unrelated volunteers-12 years of a single center experience in 3928 donors. Blood 114:3757–3763

Hölig K, Blechschmidt M, Kramer M et al (2012) Peripheral blood stem cell collection in allogeneic donors: impact of venous access. Transfusion 52(12):2600–2605

Ings SJ, Balsa C, Leverett D et al (2006) Peripheral blood stem cell yield in 400 normal donors mobilised with granulocyte colony-stimulating factor (G-CSF): impact of age, sex, donor weight and type of G-CSF used. Br J Haematol 134(5):517–525

Kim HC (2000) Therapeutic pediatric apheresis. J Clin Apher 15:129–157

Lysak D, Koza V, Jindra P (2005) Factors affecting PBSC mobilization and collection in healthy donors. Transfus Apher Sci 33:275–283

Macrae JM, Loh G, Djurdjev O et al (2005) Short and long alteplase dwells in dysfunctional hemodialysis catheters. Hemodial Int 9:189–195

Miflin G, Charley C, Stainer C, Anderson S, Hunter A, Russell N (1996) Stem cell mobilization in normal donors for allogeneic transplantation: analysis of safety and factors affecting efficacy. Br J Haematol 95:345–348

Murata M, Harada M, Kato S, Takahashi S, Ogawa H, Okamoto S, Tsuchiya S, Sakamaki H, Akiyama Y, Kodera Y (1999) Peripheral blood stem cell mobilization and apheresis: analysis of adverse events in 94 normal donors. Bone Marrow Transplant 24:1065–1071

O'Leary MF, Dunbar NM, Kim HC et al (2016) Venous access for hematopoietic progenitor cell collection: an international survey by the ASFA HPC donor subcommittee. J Clin Apher 31(6):529–534

Olson PR, Cox C, McCullough J (1977) Laboratory and clinical effects of the infusion of ACD solution during plateletpheresis. Vox Sang 33(2):79–87

Orbach D, Hojjat-Assari S, Doz F, Pacquement H, Guillaume A, Mathiot C et al (2003) Peripheral blood stem cell collection in 24 low-weight infants: experience of a single Centre. Bone Marrow Transplant 31:171–174

Pulsipher MA, Chitphakdithai P, Miller JP et al (2009) Adverse events among 2408 unrelated donors of peripheral blood stem cells: results of a prospective trial from the National Marrow Donor Program. Blood 113(15):3604–3611

Rabe C, Gramann T, Sons X et al (2002) Keeping central venous lines open: a prospective comparison of heparin, vitamin C and sodium chloride sealing solutions in medical patients. Intensive Care Med 28:1172–1176

Rowley SD, Donaldson G, Lilleby K et al (2001a) Experiences of donors enrolled in a randomized study of allogeneic bone marrow or peripheral blood stem cell transplantation. Blood 97:2541–2548

Rowley SD, Yu J, Gooley T, Heimfeld S, Holmberg L, Maloney D, Bensinger WI (2001b) Trafficking of CD34+ cells into the peripheral circulation during collection of peripheral blood stem cells by apheresis. Bone Marrow Transplant 28:649–656

Salazar E, Garcia S, Miguel R, Segura FJ, Ipe TS, Leveque C (2017) Ultrasound-guided peripheral venous access for therapeutic apheresis procedures reduces need for central venous catheters. J Clin Apher 32(4):266–269. https://doi.org/10.1002/jca.21493

Salazar-Riojas R, García-Lozano JA, Valdés-Galván M, Martínez-González O, Cantú-Rodríguez OG, González-Llano O, Gómez-De León A, Jaime-Pérez JC, Gómez-Almaguer D, Gutiérrez-Aguirre CH (2015) Effective collection of peripheral blood stem cells in children weighing 20 kilogram or less in a single large-volume apheresis procedure. J Clin Apher 30(5):281–287

Schallom ME, Prentice D, Sona C et al (2012) Heparin or 0.9% sodium chloride to maintain central venous catheter patency: a randomized trial. Crit Care Med 40:1820–1826

Schlenke P, Frohn C, Steinhardt MM, Kirchner H, Klüter H (2000) Clinically relevant hypokalaemia, hypocalcaemia, and loss of hemoglobin and platelets during stem cell apheresis. J Clin Apher 15(4):230–235

Schreiner T, Wiesneth M, Krug E, Kalinova J, Buchele H, Maccari B, Erne E, Bischof C, De Reys S (1998) Collection of allogeneic peripheral blood progenitor cells by two protocols on an apheresis system. Transfusion 38:1051–1055

Schwartz J, Padmanabhan A, Francis RO, Linenberger ML (2010) Mobilization and collection of peripheral blood hematopoietic progenitor cells. In: McCleod BC, Szczepiorkowski ZM, Weinstein R, Winters JL (eds) Apheresis: principles and practice, 3rd edition. AABB Press, Bethesda, MD

Sevilla J, Gonzalez-Vincent M, Fernandez-Plaza S et al (2004) Heparin based anticoagulation during peripheral blood stem cell collection may increase CD34 yield. Haematologica 89:249–251

Sevilla J, Gonzalez-Vincent M, Lassaletta A et al (2009) Peripheral blood progenitor cell collection adverse events for childhood allogeneic donors: variables related to the collection and safety profile. Br J Haematol 144:909–916

Concepts and Rationale for Using Predictive Algorithms for Hematopoietic Progenitor Cell Apheresis Collection

9

Michele Cottler-Fox

9.1 Introduction

Between 1985 and 1995, multiple centers reported collecting cells from peripheral blood (PB) that were used successfully in autologous hematopoietic (HPC) cell transplant; these cells were an alternative to bone marrow that avoided a trip to the operating room for harvest. Initially, collections were done in steady state, but multiple aphereses were needed, so strategies were sought to increase PB HPC concentration. Today, the process of increasing the number of these cells in blood is termed *mobilization* (see Chap. 5). As mobilization and collection are closely related processes, where collection depends to a large part but not solely on mobilization, it is important to understand mobilization before talking about collection algorithms. This chapter will present the history of mobilization and its relationship to collection in a concise but non-exhaustive manner, in order to help the reader understand how algorithms have been developed and how they can be developed and used for any collection center today.

Two main approaches were developed to increase PB HPC concentration. The first was to collect cells on recovery of white blood cells (WBC) following chemotherapy, when colony-forming assays showed that HPC increased above steady-state levels (To et al. 1984). After growth factors were developed and had been shown to shorten the time to recovery from chemotherapy, first GM-CSF and then G-CSF were routinely added to help increase the number of HPC collected, after G-CSF was shown to be more efficacious than GM-CSF (Peters et al. 1993). Eventually, when hematopoietic growth factors themselves were shown to increase the number of circulating HPC in the blood, they were used to mobilize cells for collection without preceding chemotherapy, especially if the autologous donor/

M. Cottler-Fox (✉)
University of Arkansas for Medical Sciences, Little Rock, AR, USA
e-mail: foxmicheleh@uams.edu

S. A. Abutalib et al. (eds.), *Best Practices of Apheresis in Hematopoietic Cell Transplantation*, Advances and Controversies in Hematopoietic Transplantation and Cell Therapy, https://doi.org/10.1007/978-3-319-55131-9_9

patient had no need for chemotherapy because they were in remission. Eventually, this approach was also used for healthy volunteer donors and initially related and then eventually unrelated donors once the method had been demonstrated to be safe (Nervi et al. 2006).

In the early days of HPC collection by apheresis, much effort was devoted to developing a good definition of "stem cell," but as it became apparent that this would be difficult, transplant centers settled for using surrogate markers such as $CD34^+$ cells, i.e., HPC. Many surrogates were used, starting in bone marrow (BM) harvests with total nucleated cells (TNC), followed by mononuclear cells (MNC; another problematic definition). Colony-forming unit (CFU) assays of various types were also used to evaluate hematopoietic grafts, but culture media varied greatly, the assays took weeks to complete, and readouts still are difficult to standardize. Eventually, the cell surface marker $CD34^+$ was identified as a useful surrogate, and antibodies for flow cytometry were developed (Civin et al. 1984). Flow cytometry then became the accepted technology for evaluating HPC collection, with many different approaches being proposed, until the use of $CD34^+$ cell recognition became standardized through the efforts of what was originally the International Society for Hematotherapy and Graft Engineering (ISHAGE) but is now the International Society for Cell Therapy (ISCT) (Sutherland et al. 1996).

9.2 Mobilization with Chemotherapy *Alone* for Autologous Hematopoietic Cell Transplants

Cyclophosphamide was studied early as a mobilizing agent, prior to the development of growth factors (To et al. 1984), and became the most commonly used chemotherapeutic agent for this purpose although doses were not standardized. Since then, an enormous literature has developed, with many other agents being reported as "good" or "poor" mobilizing agents based on the total number of $CD34^+$ cells collected. The assumption was that the chemotherapeutic agent was more important than how the apheresis was done and that the number of cells collected was a reflection of mobilization alone (see Chap. 5). Thus, reported information about apheresis was often brief, another assumption being that apheresis was always done in the same way by all collection sites.

However, timing of collection after chemotherapy has always been problematic for the collection site. Not every patient will recover his counts on the same day post-chemotherapy, and only a few sites were able/willing to collect on weekends. Thus, a great deal of attention was directed to looking at variables that might predict who would be a good mobilizer (Prince et al. 1996). Although a number of variables have been shown to be helpful in predicting who might be a "good" or "bad" mobilizer, none of these were universally correct and none were perfect in predicting on what day a specific person might be ready to start collection. General consensus eventually agreed that a good mobilizer was one who could collect at least 2×10^6 $CD34^+$ cells/kg of body weight in a single day of collection (see Chap. 5). It was only recently that data were shown pointing to the fact that *when* apheresis was started and *how apheresis was* done would impact the number of cells collected in a given day (Abuabdou et al. 2014). Indeed, many analyses of mobilization regimens have used the number of days of collection needed to achieve a certain cell number as the definition of a "good" or "bad" mobilization regimen while reporting only minimal information about the trigger to start collection and how apheresis was performed.

9.3 Mobilization with Chemotherapy Plus Growth Factors for Autologous Transplants: A Step Forward

Many different growth factors (Table 9.1) have been developed and tried for mobilization over the years, and not all have obtained FDA approval for mobilization, nor are all of them available at all sites (see Chap. 5). Growth factors were initially used in combination with chemotherapy, and combinations of growth factors have also been used after chemotherapy if one alone was judged to be inadequate.

The first publication to report using chemotherapy followed by a growth factor (GM-CSF) for mobilization (Gianni et al. 1989) reported starting collection as soon as WBC recovered since it was uncertain when $CD34^+$ cell mobilization would peak. As a result, this became the standard algorithm for starting collection, despite the fact that a figure in the paper demonstrated that optimal collection actually took place when WBC was closer to 10×10^9/L. Later, and with more experience, most transplant centers picked a threshold value of $CD34^+$ cell/μL blood to start collection. This threshold was most often 10 or 20/μL, although some centers would go as low as 5/μL, and it has been the de facto algorithm for collection for most centers for many years.

9.4 Mobilization with Growth Factors and/or Plerixafor for Autologous Collection: Current Practice

In many cases, a patient who does not need chemotherapy for control of their malignancy is mobilized with growth factors alone (i.e., G-CSF) as there is immediate and delayed toxicity associated with chemotherapy as a mobilization agent. Although this makes the start of collection highly predictable on day +4 or day +5 of G-CSF, many centers felt that the collections do not yield as many $CD34^+$ cells as is seen with chemotherapy followed by growth factors (Meisenberg et al. 1998).

Table 9.1 Growth factors used for mobilization

GM-CSF
G-CSF, pegylated G-CSF
Erythropoietin
Stem cell factor
FLT-3, M-CSF

While it is possible that this might depend on the underlying disease or previous treatment as much as the mobilization regimen, data have been difficult to acquire and evaluate. Mobilization without chemotherapy today generally means mobilization with G-CSF and/or plerixafor, with the understanding that at present, plerixafor is primarily used for autologous collections although it is being examined for use in the allogeneic setting.

The question of dose and frequency of G-CSF dosing to optimize mobilization has been examined by several centers. G-CSF may be given once or twice daily for mobilization; it is usual to start collection on day +4 or +5 of G-CSF. Maximum dose of G-CSF is not standard among centers, but it is commonly started at 5–10 μg/kg daily and may be increased during collection if mobilization seems suboptimal. Although it has been shown that twice daily yields better mobilization (Arbona et al. 1998; Kroger et al. 2000, 2004; Lee et al. 2000), it is more often given once daily for donor convenience. It is uncertain if once-daily timing is best done in the evening or the morning or what the optimal interval between dose and start of collection may be. In healthy donors, one center has shown that collection is better if there is a 2 h interval between morning dose of G-CSF and start of HPC collection (Bolan et al. 2003), and several centers have shown that a 15 h interval between plerixafor dose and start of collection is equivalent to a 10 h interval. However, little attention has been paid to the question of whether timing of G-CSF relative to start of apheresis may impact evaluation of a mobilization regimen based only on the total number of $CD34^+$ cells collected.

9.5 Optimizing Collection for an Individual Patient

A great deal of work in the past has been aimed at learning what the best means of predicting a good HPC collection might entail. Although patient age, prior therapy, and mobilization regimen (Morris et al. 2003) are helpful in predicting who may be a good HPC mobilizer, as are patient body size and baseline blood counts (Sandhya et al. 2015), it has been clear for some time that daily $CD34^+$ enumeration is a good predictor of daily HPC collection (Mohle et al. 1996; Ford et al. 2003). Although it is common to quantify circulating $CD34^+$ cells/μL in PB prior to collection as a means of determining mobilization failure or success, it is still not universally done on a daily basis. Reasons for not quantifying $CD34^+$ cells daily after start of G-CSF include expense, lack of personal, timing of patient visits, and in some cases the inability to guarantee that results will be available at a given time each day.

Cutoff values for initiating collection are often determined by experience at each institution (usually between 10 and 20 $CD34^+$ cells/μL). Optimizing collection for an individual patient requires an institutional algorithm, since starting too early may yield a poor or suboptimal HPC product (see text above). Most centers have attempted to predict the actual number to be collected, but as several centers working together have shown (Hosing et al. 2014), it is impossible to accurately predict exactly what everyone will collect, and therefore most centers accept a range in variability around the predicted number. Other centers use a formula validated to predict the *minimum* number of $CD34^+$ cells/kg of the recipient body weight that can be expected in a collection each day per liter of blood processed (Rosenbaum et al. 2012). This reworking of the standard apheresis device efficiency formula (CE2) is:

[(peripheral blood $CD34^+$ cells per μL) × 30%] divided by body weight in kg = minimum $CD34^+$ cells predicted to be collected per L of blood × the number of liters of blood to be processed. The value of 30% in this formula is calculated as shown in Sect. 9.7.

$$\left(\frac{\text{CD34}+\text{cells}/\mu L\times 0.3}{\text{Body wgt}(\text{kg})}=\text{CD34}+\text{Cells}/\text{L processed}\right)$$
$$\times\text{Liters}=\text{Minimum predicted collection}$$

Although formulas vary slightly, this approach has now been tested by multiple centers (Cottler-Fox et al. 2003; Pierelli et al. 2006; Costa et al. 2011a; Douglas 2012; Wuchter et al. 2017) and is finding increasing acceptance as new machines enter the field and it becomes necessary to establish their clinical baselines in each center (Lisenko et al. 2016; Cousins et al. 2015). Each center develops the % efficiency for use in the calculation, such that they are able to predict the minimum expected yield for a given volume of blood processed using the machine in whichever fashion is standard at their site. The original validation of this formula demonstrated that it works well regardless of diagnosis, mobilization regimen, day in collection sequence, how well or poorly a donor mobilizes, and what volume of blood is processed.

9.6 How Best to Use a Predictive Formula for HPC Collection and Why?

Use of a predictive formula is the first step in developing a reliable algorithm for collection. The increased general interest in recent years using a predictive formula derives not only from the advent of newer apheresis devices (Table 9.2) but from the advent of a new and expensive mobilization agent, i.e., plerixafor in the autologous transplant setting. In particular, the ability to predict the *minimum* number of $CD34^+$ cells/kg of recipient body weight a donor should collect each day not only means better products for the processing laboratory in addition to greater efficiency for the collection area but a more cost-effective use of plerixafor in the autologous setting. For example, predicting the number of $CD34^+$ cells/kg collected based on liters (L)

Table 9.2 How to evaluate performance of a new apheresis device

Performance assessment and benchmarking
Performance ratio

Table 9.3 A minimum predictive formula improves coordination for everyone

Clinicians
Apheresis
Laboratory personnel
Quality management

of blood processed means a "good mobilizer" can undergo a shorter apheresis than a "poor mobilizer" to reach the same goal with decreased resource utilization.

For example, if the formula is used to predict the *minimum* expected collection for a 30 L processed large-volume leukapheresis in a 65 kg donor with a peripheral blood CD34$^+$ cell count of 20/μL, the following result is seen:

$$20 \times 0.3 \,\text{divided by}\, 65 = 0.09 \times 30\,\text{L}$$
$$= 2.8 \times 10^6 \,\text{CD34}^+ \,\text{cells / kg of recipient body weight}$$

$$\left(\frac{20\,\mu L \times 0.3}{65\,\text{kg}} = 0.09 \right) \times 30\,\text{L} = 2.8 \times 10^6 \,\text{CD34} + \text{Cells / kg}$$

This example of the minimum predictive formula also demonstrates why those centers not using a predictive formula but who use a starting point for apheresis of 20 CD34$^+$ cells/kg have a reasonable chance of an acceptable collection if the goal is a total of 2–4 × 10^6 CD34$^+$ cells/kg of recipient body weight. The use of a predictive formula facilitates a cost-effective algorithm for plerixafor use by making it clear when a collector is unlikely to reach a goal unless plerixafor is added in the autologous setting only. Further, use of a minimum predictive formula also allows concurrent daily quality assurance (Wuchter et al. 2017) and evaluation of daily performance ratio (Table 9.3).

9.7 Developing the Institutional Minimum Predictive Formula for Hematopoietic Progenitor Cell Collection

The first step is to determine the collection efficiency to be used in the minimum predictive formula. To do this, first calculate the minimum predicted yield of a 100% efficient collection for a 30 L apheresis collection and a mobilizer with a peripheral blood CD34$^+$ cell count of 20/μL, weighing 65 kg, using the CE2 efficiency formula as follows:

$$20 \times 1 \,\text{divided by}\, 65 = 0.30 \times 30\,\text{L} = 9.2 \times 10^6 \,\text{CD34}^+ \,\text{cells / kg}$$

The actual collection of 2.8 × 10^6 CD34$^+$ cells/kg is then compared to the predicted 100% efficient collection to give the actual efficiency of the collection:

$$2.8 \,\text{divided by}\, 9.2 \times 100 = 30.4\%$$

For the best fit of a minimum predicted collection, it is important to compare collections not only for "good" or "excellent" mobilizers but for the "poor" mobilizers. Thus, for example, although the collection efficiency for the COBE Spectra and Spectra Optia at our institution is approximately 45%, we use a collection efficiency of 30% for our minimum predictive formula. As each institution has its own preferred method of utilizing the apheresis device of choice, it therefore becomes important to be sure that the collection efficiency used for the calculation best fits their own needs. Published predictive formulas have used collection efficiencies ranging from 30% (Cottler-Fox et al. 2003) to 40% (Pierelli et al. 2006) and 55% (Douglas 2016).

9.8 Developing the Institutional Algorithm

The first step is to determine the goal of a collection (Table 9.4). Thus, an algorithm for a patient for whom one wishes to collect 2×10^6 $CD34^+$ cells/kg of recipient weight would potentially be different than for a patient for whom one wishes to collect 20×10^6 $CD34^+$ cells/kg. Once there is a defined goal, it becomes simpler to decide what the minimum prediction is to start collection, how many days of collection would be acceptable before instituting use of plerixafor (autologous transplant only), and how low a prediction or collection should be allowed to go before stopping collection short of a goal. Once the algorithm is built, the only requirement is data collection and evaluation on a regular basis to be sure the algorithm is acceptable from the standpoints of efficiency and economy.

For instance, the collection goal for myeloma patients at our institution is 20×10^6 $CD34^+$ cells/kg of recipient body weight. Our algorithm therefore starts collection when the minimum predicted collection for a new patient is at least 1×10^6

Table 9.4 Adapting the minimum predictive formula for institutional use

Define goals.
Evaluate actual collection efficiency using CE2.
Determine if the actual collection efficiency is the same for all mobilizers
(poor, good, excellent).
Consider choosing a % efficiency that best predicts the minimum expected collection for the poorest mobilizers if the efficiency is not the same for all levels of mobilization.
Daily QC to see if minimum prediction is met
Consider adopting the calculated performance ratio value (Wuchter et al. 2017) (collected $CD34^+$ cells divided by the predicted $CD34^+$ cells × 100) for daily use for concurrent QA/QC (each institution decides what is acceptable for them; at our institution, we investigate each incidence of a ratio less than 100% since we use a minimum predicted collection number).

$$\text{Performance ratio} = \frac{\text{Collected}}{\text{Predicted}} \times 100$$

$CD34^+$ cells/kg and increases G-CSF from 5 μg/kg twice a day to 8 μg/kg twice a day if the prediction is no more than 1×10^6 $CD34^+$ cells/kg. Plerixafor is instituted after 2 days of collection if the collection goal will not be met by a third consecutive day of collection. Using this algorithm, approximately 70% of patients collect their goal with a mean of 2 days of collection, and a further number reach their goal with the addition of plerixafor (personal observation, unpublished data). If after starting plerixafor the collection contains less than 0.5×10^6 $CD34^+$ cells/kg, the collection is stopped even if four doses (the maximum approved by FDA) of plerixafor have not been given.

9.9 Concurrent Quality Assurance

The minimum predictive formula allows concurrent quality assurance as well as evaluation of new mobilization regimens (Table 9.5). If a collection does not meet the predicted minimum collection, the collection supervisor can immediately ask if there were issues with venous access or interface maintenance on the apheresis device or check the machine to see if there is any machine issue that had not previously been detected.

When evaluating a new mobilization regimen, if the starting rules are the same as the older regimen, it is possible to see whether the new regimen yields the same results as the older one (Table 9.6).

Table 9.5 Quality assurance

Calculate performance ratio daily ($\text{Performance ratio} = \frac{\text{Collected}}{\text{Predicted}} \times 100$) in %.
Decide whether to investigate all who undercollect or only those who undercollect by a specific % based on the *calculated performance ratio*

Table 9.6 How to use the formula to evaluate a new mobilization regimen

Starting rules for collection are defined in advance.
Defined approach to growth factor(s) used, and all changes documented
Can the goals of collection be reached with current strategy or does strategy need to be changed by increasing growth factor dose or adding a second drug?
Standard approach to how apheresis device is used
Standard approach to venous access defined in advance

9.10 Expert Point of View

Efficiency in collection is maximized by using a predictive formula to guide HPC collection. Achieving HPC collection goals is readily achieved using the minimum predictive formula based on institutional goals and determination of machine collection efficiency, using an apheresis device setup as used at a given institution (our institution and several others use 30% as it closely predicts the minimum collection in the "poorest" mobilizers). Evaluating a new mobilization regimen requires defining collection starting and stopping rules, and for publication, these need to be stated clearly for the reader, as do the mechanics of how the apheresis device is used.

9.11 Future Directions

The question of timing of the dose of a given growth factor, i.e., G-CSF, or the binding inhibitor plerixafor, or a newly developed substance, needs to be examined in the setting of a predictive formula so that data can be made on the topic for the transplant community and more uniformity of process can be developed. The use of plerixafor in the allogeneic setting needs more study. Further, it remains to find a way to use the daily calculated performance ratio to more accurately predict what a given mobilizer may likely do the following day in order to eliminate potential weekend collections and to more accurately identify a starting point for plerixafor or other new agents to rescue a poor or inadequate collection. A mathematical model for G-CSF administration after chemotherapy has been developed and deserves further attention as it may allow individualization of dose and collection (Foley and Mackey 2009). Finally, the question of whether growth factor and patient adapted use of plerixafor is superior to chemotherapy plus growth factor remains to be answered by centers using a minimum predictive formula and standardized chemotherapy protocols (Costa et al. 2011b).

References

Abuabdou A, Rosenbaum E, Usmani S et al (2014) Analysis of CD34+ cell collection using two mobilization regimens for newly diagnosed multiple myeloma patients reveals the separate impact of mobilization and collection variables. J Clin Aph 29:251–255

Arbona C, Prosper F, Benet I et al (1998) Comparison between once a day vs twice a day G-CSF fir mobilization of peripheral blood progenitor cells (PBPC) in normal donors for allogeneic PBPC transplantation. Bone Marrow Transplant 22:39–45

Bolan C, Carter C, Wesley R et al (2003) Prospective evaluation of cell kinetics, yields and donor experiences during a single large-volume apheresis versus two smaller volume consecutive day collections of allogeneic peripheral blood stem cells. Br J Haematol 120:801–807

Civin C, Straiss L, Brovall C et al (1984) Antigenic analysis of hematopoiesis. III. A hematopoietic progenitor cell surface antigen defined by a monoclonal antibody raised against KG-1a cells. J Immunol 133(1):157–165

Costa L, Alexander E, Hogan K et al (2011a) Development and validation of a decision-making algorithm to guide the use of plerixafor for autologous hematopoietic stem cell mobilization. Bone Marrow Transplant 46:64–69
Costa L, Miller A, Alexander E et al (2011b) Growth factor and patient adapted use of plerixafor is superior to CY and growth factor for autologous hematopoietic stem cell mobilization. Bone Marrow Transplant 46:523–528
Cottler-Fox M, Lapidot T, Petit I et al (2003) Stem Cell Mobilization. Blood:419–437
Cousins A, Sinclair J, Alcorn M et al (2015) HPC-A dose prediction on the Optia cell separator based on a benchmark CE2 collection efficiency: promoting clinical efficiency, minimizing toxicity, and allowing quality control. J Clin Apheresis 30:321–328
Douglas K (2012) Experience with apheresis procedures after plerixafor mobilization. How much blood to process? Dose prediction on the basis of peripheral CD34+ counts. In: Fruehauf S, Zeller WJ, Calandra G (eds) Novel developments in stem cell mobilization. Springer, New York, pp 133–164
Douglas K (2016) Algorithms to predict CD34+ cell collection with the new generation of cell separator machines. Transfus Med 26(S2):3–24
Foley C, Mackey M (2009) Mathematical model for G-CSF administration after chemotherapy. J Theoretical Biol 257:27–44
Ford C, Chan K, Reilly W, Petterson F (2003) An evaluation of predictive factors for CD34+ cell harvest yields from patients mobilized with chemotherapy and growth factors. Transfusion 43:622–625
Gianni A, Bregni M, Stern A et al (1989) Granulocyte-macrophage colony-stimulating factor to harvest circulating haematopoietic stem cells for autotransplantation. Lancet 334(8663):580–585
Hosing C, Saliba R, Hamerschlak N et al (2014) Peripheral blood stem cell yield calculated using preapheresis absolute CD34+ cell count, peripheral blood volume processed, and donor body weight accurately predicts actual yield at multiple centers. Transfusion 54:1081–1087
Kroger N, Renges H, Kruger W et al (2000) A randomized comparison of once versus twice daily recombinant human granulocyte colony-stimulating factor (filgrastim) for stem cell mobilization in healthy donors for allogeneic transplantation. Br J Haematol 111(3):761–765
Kroger N, Sonnenberg S, Cortes-Dericks L et al (2004) Kinetics of G-CSF and CD34+ cell mobilization after once or twice daily stimulation with rHu granulocyte-stimulating factor (lenograstim) in healthy volunteers: an intraindividual crossover study. Transfusion 44(1):104–110
Lee V, Li C, Chik K et al (2000) Single vs twice daily G-CSF for peripheral blood stem cells harvest in normal donors and children with non-malignant disease. Bone Marrow Transplant 25:931–935
Lisenko K, Pavel P, Brukner T et al (2016) Comparison between intermittent and continuous spectra Optia leukapheresis systems for autologous peripheral blood stem cell collection. J Clin Apher 32(1):27–34
Meisenberg B, Brehm T, Schmeckel A, Miller W, McMillan R (1998) A combination of low-dose cyclophosphamide plus colony stimulating factors is more cost-effective than granulocyte-colony stimulating factor alone to mobilize peripheral blood stem cells. Transfusion 38:209–215
Mohle R, Murea S, Pforsich M et al (1996) Estimation of the progenitor cell yield in a leukapheresis product by previous measurement of CD34+ cells in the peripheral blood. Vox Sang 71:90–96
Morris C, Siegel E, Barlogie B et al (2003) Mobilization of CD34+ cells in elderly patients with multiple myeloma: influence of age, prior therapy, platelet count and mobilization regimen. Br J Haematol 120(3):413–423
Nervi B, Link D, DiPersio J (2006) Cytokines and hematopoietic stem cell mobilization. J Cell Biochem 99:690–705
Peters W, Rosner G, Ross M et al (1993) Comparative effects of G-CFS and GM-CSF on priming peripheral blood progenitor cells for use with autologous bone marrow after high-dose chemotherapy. Blood 81:1709–1719

Pierelli L, Marasca M, Piccirillo N et al (2006) Accurate prediction of autologous stem cell apheresis yields using a double variable-dependent method assures systematic efficiency control of continuous flow collection procedures. Vox Sang 91(2):126–134

Prince H, Imrie K, Sutherland R et al (1996) Peripheral blood progenitor cell collections in multiple myeloma: predictors and management of inadequate collections. Br J Haematol 93:142–145

Rosenbaum E, O'Connell B, Cottler-Fox M (2012) Validation of a formula for predicting daily CD34+ cell collection by leukapheresis. Cytotherapy 14:461–466

Sandhya R, Yu Y, Kang E et al (2015) Mobilization characteristics and strategies to improve hematopoietic progenitor cell mobilization and collection in patients with chronic granulomatous disease and severe combined immunodeficiency. Transfusion 55(2):265–274

Sutherland D, Anderson L, Keeney M et al (1996) The ISHAGE guidelines for CD34+ cell determination by flow cytometry. J Hematother 5(3):213–226

To L, Haylock D, Kimber R, Juttner C (1984) High levels of circulating haemopoietic stem cells in very early remission from acute non-lymphoblastic leukaemia and their collection and cryopreservation. Br J Haematol 58:399–410

Wuchter P, Hundemar M, Schmitt A et al (2017) Performance assessment and benchmarking of autologous peripheral blood stem cell collection with two different apheresis devices. Transfus Med 27(1):36–42

Applications of Apheresis Devices in Processing Bone Marrow Grafts

10

Gerda C. Leitner

10.1 Introduction

Over the past half century, hematopoietic cell transplantation (HCT) using either bone marrow (BM) or peripheral blood grafts has been used with increasing frequency to treat numerous malignant and nonmalignant diseases. With the advancements in techniques, indications, and supportive therapy, the transplantation of hematopoietic progenitor cells (HPC) continues to be an advancing field in the treatment of human disease (Henig and Zuckerman 2014).

ABO blood groups antigens are inherited independently from the human leukocyte antigen (HLA) system (Rowley et al. 2000; Worel 2016). Thus, up to 50% of allogeneic HCT (allo-HCT) are performed across the blood group barrier. While PB grafts can be infused mostly without any ABO-related complication, the infusion of bone marrow requires the implementation of safety precautions to avoid acute immune-mediated hemolytic problems. BM processing techniques to remove red blood cell (RBCs), plasma, or both (MNC separation) were implemented. In addition, therapeutic approaches like plasma exchange procedures or donor ABO-type RBC transfusions were established for patients with a major ABO incompatible donor. These treatment option focuses on the removal of isohemagglutinins directed against the RBCs of the BM donor (Gale et al. 1977).

Besides allogeneic BM transplantation, in former days, autologous BM transplantation was performed. The latter started in 1955 when Barnes and Loutit successfully demonstrated cryopreservation of autologous BM grafts (Barnes and Loutit 1955). In the majority of studies, dimethylsulfoxide (DMSO) at a final concentration of 10% was used as cryoprotectant (Berz et al. 2007; Hunt 2011). DMSO

G. C. Leitner (✉)
Department for Blood Group Serology and Transfusion Medicine, Medical University Vienna, Vienna, Austria
e-mail: gerda.leitner@meduniwien.ac.at

S. A. Abutalib et al. (eds.), *Best Practices of Apheresis in Hematopoietic Cell Transplantation*, Advances and Controversies in Hematopoietic Transplantation and Cell Therapy, https://doi.org/10.1007/978-3-319-55131-9_10

has a toxic effect on HPCs at room temperature and additionally causes adverse events during infusion mostly due to histamine release. The toxicity increases with the amount of DMSO transfused (Berz et al. 2007). Thus, volume reduction of BM grafts before cryopreservation is mandatory to avoid a high amount of DMSO in the product.

The use of BM in allogeneic as well as in autologous transplantation decreased over the last 20 years in favor of peripheral blood stem cells. In children, BM is still the preferred graft source due to a lower risk of chronic graft-versus-host disease (GvHD) (Anasetti et al. 2012). Besides that, allogeneic HPC donors who do not qualify for apheresis due to various reasons (e.g., allergic reactions to G-CSF, autoimmune diseases, etc.) are candidates for a BM harvest (Worel et al. 2015). However, the decision which graft sources will be used is also dependent on the institution's preference especially in adult patients.

10.2 Volume Reduction Methods

10.2.1 Plasma Depletion of Bone Marrow Grafts

In case of minor ABO incompatibility (Table 10.1), which occurs in 20–25% of transplants, plasma depletion of BM can become necessary (Worel 2016). The infusion of donor-derived ABO-incompatible plasma with an unmanipulated BM graft can lead to acute hemolysis of recipient RBCs (Rowley 2001). The concentration of isohemagglutinins in the donors' plasma and the amount of plasma putting a patient at risk to acute hemolysis are still controversially discussed, Rowley and colleagues defined the threshold of donor-derived isohemagglutinin titers with 1:128 for IgM and/or IgG and recommended plasma depletion of products from donors with titers of >1:128 (Rowley et al. 2000; Mielcarek et al. 2000). However, most authors favor a threshold of 1:32 and recommend plasma depletion above these values (Witt et al. 2011). As known from platelet transfusions, there is no strong correlation between isohemagglutinin titers and the risk of acute hemolysis. In addition, besides the titer, also the amount of plasma in the BM graft should be considered. Thus, plasma depletion in ABO minor incompatibility should be performed whenever possible, independently of isohemagglutinin titers (Booth et al. 2013; Gajewski et al. 2008; Karafin et al. 2012; Roback et al. 2011).

Most commonly, plasma is removed by centrifugation. Centrifugation protocols vary between centers in terms of centrifugal speed and process temperature. The reported centrifugal force ranges from 400 to 4000 × *g* performed at a temperature ranging between 4 °C and room temperature (15 °C–25 °C) (Daniel-Johnson and

Table 10.1 ABO minor incompatibility

Blood group recipient	Blood group donor
A, B, AB	0
AB	A, B

Isohemagglutinins of the donor are directed against RBCs of the recipient

Schwartz 2011). Open and closed systems are reported, but closed systems should be preferred.

A common protocol is to connect product and transfer bag by sterile connection devices and centrifugation of the BM graft at 2850 × *g* centrifugal force for 30 min without brake, followed by plasma extraction using a simple plasma extractor at room temperature or 4 °C (Fig. 10.1a, b). The high centrifugation speed is necessary to induce an optimal separation of the mononuclear cell (MNC) layer in the presence of BM fat. A second centrifugation (wash procedure) can be helpful if the donor has a particularly high titer anti-ABO titer (≥1:256) (Rowley 2001). Each processing facility is required to set up a process validation protocol and to define acceptable recovery rates (Davis-Sproul et al. 2008). In general, high MNC recovery rates can be expected in this setting.

a

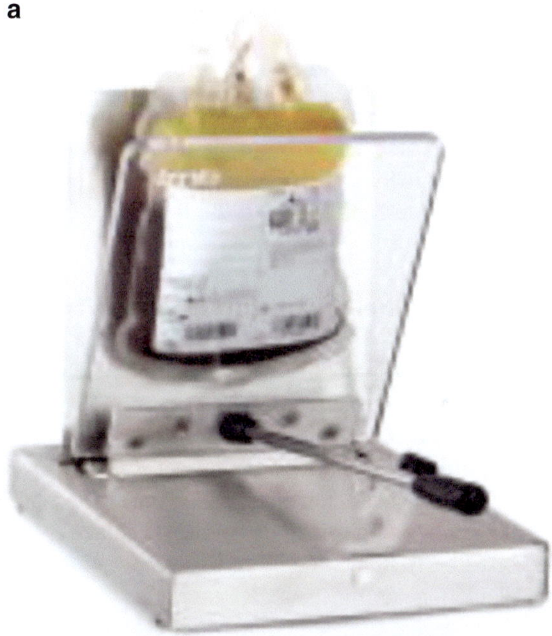

b

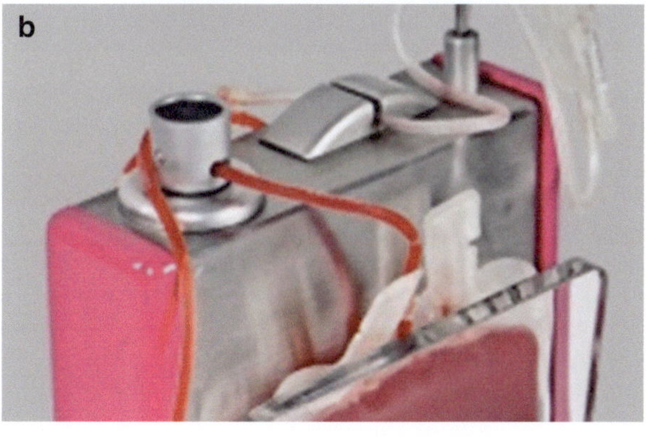

Fig. 10.1 (**a**) Manual plasma extractor; Lmb Technologie GmbH. Manual system, all kind of transfer bags can be used. (**b**) Automatic plasma extractor, Lmb Technologie GmbH. A new device, as a simple plasma extractor, it was upgraded by an automatic clamping function to standardize separation results and facilitate working processes. It ensures separation without red cell contamination and loss of BM cells

10.3 Mononuclear Cell (MNC) Separation from Bone Marrow Harvests by Red Blood Cell and Plasma Depletion

The aim of in vitro manipulation of bone marrow is to reduce (plasma) volume and RBC contamination of the BM graft while minimizing the loss of MNCs, in particular HPCs, within an acceptable time frame. The critical marker for successful MNC selection from BM is the $CD34^+$ cell recovery. A maximum volume of major ABO-incompatible RBCs is not defined. Usually, 10–30 mL of incompatible RBCs are tolerated by the recipient (Daniel-Johnson and Schwartz 2011). Some centers recommend a remaining RBC volume of <0.5 mL/kg body weight of the recipient (Curcioli and de Carvalho 2010).

10.3.1 Autologous Transplantation

BM is collected for a later transplantation and is stored after cryopreservation between −198 °C (liquid nitrogen) and −80 °C (vapor phase) until reinfusion. Cryopreservation of BM requires reduction of volume and depletion of granulocytes and RBCs. These are important features to minimize the amount of DMSO and to ensure MNC survival during storage and acceptable recovery rates after thawing (Koristek and Mayer 1999; Rowley 1992).

10.3.2 Allogeneic Hematopoietic Cell Transplantation

In allogeneic transplantation, incompatible RBCs have to be removed from the BM graft (Tables 10.2 and 10.3). In contrast to PB SC grafts, BM grafts contain high amounts of RBCs (hematocrit up to 25% to 35%) (Rowley 2001). This is equivalent to the erythrocyte mass of 2–3 units of RBCs, respectively. In major and bidirectional ABO-mismatch transplantation, transfusion of unmanipulated BM can cause life-threatening complications leading to fatal hemolysis. Since BM manipulation methods like RBC depletion and volume reduction have been implemented, BM transplantation across the ABO barrier is feasible without an increased risk for hemolysis during graft infusion.

Another possibility to reduce the risk of hemolysis is to reduce recipient-derived anti-donor isohemagglutinins by plasma exchange, double-filtration plasmapheresis, or immunoadsorption therapy. Also, pretransplant donor-type RBC transfusion is an option to reduce anti-donor isohemagglutinin titers and enables a safe infusion

Table 10.2 ABO major incompatibility

Blood group recipient	Blood group donor
0	A, B, AB
A, B	AB

Isohemagglutinins of the recipient are directed against RBCs of the donor

Table 10.3 ABO bidirectional incompatibility

Blood group recipient	Blood group donor
A	B
B	A

Isohemagglutinins of the donor are directed against RBCs of the recipient and vice versa

of unmanipulated major ABO-incompatible BM graft. However, these methods have limitations and are probably not effective enough in all cases (Daniele et al. 2014; Nussbaumer et al. 1995; Rabitsch et al. 2003). Thus, various techniques to remove RBC simultaneously with plasma from BM grafts have been developed.

10.3.3 Red Blood Cell Depletion and Volume Reduction Methods

In the 1980s, in vitro manipulation of BM was performed manually by gravity sedimentation with and without sedimentation agents, by density gradient centrifugation using density gradient reagents (i.e., Ficoll-Hypaque) (Daniel-Johnson and Schwartz 2011; Koristek and Mayer 1999; Daniele et al. 2014; Gilmore et al. 1982; Warkentin et al. 1985; Wells et al. 1979), by using double centrifugation mode, or by apheresis technology with either an intermittent-flow cell separator (i.e., H30, Haemonetics) or continuous-flow systems (i.e., Aminco Celltrifuge) (Linch et al. 1982). A very time-consuming method (4–5 h) was described by Falkenburg and colleagues who were able to remove up to 99% of incompatible RBCs from the BM graft. The success of this procedure was highly associated with the operator's experience (Falkenburg et al. 1985). At that time, most of the manual methods were superior to the apheresis systems in RBC depletion and/or HPC recovery (Linch et al. 1982). However, manual separation techniques were partly performed with reagents at risk to cause in vitro cell injury (e.g., Ficoll-Hypaque) or with their exposure to the recipient (i.e., HES), respectively (Koristek and Mayer 1999).

Advances in apheresis technology simplified BM processing with regard to man power, time consumption, and risk of bacterial contamination and lead to reproducibility of results (RBC and volume depletion as well as MNC and CD34$^+$ cell recovery). Over the last two decades, a variety of cell separators, i.e., Dideco T90® (*Dideco, Mirandola, Italy*), CS3000™/CS3000plus™ (*Baxter, Deerfield, IL, USA; Fenwal, Lake Zurich, IL, USA*), AS 104® (*Fresenius HemoCare, Germany*), Cobe 2991®, Cobe 2997®, Cobe Spectra® (*COBE BCT, Inc., Lakewood, Co, USA*), Amicus™ (*Fenwal, Zaventem, Belgium*), Biosafe Sepax (*automated cell processing; Haemotec Inc., Vaudreuil-Dorion, Canada*), and Spectra Optia® (*Terumo BCT, Denver, USA*), were investigated concerning their usability in this field (Daniele et al. 2014).

The application of continuous-flow technology for BM processing follows the same principles as collection of grafts from PB (see Chaps. 5, 6, 8, and 9). The main difference is the graft source which contributes to differences in quantity and composition of cells and differences in proteins, lipids, and product viscosity. These issues, as well as the underlying disease of the individual (patient, healthy donor), were thought to probably influence MNC and progenitor cell recovery. Hester and colleagues investigated the ***Cobe Spectra***® apheresis device, which was newly introduced for this purpose in the 1990s for factors possibly influencing cell recovery in BM processing (Hester et al. 1995). The ***Cobe Spectra***® is a half-automated device requiring operator control. The relevant factors influencing the quality of products were identified to be procedure related as an instable interface or difficulties in adjusting the hematocrit of the collection line and the human (operator) factor. However, the final HCT in BM was in mean 4%, and the correlation coefficient for $CD34^+$ cell recovery was 0.82. Koristek and Mayer (Koristek and Mayer 1999) stated that the ***Cobe Spectra***® can be used effectively for volume reduction and MNC and $CD34^+$ cell enrichment of BM but observed a wide range in the recovery of $CD34^+$ cells. In 150 procedures, a recovery for $CD34^+$ cells of >77% (range 8.3 to 260) and a reduction of RBCs of >98% were observed. An important issue for optimal results is a prompt processing after collection, which means a short transit time between collection facility and processing facility. If an overnight storage is unavoidable, the BM should be stored in a refrigerator (4 °C ± 2) until further manipulation (Guttridge et al. 2006; Leemhuis et al. 2014).

The ***Amicus***™ (nowadays Fresenius Kabi, Germany), a cell separator, is the succeeding model of the CS3000 plus™ (former *Baxter, Deerfield, IL, USA).* The ***CS3000 plus***™ was an automated system which provided pediatric (50 mL) and adult (200 mL) volume products of high quality. Depletion of RBCs as well as CD34 recovery was >96%, $n = 99$ (Gonzalez-Campos et al. 2000). The Amicus™ lacks a designated BM processing program until now, but Witt et al. demonstrated that using the preinstalled MNC collection program (used for peripheral blood HPC collection), when adjusted for BM processing, reveals similar results in RBC depletion and $CD34^+$ cell recovery as **CS3000**™ (forerunner of CS3000 plus™) (Witt et al. 2011). With both devices, the hematocrit was relatively high (mean 10% for Amicus™ and 12% for CS3000™, respectively), but the absolute RBC volume was below 20 mL (cumulative threshold for major ABO-incompatible BM infusion in children (Witt et al. 2011)). All graft infusions ($n = 22$) were well tolerated.

The latest development in this field is the cell separator ***Spectra Optia***® (*Terumo BCT, Denver, USA),* the succeeding model of *Cobe Spectra*®. It eases the BM processing procedure; requires less operator supervision, as the system continuously monitors and adjusts the interface; reduces man power; and provides robust and reproducible results with regard to progenitor cell ($CD34^+$ cells) recovery (median > 90%), RBC depletion (median > 97%), and volume reduction (median > 93%) (Guttridge et al. 2016; Sorg et al. 2015). In case of extended transit time (up to 24 h), BM should be kept cooled (2 °C–6 °C) to ensure optimal processing results (Guttridge et al. 2006, 2016; Leemhuis et al. 2014).

Since more than 30 years, the ***COBE 2991***® cell processor (*Terumo BCT, Denver, USA*) is a reliable tool for a variety of cell processing applications. Two protocols for BM processing are available, "bone marrow concentration" and "bone marrow processing" using a density gradient separation medium. The latter achieves RBC depletion and MNC recovery of >97% (Gilmore et al. 1982; Sorg et al. 2015). The bone marrow concentration protocol is lacking of data, and the density gradient protocol uses Ficoll-Hypaque and thus bears the risk of MNC injury (Posel et al. 2012).

A versatile technology platform, the new ***Biosafe Sepax 2*** (*Haemotec, South Africa*), is a fully automated, mobile, GMP-compliant system for efficient and reproducible processing of CB and BM (Babic and Regan 2014). This device is well established in cell therapy procedures and is suitable for small-volume products) (Sorg et al. 2015).

10.4 Principles of Cell Separation and Collection

Centrifugation is a technique used to process whole blood in order to separate the blood into its various components by stratifying the particular blood components into layers according to their specific density. The separation factor (SF) is a combination of centrifugal force (g) and dwelling time. A thin mononuclear (MNC) layer is formed at the interface of RBCs and plasma. Accumulation of RBCs (cells with the highest density) results in building a stable interface for optimal collection.

10.5 Apheresis Devices Currently in Use

10.5.1 *Cobe Spectra® (Terumo BCT)* (Is Still in Use in the USA and in Some European Countries)

The Cobe Spectra® is a continuous-flow, functionally closed cell separator. The MNCs (including CD34$^+$ cells) are enriched in a buffy layer by centrifugation. The separation of the cells is based on their different density and size. The collection of the desired cell fraction is enabled via configuration of the channel and adjusted by the appropriate plasma flow. The BM processing (BMP) program works on a semi-automated basis and requires continuous visual control of the collection line. The double-bag set needs a manual reverse of the flow multiple times during the procedure (Fig. 10.2). The minimal volume of BM, which can be processed, is 300 mL, and the minimal RBC content of the BM is 125 mL. Small BM volumes have to be adjusted with compatible crossmatched RBCs. This procedure is important in the pediatric setting. Routinely, three to four times of the initial BM volume should be processed to achieve an efficient volume reduction, RBC depletion, and MNC and CD34$^+$ cell recovery during approximately 90 min procedure time (TerumoBCT n.d.-a) (Fig. 10.3a, b).

10.5.2 Spectra Optia® (Terumo BCT)

This advanced system is an automated, functionally closed blood cell separator, using a continuous-flow centrifugation and an optical detection technology.

Fig. 10.2 Cobe Spectra bone marrow processing set

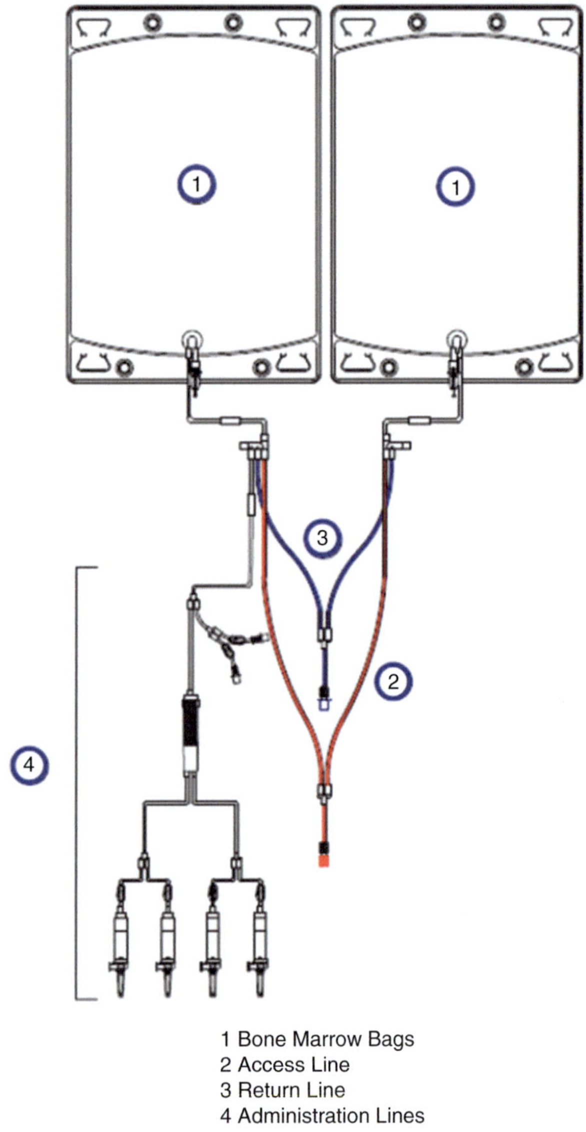

The procedures are controlled with real-time interface monitoring by interpretation and adjustment with the automated interface management (AIM) system (Fig. 10.4). Through helpful on-screen guidance and a single-bag approach (to allow the BM aspirate to be recirculated as it is processed) (Fig. 10.5), the Spectra Optia system simplifies the BMP procedure and requires less operator supervision by continuous interface monitoring using a unique optical detection software (Leitner et al. 2015). To optimize the MNC selection, the collection preference should be adjusted by the operator. Initially, a collection preference

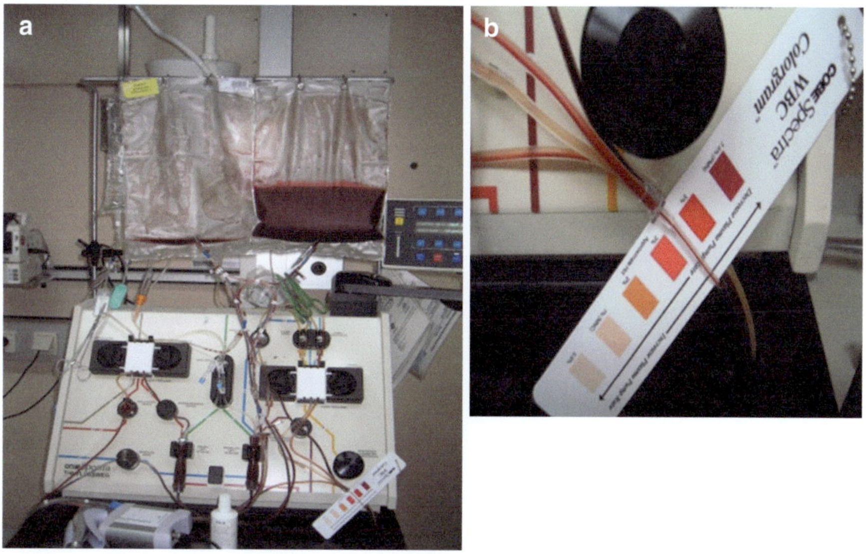

Fig. 10.3 (**a**, **b**) Provided by Dept. of Blood Group Serology and Transfusion Medicine, Medical University Vienna, Vienna, Austria. (**b**) The color of collection line is controlled visually (indicating the hematocrit level). Bone marrow processing set: The product is transferred from one bag to the other, the inlet line switches between both bags, and the clamps are set manually

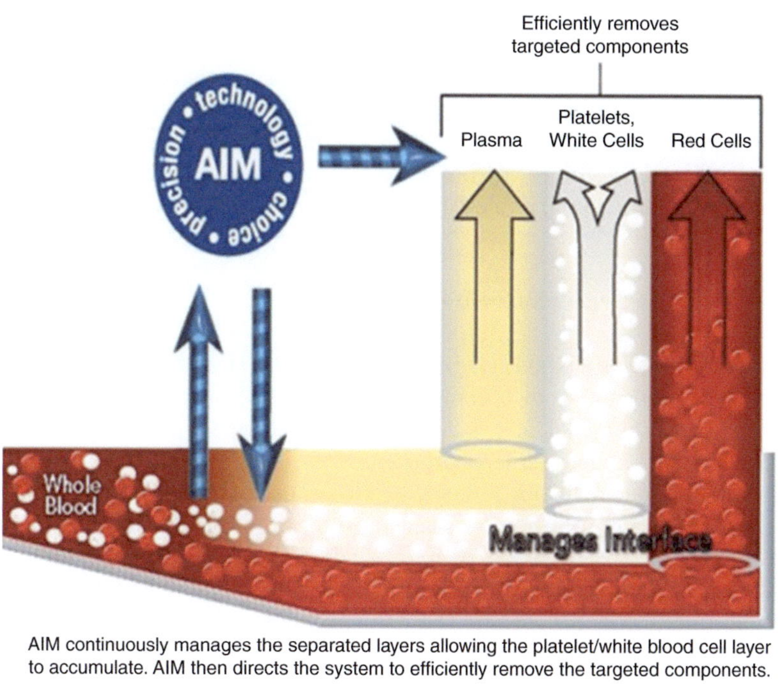

Fig. 10.4 Automated interface monitoring (AIM) Spectra Optia avoids visual control of the collection line

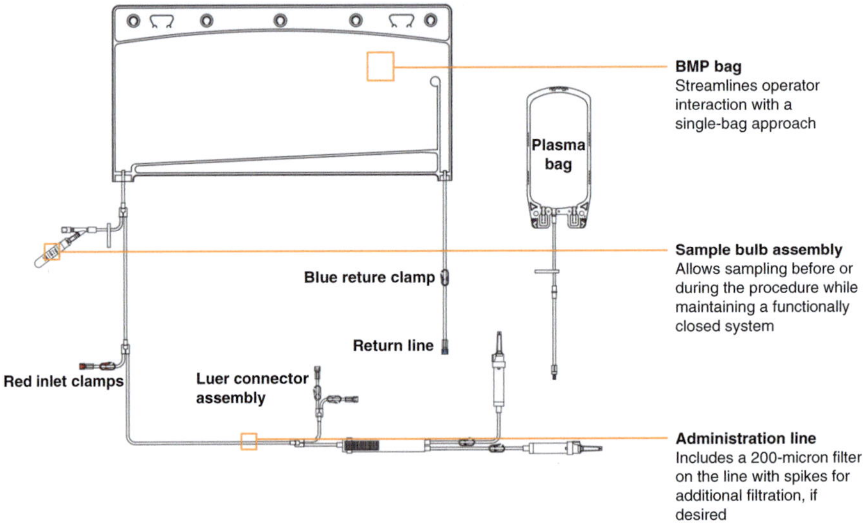

Fig. 10.5 Only one single bone marrow processing (BMP) bag, allowing automatic recirculation of BM during processing

of 50 is selected (ranges between 10 and 90). Higher collection preferences induce lower MNC concentration. Equal restrictions to the total BM volume and the RBC volume (125 mL) like with *Cobe Spectra®* have to be taken into account. The BM is processed multiple times to ensure high recovery and a sufficient depletion of contaminating cells. The number of times the BM is processed depends on the RBC volume of the graft: The higher the number of RBCs in the BM product, the fewer times the device needs to process the graft to efficiently remove incompatible RBCs (Fig. 10.6) (TerumoBCT n.d.-b).

10.5.3 Biosafe Sepax System (Haemotec)

The *SEPAX system* is a blood cell processing system intended for laboratory use in exclusive combination with a compatible single-use separation kit supplied by Biosafe. The *Sepax system* allows the fast, automated, and reproducible separation of blood in a closed and sterile environment. It is not intended for use at bedside. The generic volume reduction protocol (GVR protocol, without Ficoll-Hypaque or density gradient centrifugation) was generated for the volume reduction of generic products (BM, peripheral blood, or cord blood). This protocol is designed for volumes between 30 mL and approximately 800 mL and gives an option for very small BM collections (collected predominately from very young donors) (Haemotec n.d.). Of note, this device is generally not used in hospital-based transfusion centers, which usually process BM. This device is predominantly used for cord blood processing and washing of thawed DMSO-preserved HPC units (Scerpa et al. 2011).

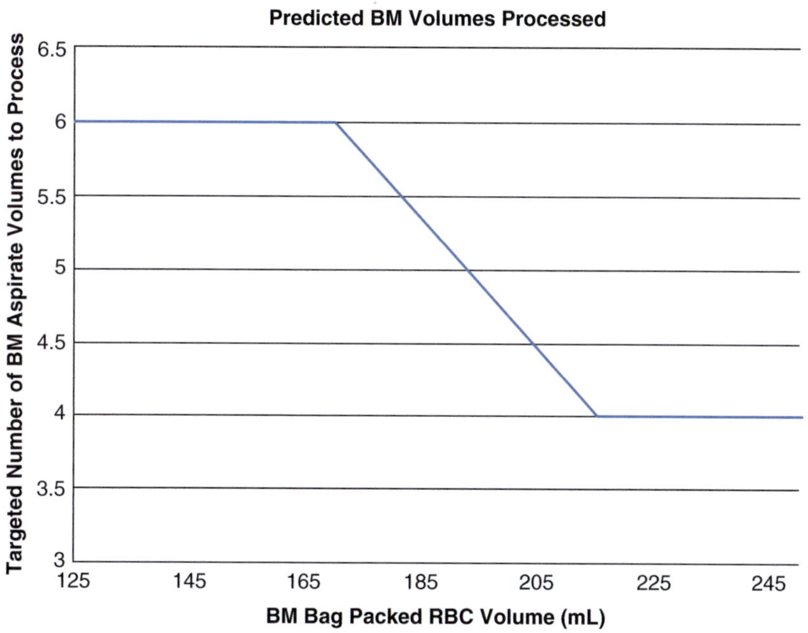

Fig. 10.6 Spectra Optia: A small RBC volume in the bone marrow graft requires a higher process volume; this is in general true for all physical RBC depletion techniques

10.5.4 Amicus™ (Fresenius Kabi)

This apheresis system works like the previously mentioned systems. The Amicus is a continuous-flow, functionally closed, fully automated cell separator designed for therapeutic and preparative use. It is lacking of a defined BMP protocol, but Witt and colleagues showed that efficient BM processing is feasible by manipulating the preinstalled MNC collection program (Witt et al. 2011). In face of the existence of special programs and special installation kits and processing sets, this program should only be used in centers where the operators are experienced with this individual technique.

10.6 Processing of Small Bone Marrow Volumes by Apheresis

Small BM volume is defined as a total volume below 300 mL and an RBC volume below 125 mL.

As the BM product is being drawn into the system, RBCs are accumulating in the connector to build the interface for optimal cell collection. The more RBCs are available, the faster the interface is build and the quicker the target cells get to the collect port. When the RBC volume is low, the efficient removal of the target cells takes longer (Fig. 10.6). Below the threshold of 300 mL of BM and/or 125 mL RBCs, an efficient MNC and progenitor separation and RBC depletion cannot be guaranteed. Thus, it is necessary to increase the RBC volume with compatible and BM donor crossmatched RBC units in the autologous as well as in the allogeneic setting. This can be performed either by adding the RBC unit directly to the BM graft or by priming the tubing set of the apheresis device (Witt et al. 2007, 2011). Both methods are suitable to enable optimal processing results.

10.7 Time Frame from Collection to Processing

For an acceptable cell recovery and RBC depletion (both greater than 90%), it is important to keep the elapsed time between the BM collection in the operation theater and the BM processing facility as short as possible. Overnight storages should take place in the cold (4 °C ± 2). Guttridge and colleagues describe that a median transit time from the collection to processing facility exceeding 6 h is associated with a lower MNCs and $CD34^+$ recovery. Cold storage (2–6 °C) until processing had no negative impact on the processing results for the relevant parameters (MNCs, $CD34^+$, RBC, and volume reduction) (Guttridge et al. 2006, 2016).

10.8 Expert Point of View

For BM processing, automated apheresis devices with a dedicated installed BM programs, without using sedimentation agents (HES) or density gradient reagents (Ficoll-Hypaque), should be preferred.

However, each center should use the device and program where the operators are most experienced with.

Technical regulations concerning process limitations, like small volumes, have to be kept in mind.

Long transit times should be avoided. In-between storage in a refrigerator (4 °C ± 2 °C) is strongly recommended. Post-process quality control measures are warranted.

References

Anasetti C, Logan BR, Lee SJ, Waller EK, Weisdorf DJ, Wingard JR et al (2012) Peripheral-blood stem cells versus bone marrow from unrelated donors. New Engl J Med 367(16):1487–1496

Babic A, Regan D (2014) Umbilical cord blood banking. American Association of Blood Banks (AABB), Bethesda. 729 p

Barnes DWH, Loutit JF (1955) Radiation recovery factor and preservation by the Polge Smith Parkes Parkes technique. J Natl Cancer Inst 15:901–905

Berz D, McCormack EM, Winer ES, Colvin GA, Quesenberry PJ (2007) Cryopreservation of hematopoietic stem cells. Am J Hematol 82(6):463–472

Booth GS, Gehrie EA, Bolan CD, Savani BN (2013) Clinical guide to ABO-incompatible allogeneic stem cell transplantation. Biol Blood Marrow Transplant 19(8):1152–1158

Curcioli AC, de Carvalho EC (2010) Infusion of hematopoietic stem cells: types, characteristics, adverse and transfusion reactions and the implications for nursing. Rev Lat Am Enfermagem 18(4):716–724

Daniele N, Scerpa MC, Rossi C, Lanti A, Adorno G, Isacchi G et al (2014) The processing of stem cell concentrates from the bone marrow in ABO-incompatible transplants: how and when. Blood Transfus 12(2):150–158

Daniel-Johnson J, Schwartz J (2011) How do I approach ABO-incompatible hematopoietic progenitor cell transplantation? Transfusion 51(6):1143–1149

Davis-Sproul J, Haley NR, McMannis J (2008) Collecting and processing marrow products for transplantation. 16th edition. S Karger AG, Basel. 765 p

Falkenburg JH, Schaafsma MR, Jansen J, Brand A, Goselink HM, Zwaan FE et al (1985) Recovery of hematopoiesis after blood-group-incompatible bone marrow transplantation with red-blood-cell-depleted grafts. Transplantation 39(5):514–520

Gajewski JL, Johnson VV, Sandler SG, Sayegh A, Klumpp TR (2008) A review of transfusion practice before, during, and after hematopoietic progenitor cell transplantation. Blood 112(8):3036–3047

Gale RP, Feig S, Ho W, Falk P, Rippee C, Sparkes R (1977) ABO blood group system and bone marrow transplantation. Blood 50(2):185–194

Gilmore MJ, Prentice HG, Blacklock HA, Janossy G, Hoffbrand AV (1982) A technique for rapid isolation of bone marrow mononuclear cells using Ficoll-Metrizoate and the IBM 2991 blood cell processor. Br J Hematol 50(4):619–626

Gonzalez-Campos J, Carmona-Gonzalez M, Rodriguez-Fernandez JM, Mellado-Damas N, de Luis-Navarro J (2000) Bone marrow processing using the fenwal CS-3000 plus blood cell separator: results of 99 procedures. J Hematother Stem Cell Res 9(1):83–88

Guttridge MG, Sidders C, Booth-Davey E, Pamphilon D, Watt SM (2006) Factors affecting volume reduction and red blood cell depletion of bone marrow on the COBE Spectra cell separator before haematopoietic stem cell transplantation. Bone Marrow Transplant 38(3):175–181

Guttridge MG, Bailey C, Sidders C, Nichols J, Bromham J, Watt SM (2016) Human bone marrow processing using a new continuous-flow cell separation device. Transfusion 56(4):899–904

Haemotec. Biosafe Sepax Automated Cell Processing. Operators manual

Henig I, Zuckerman T (2014) Hematopoietic stem cell transplantation-50 years of evolution and future perspectives. Rambam Maimonid Med J 5(4):e0028

Hester JP, Rondon G, Huh YO, Lauppe MJ, Champlin RE, Deisseroth AB (1995) Principles of bone marrow processing and progenitor cell/mononuclear cell concentrate collection in a continuous flow blood cell separation system. J Hematother 4(4):299–306

Hunt CJ (2011) Cryopreservation of human stem cells for clinical application: a review. Transfus Med Hemother 38(2):107–123

Karafin MS, Blagg L, Tobian AA, King KE, Ness PM, Savage WJ (2012) ABO antibody titers are not predictive of hemolytic reactions due to plasma-incompatible platelet transfusions. Transfusion 52(10):2087–2093

Koristek Z, Mayer J (1999) Bone marrow processing for transplantation using the COBE spectra cell separator. J Hematother Stem Cell Res 8(4):443–448

Leemhuis T, Padley D, Keever-Taylor C, Niederwieser D, Teshima T, Lanza F et al (2014) Essential requirements for setting up a stem cell processing laboratory. Bone Marrow Transplant 49(8):1098–1105

Leitner GC, Kolovratova V, Horvath M, Worel N (2015) Granulocyte collection using a novel apheresis system eases the procedure and provides concentrates of high quality. Transfusion 55(5):991–995

Linch DC, Knott LJ, Patterson KG, Cowan DA, Harper PG (1982) Bone marrow processing and cryopreservation. J Clin Pathol 35(2):186–190

Mielcarek M, Leisenring W, Torok-Storb B, Storb R (2000) Graft-versus-host disease and donor-directed hemagglutinin titers after ABO-mismatched related and unrelated marrow allografts: evidence for a graft-versus-plasma cell effect. Blood 96(3):1150–1156

Nussbaumer W, Schwaighofer H, Gratwohl A, Kilga S, Schonitzer D, Nachbaur D et al (1995) Transfusion of donor-type red cells as a single preparative treatment for bone marrow transplants with major ABO incompatibility. Transfusion 35(7):592–595

Posel C, Moller K, Frohlich W, Schulz I, Boltze J, Wagner DC (2012) Density gradient centrifugation compromises bone marrow mononuclear cell yield. PLoS One 7(12):e50293

Rabitsch W, Knobl P, Greinix H, Prinz E, Kalhs P, Horl WH et al (2003) Removal of persisting isohaemagglutinins with Ig-Therasorb immunoadsorption after major ABO-incompatible non-myeloablative allogeneic haematopoietic stem cell transplantation. Nephrol Dial Transplant 18(11):2405–2408

Roback JD, Grossman BJ, Harris T, Hillyer CD (2011) American Association of Blood Banks

Rowley SD (1992) Hematopoietic stem cell cryopreservation: a review of current techniques. J Hematother 1(3):233–250

Rowley SD (2001) Hematopoietic stem cell transplantation between red cell incompatible donor-recipient pairs. Bone Marrow Transplant 28(4):315–321

Rowley SD, Liang PS, Ulz L (2000) Transplantation of ABO-incompatible bone marrow and peripheral blood stem cell components. Bone Marrow Transplant 26(7):749–757

Scerpa MC, Daniele N, Landi F, Caniglia M, Cometa AM, Ciammetti C et al (2011) Automated washing of human progenitor cells: evaluation of apoptosis and cell necrosis. Transfus Med 21(6):402–407

Sorg N, Poppe C, Bunos M, Wingenfeld E, Hummer C, Kramer A et al (2015) Red blood cell depletion from bone marrow and peripheral blood buffy coat: a comparison of two new and three established technologies. Transfusion 55(6):1275–1282

TerumoBCT. Cobe Spectra Apheresis Systems. Technical guide

TerumoBCT. Spectra Optia® Apheresis System Protocols. Technical guide

Warkentin PI, Hilden JM, Kersey JH, Ramsay NK, McCullough J (1985) Transplantation of major ABO-incompatible bone marrow depleted of red cells by hydroxyethyl starch. Vox Sang 48(2):89–104

Wells JR, Sullivan A, Cline MJ (1979) A technique for the separation and cryopreservation of myeloid stem cells from human bone marrow. Cryobiology 16(3):201–210

Witt V, Beiglbock E, Ritter R, Wurth M, Peters C, Ladenstein R et al (2007) Performance of a new separator system for routine autologous hematopoietic progenitor cell collection in small children. J Clin Apher 22(6):306–313

Witt V, Beiglbock E, Fritsch G (2011) Bone marrow processing with the AMICUS separator system. J Clin Apher 26(4):195–199

Worel N (2016) ABO-mismatched allogeneic hematopoietic stem cell transplantation. Transfus Med Hemother 43(1):3–12

Worel N, Buser A, Greinix HT, Hagglund H, Navarro W, Pulsipher MA et al (2015) Suitability criteria for adult related donors: a consensus statement from the worldwide network for blood and marrow transplantation standing committee on donor issues. Biol Blood Marrow Transplant 21(12):2052–2060

Therapeutic Plasma Exchange and Immunoadsorption: Indications and Implementation

11

Ammon Handisurya, Christof Aigner, Benjamin Schairer, and Kurt Derfler

11.1 Introduction

The term apheresis comprises a variety of extracorporeal treatment modalities, which enable the removal of pathogenic components with or without replacement fluid. The following chapter will focus on plasma exchange and immunoadsorption, which was initially reported as an option to treat Waldenström's macroglobulinemia by Solomon and Fahey (1963).

11.1.1 Therapeutic Plasma Exchange

Therapeutic plasma exchange (TPE) is based on a rather simple mechanism: plasma is separated from corpuscular blood elements and, thereafter, discarded and replaced by substitution fluids, e.g., plasma or human albumin 5%. By this rather unspecific procedure, circulating immunoglobulins (antibodies and autoantibodies) and immune complexes are removed from circulation. However, the concomitant loss of other plasma proteins like coagulation factors, fibrinogen, electrolytes, or

A. Handisurya (✉)
Apheresis Unit, Division of Nephrology and Dialysis, Department of Medicine III, Medical University of Vienna, Vienna, Austria

1st Medical Department,
Hanusch Hospital, Vienna, Austria
e-mail: ammon.handisurya@wgkk.at

C. Aigner · B. Schairer · K. Derfler
Apheresis Unit, Division of Nephrology and Dialysis, Department of Medicine III, Medical University of Vienna, Vienna, Austria
e-mail: christof.aigner@meduniwien.ac.at; benjamin.schairer@meduniwien.ac.at; kurt.derfler@meduniwien.ac.at

S. A. Abutalib et al. (eds.), *Best Practices of Apheresis in Hematopoietic Cell Transplantation*, Advances and Controversies in Hematopoietic Transplantation and Cell Therapy, https://doi.org/10.1007/978-3-319-55131-9_11

protein-bound drugs as well as the diminish of return effect limits the plasma volume processed during a single treatment (Zöllner et al. 2014; Chirnside et al. 1981). In general, the continuous substitution of plasma by an isovolemic, iso-osmotic, and iso-oncotic fluid is mandatory during TPE, and the 1.0–1.5 times estimated plasma volume is usually processed during a single treatment (Fig. 11.1, Table 11.1) (Schwartz et al. 2016).

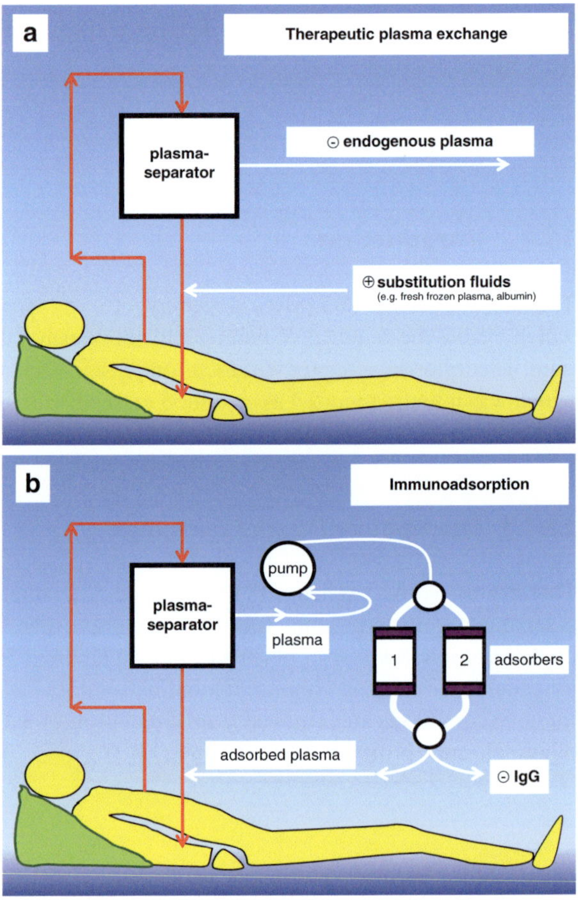

Fig. 11.1 Schematic presentation of therapeutic plasma exchange (**a**) and immunoadsorption (**b**)

Table 11.1 Recommended treatment volume in therapeutic plasma exchange and immunoadsorption

Apheresis modality	Recommended treatment volume [L]
Immunoadsorption	2.5–3.0 times estimated plasma volume
Therapeutic plasma exchange	1.0–1.5 times estimated plasma volume
Estimated plasma volume [mL, simplified formula] = 70 × body weight [kg] × (1-HCT (in decimal number))	

11.1.2 Immunoadsorption

Immunoadsorption (IA) has first gained clinical acceptance as therapeutic option to remove atherogenic lipoproteins in patients with familial hypercholesterolemia. Based on the experience derived from hyperlipidemic subjects, IA was subsequently also employed to remove immunoglobulins, immune complexes, and circulating alloantibodies (i.e., antibodies directed against antigens from a genetically distinct member of the same species) in a wide variety of different autoimmune diseases. During IA, plasma is separated from blood cells but, in contrast to TPE, thereafter, loaded in two reusable adsorber columns, where specifically immunoglobulins are adsorbed and, consecutively, removed. From immunoglobulins depleted endogenous plasma is then retransferred to the patient together with the previously separated blood cells. Thus, IA does not require any substitution fluid, and also the processed treatment volume is theoretically unlimited as IA, in contrast to TPE, does not usually cause losses of electrolytes or plasma proteins other than immunoglobulins. Due to antibody kinetics, 2.5–3.0 times estimated plasma volume is usually processed during a single IA treatment (Table 11.1). Of note, IA is not FDA cleared in the USA.

11.2 Methods

11.2.1 Vascular Access

In theory, all types of vascular access including native peripheral veins are eligible for apheresis (Fig. 11.2). Due to the significantly lower risk of infectious complications, a peripheral vascular access should be favored over central venous catheters. Insufficient peripheral veins and high need for an immediate initiation of apheresis, however, often necessitate central venous catheters. In a chronic setting, when apheresis treatments over a longer period of time are anticipated, a conversion to peripheral venous access including the surgical creation of a hemodialysis fistula should be considered. At our center, 95% of all chronic apheresis treatments (n = approx. 2800/year) are performed via native peripheral veins using 16–18 gauge dialysis cannulas, one at each arm (for withdrawal and return of blood).

11.2.2 Anticoagulation

Due to the extracorporeal circuit, anticoagulation is compulsory to prevent clotting of blood. While the sole use of citrate, anticoagulant citrate dextrose, formula A (ACD-A, Baxter®, Munich, Germany), may be sufficient in TPE, IA is usually performed using citrate in combination with heparin administered as an initial bolus of 1000–4000 IE followed by a continuous infusion of approximately 20 units/min (max. total dose 6000 IE/treatment). The combination of two anticoagulants during IA, where reusable IA adsorbers are employed, improves the quality of the separated plasma and ensures a higher reduction of eliminated immunoglobulins per IA over a longer period of time. The ratio of citrate to whole blood flow is kept at 1:20 to 1:30.

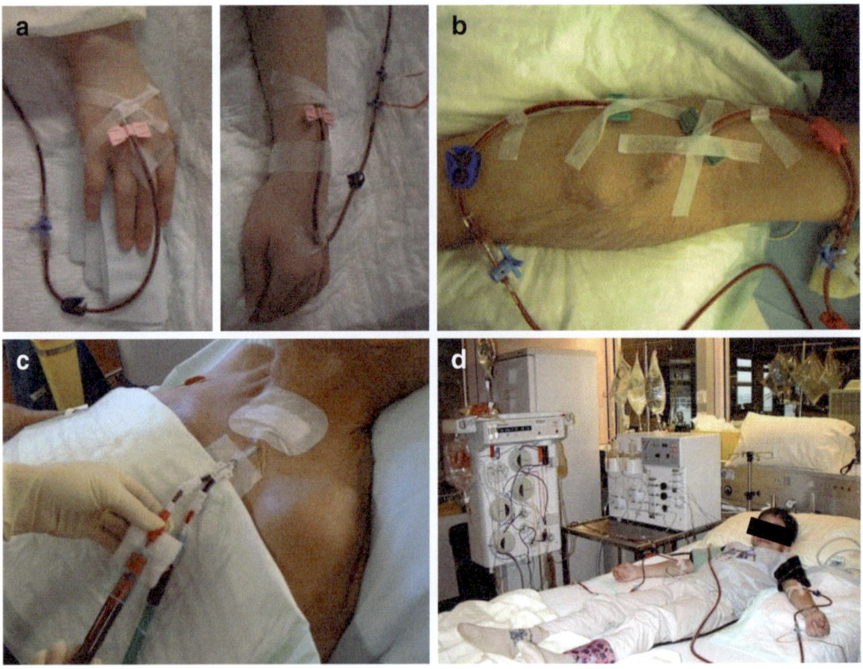

Fig. 11.2 Eligible types of vascular access: (**a**) native peripheral veins (venovenous access), (**b**) arteriovenous fistula, (**c**) central venous catheter, (**d**) example of a venovenous treatment in a 6 years old boy

11.2.3 Devices

For initial plasma separation, necessary for both TPE and IA, blood is drawn via above mentioned 16–18 gauge dialysis cannula at a flow rate of 70–100 mL/min assuring a plasma flow rate of 25–50 mL/min. IgG-plasmapheresis is routinely performed using an automated double-needle, continuous-flow operation system, consisting of a plasma separator and, for IA, the additionally connected adsorption-desorption-automate (ADASORB; Medicap, Ulrichstein, Germany), to which the two IA adsorber columns are attached. The ADASORB regulates the loading of the two IA adsorbers in alternate cycles with (1) plasma for adsorption of immunoglobulins or (2) regeneration solutions for desorption, i.e., elimination of adsorbed immunoglobulins. Of note, none of the IA device is FDA cleared in the USA.

Three different IA adsorber columns are used at our department (>24,000 treatments within 24 years):

1. Ig-Therasorb® (Miltenyi Biotec, Bergisch Gladbach, Germany): Each adsorber column contains 150 mL Sepharose coupled with polyclonal sheep antibodies to human IgG heavy and light chains and has an immunoglobulin-binding capacity of approximately 4.0 g.

2. Immunosorba® and LIGASORB® (Fresenius Medical Care, Bad Homburg, Germany): Reusable protein A-based adsorber columns, which remove IgG-subclasses 1,2,4 and to a smaller degree IgG-3 (Süfke et al. 2017; Koefoed-Nielsen et al. 2017). The removal rate of IgG-3, however, is comparable when high plasma volumes are processed.
3. Globaffin® and Coraffin® (Fresenius Medical Care, Bad Homburg, Germany): More recently developed reusable broadband adsorbers based on synthetic peptides (GAM®) covalently coupled to Sepharose CL-4B (Stummvoll et al. 2017; Dandel et al. 2015).

11.3 Indications for Therapeutic Plasma Exchange and Immunoadsorption

Several indications for both plasmapheresis modalities have been established in numerous autoimmune diseases and in the peri-transplant setting (Schwartz et al. 2016). However, TPE and IA most commonly do not represent first-line therapy but are rather initiated when conventional treatment either fails or elicits inadequately delayed effects in a clinically critical condition (Schwartz et al. 2016; Süfke et al. 2017; Koefoed-Nielsen et al. 2017; Stummvoll et al. 2017; Dandel et al. 2015; Clark et al. 2016; Azoulay et al. 2017; Rock et al. 2017; Raval et al. 2017).

A summary of the indications according to the American Society for Apheresis (Schwartz et al. 2016) is shown in Table 11.2. The system used for categorization and grading is given in an abbreviated version (Schwartz et al. 2016) in Table 11.3.

Here we will focus on three hematological entities with, in part, imminent treatment character.

Table 11.2 Hematological and hemostasiological indications for plasmapheresis according the Writing Committee of the American Society for Apheresis

Disease	Indication	Modality	Category	Grade
Amyloidosis, systemic		TPE	IV	2C
Aplastic anemia		TPE	III	2C
Pure red cell aplasia		TPE	III	2C
Autoimmune hemolytic anemia	– Warm antibody, severe	TPE	III	2C
	– Cold agglutinin disease, severe	TPE	II	2C
Catastrophic antiphospholipid syndrome		TPE	II	2C
Coagulation factor inhibitors	– Alloantibody	TPE	IV	2C
	– Autoantibody	TPE	III	2C
	– Alloantibody	IA	III	2B
	– Autoantibody	IA	III	1C
Cryoglobulinemia	– Symptomatic, severe	TPE	II	2A
	– Symptomatic, severe	IA	II	2B

(continued)

Table 11.2 (continued)

Disease	Indication	Modality	Category	Grade
Erythropoietic porphyria, liver disease		TPE	III	2C
Hematopoietic stem cell transplantation	– Major HPC, marrow	TPE	II	1B
	– Major HPC, apheresis	TPE	II	2B
	– HLA desensitization	TPE	III	2C
Hemophagocytic lymphohistiocytosis, hemophagocytic syndrome, macrophage activation syndrome		TPE	III	2C
Heparin-induced thrombocytopenia and thrombosis	– Pre-cardiopulmonary bypass	TPE	III	2C
	– Thrombosis	TPE	III	2C
Hyperviscosity in monoclonal gammopathies	– Symptomatic	TPE	I	1B
	– Prophylaxis for rituximab	TPE	I	1C
Immune thrombocytopenia	– Refractory	TPE	III	2C
	– Refractory	IA	III	2C
Multiple myeloma	– Cast nephropathy	TPE	II	2B
	– Paraproteinemic demyelinating neuropathies	TPE	III	2C
Paraneoplastic neurological syndromes		TPE	III	2C
		IA	III	2C
Posttransfusion purpura		TPE	III	2C
Red cell alloimmunization in pregnancy	– Prior to IUT availability	TPE	III	2C
Thrombotic microangiopathy	– Coagulation-mediated THBD mutation	TPE	III	2C
	– Complement-mediated complement factor gene mutations	TPE	III	2C
	– Complement-mediated factor H autoantibodies	TPE	I	2C
	– Complement-mediated MCP mutations	TPE	III	1C
	– Drug-associated ticlopidine	TPE	I	2B
	– Drug-associated clopidogrel	TPE	III	2B
	– Drug-associated calcineurin inhibitors	TPE	III	2C
	– Drug-associated gemcitabine	TPE	IV	2C
	– Drug-associated quinine	TPE	IV	2C

Table 11.2 (continued)

Disease	Indication	Modality	Category	Grade
	– Hematopoietic stem cell transplantation associated	TPE	III	2C
	– Shiga toxin-mediated severe neurological symptoms	TPE/IA	III	2C
	– Thrombotic thrombocytopenic purpura	TPE	I	1A

Table 11.3 Categorization and grading system of the Writing Committee of the American Society for Apheresis

Category	*Description*
I	Apheresis as first-line therapy, either stand-alone or with other modes of treatment
II	Apheresis as second-line therapy, either stand-alone or with other modes of treatment
III	Optimum role of apheresis not established, individualized decision making
IV	Published evidence for ineffectiveness or harmfulness of apheresis
Grade	*Description*
1A	Strong recommendation, high-quality evidence
1B	Strong recommendation, moderate evidence
1C	Strong recommendation, low- to very low-quality evidence
2A	Weak recommendation, high-quality evidence
2B	Weak recommendation, moderate evidence
2C	Weak recommendation, low- to very low-quality evidence

11.3.1 Thrombotic Microangiopathy

Thrombotic microangiopathies (TMAs), which may be categorized in inherited and acquired forms (Table 11.4), are a combination of symptoms characterized by acute and chronic thrombotic occlusion of arterioles and arteries (Caprioli et al. 2003; George and Nester 2014). The classical clinical and laboratory signs indicating TMA are Coombs negative, mechanical hemolysis, and thrombocytopenia. Acute kidney injury or neurological symptoms may also be present.

Inherited TMAs: Complement-mediated TMA results from an impaired regulation of the alternative complement pathway caused by mutations in complement regulatory proteins or in complement protein C3. The most frequent mutations occur in complement factor (CF) H, CFI, and CD46, followed by mutations in C3, CFB, and the factor H-related proteins 1–5. Notably, CD46 is a membrane-bound protein, whereas all other are circulating factors. Previously, mutations in 40–60%

Table 11.4 Syndromes of TMA (modified after (George and Nester 2014))

Name	Cause	Clinical features	Initial management
Inherited disorders			
ADAMTS13 deficiency-mediated TMA (TTP)	Mutations in *ADAMTS13*	Neurological symptoms	PI
Complement-mediated TMA	Mutations in *CFH*, *CFI*, *CFB*, *MCP*, and *C3*, leading to uncontrolled AP activation	AKI or CKD, optional: involvement of other organs	PI, TPE, complement inhibition
Metabolism-mediated TMA	Homozygous mutations in *MMACHC*	Often in children <1 year; sometimes in adolescents and adults	Vitamin B12, betaine, folic acid
Coagulation-mediated TMA	Homozygous and compound heterozygous mutations in *DGKE*, *THBD*; (PLG)	Typically AKI in children <1 year	PI
Acquired disorders			
ADAMTS13 deficiency-mediated TMA (TTP)	Autoantibodies directed against ADAMTS13	Neurological symptoms, uncommon in children	TPE, immunosuppression
Shiga toxin-mediated TMA (STEC-HUS)	Infection with toxin-producing strains of *E. coli* or *Shigella*	Most common in small children. Usually sporadic, but large outbreaks may occur	Supportive treatment
Drug-mediated TMA	Immune reactions (i.e., in quinine) or dose-dependent toxicity (i.e., in tacrolimus)	Immune: sudden onset, often with anuric AKI	Removal of drug, supportive treatment
		Dose: gradual onset of AKI over weeks	TPE
Complement-mediated TMA	Autoantibodies directed against CFH. Association with deletion in *CFHR*	AKI in children and adults.	TPE, immunosuppression, complement inhibition

ADAMTS13 a disintegrin and metalloproteinase with a thrombospondin motif 13, *TTP* thrombotic thrombocytopenic purpura, *PI* plasma infusions, *TMA* thrombotic microangiopathy, *CFH*, *CFI*, *CFB* complement factor H, I, B, *MCP* membrane cofactor protein, *C3* complement protein 3, *THBD* thrombomodulin, *AP* alternative pathway, *AKI* acute kidney injury, *CKD* chronic kidney disease, *TPE* therapeutic plasma exchange, *MMACHC* methylmalonic aciduria and homocystinuria type C protein, *DGKE* diacylglycerol kinase epsilon, *PLG* plasminogen, *CFHR* complement factor H-related protein

of patients with a disease penetrance of 50% among the carriers were reported (Noris et al. 2010; Fremeaux-Bacchi et al. 2013; Bu et al. 2016).

The coagulation-mediated TMA is caused by mutations in diacylglycerol kinase epsilon (DGKE) and thrombomodulin (THBD). In case of DGKE mutations, patients do not show any abnormalities in extended complement component workup, while patients with THBD might show signs of systemic complement dysregulation (Lemaire et al. 2013; Delvaeye et al. 2009).

Some syndromes associated with TMA can be attributed to metabolic dysregulation. Cobalamin C disease is a rare autosomal inherited disease caused by mutations in the methylmalonic aciduria and homocystinuria type C protein *(MMACHC)* gene and usually manifests in the first year of life with developmental delays and muscular hypotonia (Cornec-Le Gall et al. 2014).

Acquired TMAs: Secondary causes of TMA are manifold and include drug reactions, systemic diseases, and infections (Campistol et al. 2013). Drug-associated TMAs can be attributed to dose-dependent adverse drug reactions or immune-mediated reactions, e.g., quinine. The therapy for drug-induced TMA is the discontinuation or the dose reduction of the causal agent. However, in case of ticlopidine-associated TMA, ADAMTS13 levels are often diminished and inhibitors can be detected (Reese et al. 2015). In this case, TPE can be considered, as recommended by the American Society of Apheresis (Schwartz et al. 2016).

In acquired complement-mediated TMA, complement dysregulation is caused by autoantibodies against CFH (Józsi et al. 2008). In 90% of these cases, a homozygous deletion in *CFHR1* and *CFHR3* can be diagnosed. Treatment of these cases often requires immunosuppression. Anticomplement therapy is the definite therapy (Sana et al. 2014).

Shiga toxin-mediated TMA (formerly called classic HUS) results from acute infection with certain members of the *E. coli* family after ingestion of contaminated food or water. Symptoms are bloody diarrhea, followed by hemolytic anemia, thrombocytopenia, and acute kidney injury. Children under the age of 1 year are most commonly affected. Treatment of choice is supportive treatment (Campistol et al. 2013).

Thrombotic Thrombocytopenic Purpura: ADAMTS13 deficiency-mediated TMA, or formerly called thrombotic thrombocytopenic purpura (TTP), is diagnosed by the detection of decreased levels of ADAMTS13, a disintegrin and metalloproteinase with a thrombospondin motif 13, which cleaves von Willebrand factor (vWF) into small multimers. vWF is essential for homeostasis as it induces platelet aggregation and thrombus formation on damaged endothelium. Severe ADAMTS13 deficiency (<5–10% of normal enzyme activity) is diagnostic of TTP in the right clinical scenario. In contrast to the other forms of TMA, TTP predominantly affects the central nervous system, and renal involvement is not typical (George and Nester 2014). Acquired TTP is more common than the hereditary form, which is caused by mutations in the ADAMTS13 gene and is commonly associated with a neonatal onset. Acquired TTP is caused by autoantibodies against ADAMTS13, which inhibit the enzyme function. The autoantibodies tend to disappear during remission, which suggests a transient immune reaction. Recently, a monoclonal antibody against vWF, caplacizumab, has shown promising results in the treatment of acquired TTP in a phase 2 trial (Peyvandi et al. 2016).

Treatment strategies depend on the underlying cause of TMA. Of note, some form of therapy is, however, required even before the final diagnosis, i.e., the type of TMA, is established. Consensus guidelines recommend the emergent initiation of

TPE or, if TPE is unavailable, of plasma infusions after (preliminary) diagnosis of TMA. The effectiveness of TPE depends on the form of TMA and, in inherited complement-mediated TMA, on the underlying mutation. The rationale of TPE in TMA is to supplement functioning complement (regulatory) proteins such as CFH, CFI, and CFB while removing dysfunctional complement (regulatory) proteins and other potential disease-causing factors. If mutations of membrane-bound proteins, i.e., CD46, are present, TPE does not positively influence patient outcomes (Bresin et al. 2013). In contrast, TPE in combination with immunosuppressive agents remains a standard treatment approach in case of autoantibody-mediated TMA as underlying circulating autoantibodies are effectively removed (Sana et al. 2014). Alternatively, anticomplement agents should be considered, especially in cases with limited response to TPE (Legendre et al. 2013).

11.3.2 Acquired Coagulation Inhibitors

Coagulation inhibitors may occur spontaneously in seriously ill patients with previously normal coagulation and lead to varying degrees of hemorrhagic diathesis. In most cases, these autoantibodies are directed against factor VIII (so-called acquired hemophilia A) and far less frequent against coagulation factors II, IIa, or V (inhibitors of other coagulation factors are extremely rare) (Cugno et al. 2014; Franchini and Mannucci 2013).

Treatment of bleeding complications caused by acquired coagulation inhibitors against factor VIII comprises (1) the control over active bleeding by administration of desmopressin and substitution of factor concentrates and (2) the elimination of the inhibitor (Franchini and Mannucci 2013; Kruse-Jarres et al. 2017). The choice of factor concentrates is determined by the severity of bleeding and the titer of the coagulation inhibitor, usually measured in Bethesda units (BU). While high doses of human factor VIII concentrates may be sufficient in cases with low factor VIII inhibitor titer (<5 BU), activated prothrombin complex concentrates, recombinant porcine factor VIII, or recombinant human factor VIIa are necessary in those subjects with a titer >5 BU. As most of these factor concentrates are rather expensive, the expenses may exceed 90.000€/day. Further, even after diagnosis of the acquired coagulation inhibitor, this state represents a life-threatening condition as the response to conservative pharmaceutical immunosuppressive treatment used to eliminate the inhibitor, i.e., corticosteroids, cyclophosphamide, and rituximab, is often delayed, and the administration of the mentioned factor concentrates is insufficient to control the bleeding especially in postsurgical setting (Kruse-Jarres et al. 2017; Goldmann et al. 2015).

IA has been demonstrated to provide a rapid reduction of circulating inhibitors (Jansen et al. 2001). The mean reduction of acquired anti-factor VIII autoantibodies by a single IA session, desorbing about 2.5-fold the calculated plasma volume, was 71.9 ± 19.4% (range 50.0–97.1%). The level of total serum IgG was reduced by 68.7 ± 10.1%, of total serum IgA by 55.7 ± 12.7%, and of total serum IgM level by 48.6 ± 11.1% per IA session (Jansen et al. 2001). In mean 8.1 ± 5.1 IA treatments, concomitant to the substitution of human factor VIII, had to be performed until sufficient response without further bleedings was achieved (Jansen et al. 2001). These findings were corroborated by data of Goldmann et al. (2015) suggesting an IA-based protocol including immunosuppressive treatment to be considered as first-line therapy or even as salvage strategy. As IA was able to significantly reduce or even avoid substitution of coagulation factors, a dramatic reduction in the treatment costs of these patients might be achieved (Freedman et al. 2003).

11.3.3 Prolonged Red Cell Aplasia After Major ABO-Incompatible Allogenic Hematopoietic Cell Transplantation

Allogenic hematopoietic cell transplantation (HCT) is widely used to treat patients with malignant and nonmalignant hematological and autoimmune diseases. While compatibility in the major human leucocyte antigens (HLA) system is essential for short- and long-term outcome after transplantation, ABO-incompatible (ABO-I) HCT is regarded feasible and affects approximately 30–50% of all HCT patients (Worel 2016). A complication following major ABO incompatibility is pure red cell aplasia (PRCA), which is associated with higher peri-transplant and long-term mortality due to iron overload related to poly-transfusion (Worel 2016). The underlying mechanism of PRCA is not fully understood, but the persistence of memory B lymphocytes of the recipient, which continuously produce hemagglutinins against the ABO antigens on donor erythrocytes, or the persistence of preformed host isohemagglutinins, which suppress the donor erythropoiesis, is held responsible for this complication of ABO-I HCT (Worel 2016; Rabitsch et al. 2003a, b). Only limited experience on the prevention of PRCA is available. Some investigators reported a beneficial effect of pretransplant TPE, but further studies are clearly warranted (Worel 2016; Dellacasa et al. 2015).

Apart from supportive measures including erythropoietin-stimulating agents and transfusion of RBCs, treatment options consist of immunosuppressive treatment with corticosteroids, antithymocyte globulin, rituximab, or apheresis modalities like TPE and IA. In two case series, we reported on, in total, eight patients with PRCA after ABO-I HCT, who were treated with IA (Rabitsch et al. 2003a, b). To achieve maximal elimination of preformed and potentially reproduced circulating isohemagglutinins, the 2.5–3.0-fold of the estimated plasma volume was desorbed during each IA, and five IA treatments per week were performed initially. In the second larger case series (Rabitsch et al. 2003b), all five patients became transfusion independent after a median of 17 IA treatments (range 9–25). Of note, three of the included HCT recipients have been ineffectively treated with TPE before.

Despite the missing prospective, multicenter study, IA seems to be a promising therapeutic method for rapid, efficient, and safe elimination of persisting isohemagglutinins in patients with PRCA after ABO-I HCT.

11.4 Complications of Therapeutic Plasma Exchange and Immunoadsorption

Both forms of apheresis are usually well tolerated and associated with a low rate of adverse events. However, monitoring of vital signs during the treatment as well as routine laboratory tests, such as complete blood count, electrolytes, and coagulation markers, including fibrinogen is mandatory.

TPE-related side effects are mainly caused by the choice of the substitution fluid. For example, albumin 5% does not compensate for the loss of fibrinogen and coagulations factors caused by the removal of endogenous plasma (Chirnside et al. 1981), and plasma may cause anaphylactic and/or other transfusion-reacted reactions. Of note, fibrinogen loss may be significant even after only one TPE session, which may result in significant bleeding complications as was shown by Zoellner et al. (Fig. 11.3) (Zöllner et al. 2014). Thus, the combination of human albumin 5% and plasma or the exclusive use of plasma, especially in patients with hemorrhagic diathesis, is recommended.

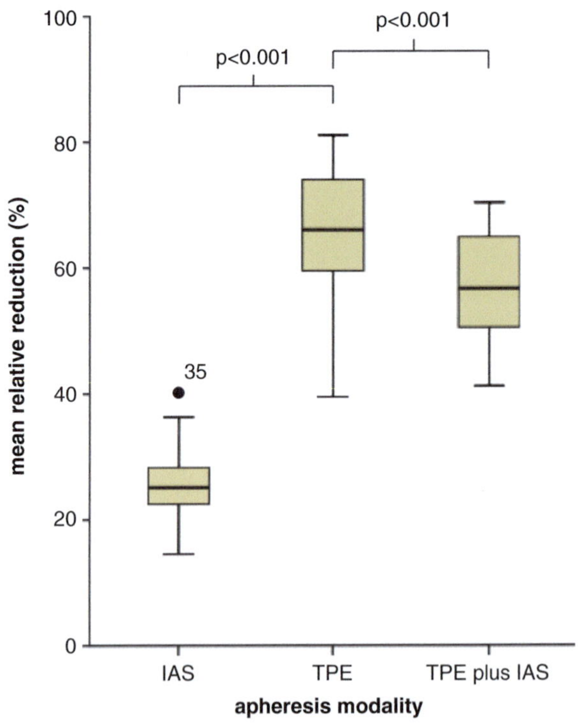

Fig. 11.3 Mean relative reduction (%) of plasma fibrinogen in relation to apheresis modality (adapted from (Zöllner et al. 2014))

Due to the unspecific removal of total IgG and also IgM, the rate of infectious complications may be increased irrespective of the apheresis modality, especially if concomitant immunosuppressive medication is needed (Stummvoll et al. 2012). Infection complications related to central venous catheters are well established and are not discussed in this chapter.

In addition, iron loss is frequent, and anemia requiring iron substitution develops in approximately 25% of subjects undergoing chronic apheresis.

Patients on ACE inhibitors may have facial flushing or hypotension. This reaction has been observed in patients taking an ACE inhibitor who undergo treatments involving an extracorporeal circuit, including IA, LDL apheresis, and TPE procedures. The hypotheses explaining this reaction involve the generation and accumulation of excess bradykinin (a potent vasodilator). One hypothesis suggested the reaction might be due to activation of the contact pathway in the extracorporeal circuit, which generates bradykinin. Others postulated that these reactions are secondary to the presence of prekallikrein activator in the albumin, which is activated to bradykinin. However, the relationship between hypotension during apheresis procedure and prekallikrein activator in the albumin has never been confirmed by actual measurements. Some experts prefer ACE inhibitor therapy to be discontinued 24–48 h prior to the start of apheresis procedures, if possible. If the procedure must be done, the decision of how to proceed is based on the emergent nature of the procedure and the risks/benefits for the individual patient.

A major issue is the effect of apheresis, especially of TPE, on drug levels. Literature on the elimination of specific drugs by TPE is scarce. In general, substances with high plasma protein affinity and low distribution volume are more susceptible to the removal by TPE (Cheng et al. 2017; Ibrahim et al. 2007). However, several other factors may also account for TPE-related changes in pharmacokinetics, including drug distribution or drug half-life (Cheng et al. 2017; Ibrahim et al. 2007). For example, plasma levels of rituximab, a chimeric anti-CD20 monoclonal antibody employed in several hematological and autoimmune diseases, are decreased by approximately 50%, if TPE is performed within 72 h after rituximab infusion (Puisset et al. 2013). In contrast, calcineurin inhibitors cyclosporine A and tacrolimus levels, used, e.g., for prophylaxis of graft-vs-host disease after HCT, are hardly altered by TPE (Ibrahim et al. 2007).

References

Azoulay E, Knoebl P, Garnacho-Montero J, Rusinova K, Galstian G, Eggimann P, Abroug F, Benoit D, von Bergwelt-Baildon M, Wendon J, Scully M (2017) Expert statements on the standard of care in critically ill adult patients with atypical hemolytic uremic syndrome. Chest 152(2):424–434

Bresin E, Rurali E, Caprioli J, Sanchez-Corral P, Fremeaux-Bacchi V, Rodriguez de Cordoba S, Pinto S, Goodship TH, Alberti M, Ribes D, Valoti E, Remuzzi G, Noris M (2013) European working party on complement genetics in renal diseases. Combined complement gene mutations in atypical hemolytic uremic syndrome influence clinical phenotype. J Am Soc Nephrol 24(3):475–486

Bu F, Borsa NG, Jones MB, Takanami E, Nishimura C, Hauer JJ, Azaiez H, Black-Ziegelbein EA, Meyer NC, Kolbe DL, Li Y, Frees K, Schnieders MJ, Thomas C, Nester C, Smith RJ (2016) High-throughput genetic testing for thrombotic microangiopathies and C3 glomerulopathies. J Am Soc Nephrol 27(4):1245–1253

Campistol JM, Arias M, Ariceta G, Blasco M, Espinosa M, Grinyó JM, Praga M, Torra R, Vilalta R, Rodríguez de Córdoba S (2013) An update for atypical haemolytic uraemic syndrome: diagnosis and treatment. A consensus document. Nefrologia 33(1):27–45

Caprioli J, Castelletti F, Bucchioni S, Bettinaglio P, Bresin E, Pianetti G, Gamba S, Brioschi S, Daina E, Remuzzi G, Noris M, International Registry of Recurrent and Familial HUS/TTP (2003) Complement factor H mutations and gene polymorphisms in haemolytic uraemic syndrome: the C-257T, the A2089G and the G2881T polymorphisms are strongly associated with the disease. Hum Mol Genet 12(24):3385–3395

Cheng CW, Hendrickson JE, Tormey CA, Sidhu D (2017) Therapeutic plasma exchange and its impact on drug levels: an ACLPS critical review. Am J Clin Pathol 148(3):190–198

Chirnside A, Urbaniak SJ, Prowse CV, Keller AJ (1981) Coagulation abnormalities following intensive plasma exchange on the cell separator. II. Effects on factors I, II, V, VII, VIII, IX, X and antithrombin III. Br J Haematol 48(4):627–634

Clark WF, Huang SS, Walsh MW, Farah M, Hildebrand AM, Sontrop JM (2016) Plasmapheresis for the treatment of kidney diseases. Kidney Int 90(5):974–984

Cornec-Le Gall E, Delmas Y, De Parscau L, Doucet L, Ogier H, Benoist JF, Fremeaux-Bacchi V, Le Meur Y (2014) Adult-onset eculizumab-resistant hemolytic uremic syndrome associated with cobalamin C deficiency. Am J Kidney Dis 63(1):119–123

Cugno M, Gualtierotti R, Tedeschi A, Meroni PL (2014) Autoantibodies to coagulation factors: from pathophysiology to diagnosis and therapy. Autoimmun Rev 13(1):40–48

Dandel M, Englert A, Wallukat G, Riese A, Knosalla C, Stein J, Hetzer R (2015) Immunoadsorption can improve cardiac function in transplant candidates with non-ischemic dilated cardiomyopathy associated with diabetes mellitus. Atheroscler Suppl 18:124–133

Dellacasa CM, D'Ardia S, Allione B, Aydin S, Tassi V, Francisci T, Pecoraro C, Busca A (2015) Efficacy of plasmapheresis for the treatment of pure red blood cell aplasia after allogeneic stem cell transplantation. Transfusion 55(12):2979–2982

Delvaeye M, Noris M, De Vriese A, Esmon CT, Esmon NL, Ferrell G, Del-Favero J, Plaisance S, Claes B, Lambrechts D, Zoja C, Remuzzi G, Conway EM (2009) Thrombomodulin mutations in atypical hemolytic-uremic syndrome. N Engl J Med 361(4):345–357

Franchini M, Mannucci PM (2013) Acquired haemophilia A: a 2013 update. Thromb Haemost 110(6):1114–1120

Freedman J, Rand ML, Russell O, Davis C, Cheatley PL, Blanchette V, Garvey MB (2003) Immunoadsorption may provide a cost-effective approach to management of patients with inhibitors to FVIII. Transfusion 43(11):1508–1513

Fremeaux-Bacchi V, Fakhouri F, Garnier A, Bienaimé F, Dragon-Durey MA, Ngo S, Moulin B, Servais A, Provot F, Rostaing L, Burtey S, Niaudet P, Deschênes G, Lebranchu Y, Zuber J, Loirat C (2013) Genetics and outcome of atypical hemolytic uremic syndrome: a nationwide French series comparing children and adults. Clin J Am Soc Nephrol 8(4):554–562

George JN, Nester CM (2014) Syndromes of thrombotic microangiopathy. N Engl J Med 371(7):654–666

Goldmann G, Marquardt N, Horneff S, Oldenburg J, Zeitler H (2015) Treatment of minor severe acquired haemophilia. Is there a rationale for immunoadsorption? Atheroscler Suppl 18:74–79

Ibrahim RB, Liu C, Cronin SM, Murphy BC, Cha R, Swerdlow P, Edwards DJ (2007) Drug removal by plasmapheresis: an evidence-based review. Pharmacotherapy 27(11):1529–1549

Jansen M, Schmaldienst S, Banyai S, Quehenberger P, Pabinger I, Derfler K, Hörl WH, Knöbl P (2001) Treatment of coagulation inhibitors with extracorporeal immunoadsorption (Ig-Therasorb). Br J Haematol 112(1):91–97

Józsi M, Licht C, Strobel S, Zipfel SL, Richter H, Heinen S, Zipfel PF, Skerka C (2008) Factor H autoantibodies in atypical hemolytic uremic syndrome correlate with CFHR1/CFHR3 deficiency. Blood 111(3):1512–1514

Koefoed-Nielsen P, Bistrup C, Christiansen M (2017) Protein a immunoadsorption may hamper the decision to transplant due to interference with CDC crossmatch results. J Clin Apher 32(3):163–169

Kruse-Jarres R, Kempton CL, Baudo F, Collins PW, Knoebl P, Leissinger CA, Tiede A, Kessler CM (2017) Acquired hemophilia A: updated review of evidence and treatment guidance. Am J Hematol 92(7):695–705

Legendre CM, Licht C, Muus P, Greenbaum LA, Babu S, Bedrosian C, Bingham C, Cohen DJ, Delmas Y, Douglas K, Eitner F, Feldkamp T, Fouque D, Furman RR, Gaber O, Herthelius M, Hourmant M, Karpman D, Lebranchu Y, Mariat C, Menne J, Moulin B, Nürnberger J, Ogawa M, Remuzzi G, Richard T, Sberro-Soussan R, Severino B, Sheerin NS, Trivelli A, Zimmerhackl LB, Goodship T, Loirat C (2013) Terminal complement inhibitor eculizumab in atypical hemolytic-uremic syndrome. N Engl J Med 368(23):2169–2181

Lemaire M, Frémeaux-Bacchi V, Schaefer F, Choi M, Tang WH, Le Quintrec M, Fakhouri F, Taque S, Nobili F, Martinez F, Ji W, Overton JD, Mane SM, Nürnberg G, Altmüller J, Thiele H, Morin D, Deschenes G, Baudouin V, Llanas B, Collard L, Majid MA, Simkova E, Nürnberg P, Rioux-Leclerc N, Moeckel GW, Gubler MC, Hwa J, Loirat C, Lifton RP (2013) Recessive mutations in DGKE cause atypical hemolytic-uremic syndrome. Nat Genet 45(5):531–536

Noris M, Caprioli J, Bresin E, Mossali C, Pianetti G, Gamba S, Daina E, Fenili C, Castelletti F, Sorosina A, Piras R, Donadelli R, Maranta R, van der Meer I, Conway EM, Zipfel PF, Goodship TH, Remuzzi G (2010) Relative role of genetic complement abnormalities in sporadic and familial aHUS and their impact on clinical phenotype. Clin J Am Soc Nephrol 5(10):1844–1859

Peyvandi F, Scully M, Kremer Hovinga JA, Cataland S, Knöbl P, Wu H, Artoni A, Westwood JP, Mansouri Taleghani M, Jilma B, Callewaert F, Ulrichts H, Duby C, Tersago D, Investigators TITAN (2016) Caplacizumab for acquired thrombotic thrombocytopenic purpura. N Engl J Med 374(6):511–522

Puisset F, White-Koning M, Kamar N, Huart A, Haberer F, Blasco H, Le Guellec C, Lafont T, Grand A, Rostaing L, Chatelut E, Pourrat J (2013) Population pharmacokinetics of rituximab with or without plasmapheresis in kidney patients with antibody-mediated disease. Br J Clin Pharmacol 76(5):734–740

Rabitsch W, Knöbl P, Greinix H, Prinz E, Kalhs P, Hörl WH, Derfler K (2003a) Removal of persisting isohaemagglutinins with Ig-Therasorb immunoadsorption after major ABO-incompatible non-myeloablative allogeneic haematopoietic stem cell transplantation. Nephrol Dial Transplant 18(11):2405–2408

Rabitsch W, Knöbl P, Prinz E, Keil F, Greinix H, Kalhs P, Worel N, Jansen M, Hörl WH, Derfler K (2003b) Prolonged red cell aplasia after major ABO-incompatible allogeneic hematopoietic stem cell transplantation: removal of persisting isohemagglutinins with Ig-Therasorb immunoadsorption. Bone Marrow Transplant 32(10):1015–1019

Raval JS, Mazepa MA, Whinna HC, Park YA (2017) Monitoring therapeutic apheresis utilization: database versus registry. J Clin Apher 32(3):208–209

Reese JA, Bougie DW, Curtis BR, Terrell DR, Vesely SK, Aster RH, George JN (2015) Drug-induced thrombotic microangiopathy: experience of the Oklahoma registry and the BloodCenter of Wisconsin. Am J Hematol 90(5):406–410

Rock G; Members of the Canadian Apheresis Group (2017) The Canadian apheresis group registry. Transfus Apher Sci 56(1):86–88

Sana G, Dragon-Durey MA, Charbit M, Bouchireb K, Rousset-Rouvière C, Bérard E, Salomon R, Frémeaux-Bacchi V, Niaudet P, Boyer O (2014) Long-term remission of atypical HUS with anti-factor H antibodies after cyclophosphamide pulses. Pediatr Nephrol 29(1):75–83

Schwartz J, Padmanabhan A, Aqui N, Balogun RA, Connelly-Smith L, Delaney M, Dunbar NM, Witt V, Wu Y, Shaz BH (2016) Guidelines on the use of therapeutic apheresis in clinical practice-evidence-based approach from the writing Committee of the American Society for apheresis: the seventh special issue. J Clin Apher 31(3):149–162

Solomon A, Fahey JL (1963) Plasmapheresis therapy in macroglobulinemia. Ann Intern Med 58:789–800

Stummvoll GH, Schmaldienst S, Smolen JS, Derfler K, Biesenbach P (2012) Lupus nephritis: prolonged immunoadsorption (IAS) reduces proteinuria and stabilizes global disease activity. Nephrol Dial Transplant 27(2):618–626

Stummvoll G, Aringer M, Handisurya A, Derfler K (2017) Immunoadsorption in autoimmune diseases affecting the kidney. Semin Nephrol 37(5):478–487

Süfke S, Lehnert H, Uhlenbusch-Körwer I, Gebauer F (2017) Safety aspects of immunoadsorption in IgG removal using a single-use, multiple-pass protein a immunoadsorber (LIGASORB): clinical investigation in healthy volunteers. Ther Apher Dial 21(4):405–413

Worel N (2016) ABO-mismatched allogeneic hematopoietic stem cell transplantation. Transfus Med Hemother 43(1):3–12

Zöllner S, Pablik E, Druml W, Derfler K, Rees A, Biesenbach P (2014) Fibrinogen reduction and bleeding complications in plasma exchange, immunoadsorption and a combination of the two. Blood Purif 38(2):160–166

Red Blood Cell Exchange: When and Why?

12

Georg Stussi, Andreas Buser, and Andreas Holbro

12.1 Introduction

Red blood cell (RBC) exchange is the replacement of patient's RBC with allogeneic donor RBC and can be performed either manually or automated. It has the advantage over simple transfusions that patient's RBCs are replaced without increasing the hematocrit or exposing the patient to the risk of fluid overload. RBC depletion describes an ex vivo procedure where RBCs are removed and replaced with crystalloid or colloid solution, when necessary. Typically, RBC depletion is used for bone marrow processing in the context of ABO-incompatible hematopoietic cell transplantation (HCT). This can be performed using different techniques, including sedimentation and apheresis. Erythrocytapheresis is an in vivo procedure in which RBCs are removed from the whole blood of the patient during the apheresis procedure and replaced by crystalloid or colloid solution (Padmanabhan et al. 2019). Although the terms RBC exchange, RBC depletion, and erythrocytapheresis in the medical literature are often used interchangeably, they describe different therapeutic procedures.

Manual RBC exchange implies sequential phlebotomies and isovolemic replacement with crystalloids and/or donor RBC. It has been frequently used in the past. However, with the introduction of automated cell separators, it has lost its importance but still might be applied in selected situations (Kuo et al. 2015; Swerdlow

G. Stussi (✉)
Division of Hematology, Oncology Institute of Southern Switzerland, Bellinzona, Switzerland
e-mail: Georg.stuessi@eoc.ch

A. Buser · A. Holbro
Regional Transfusion Service, Swiss Red Cross, Basel, Switzerland

Division of Hematology, University Hospital Basel, Basel, Switzerland
e-mail: Andreas.Buser@usb.ch; andreas.holbro@usb.ch

S. A. Abutalib et al. (eds.), *Best Practices of Apheresis in Hematopoietic Cell Transplantation*, Advances and Controversies in Hematopoietic Transplantation and Cell Therapy, https://doi.org/10.1007/978-3-319-55131-9_12

2006). Automated RBC exchange is based on an apheresis procedure that separates RBCs from other blood components. The RBCs are subsequently selectively removed and replaced with donor RBCs alone and/or crystalloids/colloid solutions (Padmanabhan et al. 2019). Automated apheresis instruments have substantially facilitated the collection and replacement procedures. Based on clinical data such as body weight, height, gender, age, initial and final hematocrit, as well as average replacement fluid hematocrit and the fluid balance, the instruments calculate the exchange volumes. Moreover, automated systems allow to determine the percentage of remaining patient's erythrocytes (fraction of the remaining cells), which is of particular interest for the calculation of the remaining pathological erythrocytes not only in patients with sickle cell disease but also in malaria and babesiosis. The introduction of automated RBC exchange procedures has substantially improved the standardization and has reduced the manipulations by the operator, and by that, it has become better applicable in clinical routine. Nevertheless, RBC exchange is still associated with some procedural risks as shown in Table 12.1, and the indications should therefore be carefully evaluated.

Table 12.1 Complications of RBC exchange

Complications
Central venous catheter
Hematomas
Infections
Thrombosis
Arterial puncture
Pneumothorax/hemothorax (subclavian/jugular)
Arteriovenous fistula (femoralis)
Apheresis
Catheter occlusion
Catheter leakage
Air embolism
Extracorporal circulation/anticoagulation
Vasovagal reactions
Citrate toxicity
Cytopenias
Thrombocytopenia
Leukopenia
Immune hematological complication
Alloimmunization including HLA
Febrile nonhemolytic transfusion reaction
Allergic transfusion reactions
Others

While plasmapheresis is quite frequently used in allogeneic HCT, there are few indications for RBC exchange or depletion mainly in the context of bone marrow processing. The indication for RBC exchange and depletion will be discussed in the following chapters.

12.2 ABO-Incompatible Hematopoietic Stem Cell Transplantation

Due to the fact that HLA and ABO antigens are independently inherited, 40–50% of all allogeneic HCT are performed across the ABO blood group barrier (Stussi et al. 2006; Klumpp 1991). As shown in Fig. 12.1, three groups of ABO mismatch can be distinguished in HCT: minor, major, and bidirectional ABO incompatibility. Minor ABO incompatibility, e.g., from an O-type donor to an A-type recipient, is characterized by the ability of donor B-lymphocytes to produce anti-recipient isohemagglutinins. In contrast, major ABO-incompatible HCT, e.g., from an A-type donor to an O-type recipient, is characterized by the presence of preformed anti-donor isohemagglutinins. In bidirectional ABO incompatibility, e.g., A-type donor to a B-type recipient, a combination of both the major and minor ABO blood group barriers must be overcome (Holbro and Passweg 2015). Although the overall outcome of patients undergoing ABO-incompatible HCT is not affected, several immunohematological complications such as hemolysis and pure red cell aplasia may arise in the posttransplant course (Worel 2016).

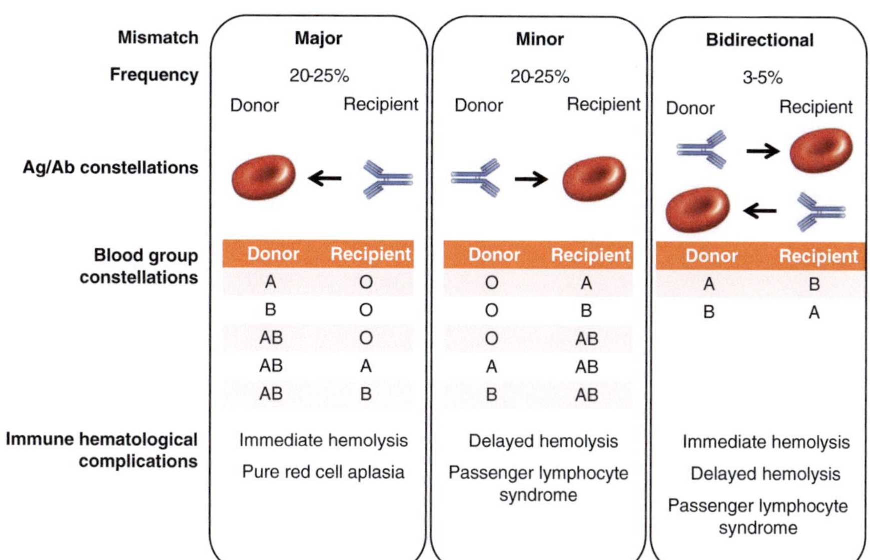

Fig. 12.1 ABO incompatibility in allogeneic HCT

12.3 Hemolysis After Hematopoietic Stem Cell Transplantation

Hemolysis is a frequent complication after allogeneic HCT, but fortunately, most patients present with relatively mild and transient symptoms (Sokol et al. 2002). The most important causes of posttransplant hemolysis are shown in Fig. 12.2. Hemolysis can be classified by the onset of the symptoms into immediate and delayed hemolysis (Holbro and Passweg 2015). Immunological causes should be differentiated from nonimmune causes and microangiopathic hemolytic anemias. A thorough anamnesis including detailed drug history, as well as laboratory analysis to further characterize the nature of the hemolysis, is essential for the correct diagnosis. The Coombs test, elution techniques, and a morphological search for schistocytes on the blood film provide important diagnostic clues and should always be performed in patients presenting with hemolysis after allogeneic HCT.

Immune hematological complications such as antibody-mediated posttransplant hemolysis often, but not always, arise in the context of ABO-mismatched transplantations. Patients with a major ABO barrier are at risk for immediate hemolysis and later on delayed RBC engraftment or pure red cell aplasia, while patients with a minor ABO barrier are at risk for delayed hemolysis due to a passenger lymphocyte syndrome (PLS) (Fig. 12.1).

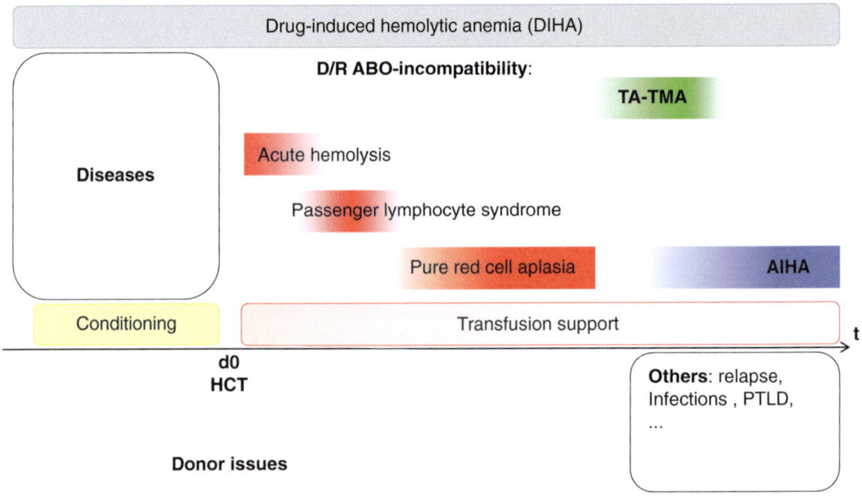

Fig. 12.2 Hemolysis in the context of allogeneic HCT

12.4 Management of Immediate Hemolysis

Acute immune hemolysis arising immediately after the infusion of the stem cell product is caused by preexisting isohemagglutinins of the recipient that bind to and eventually eliminate transplanted donor erythrocytes. Stem cell products collected by peripheral blood apheresis usually contain small amounts of donor erythrocytes, and further processing is recommended only if the erythrocyte content in the product is more than or equal to 20 mL and the isohemagglutinins of the patient are equal to or higher than 1:32 (Fig. 12.3) (Rowley et al. 2011). In contrast, bone marrow-derived stem cell products contain approximately 25–35% donor erythrocytes; thus, prevention of immediate hemolysis is mandatory prior to HCT. Since many products contain 1–1.5 L non-manipulated bone marrow, the equivalent of one RBC unit or even more can be present in the product.

Two strategies can be applied to reduce the risk of acute hemolysis. First, isohemagglutinins can be removed from the recipient prior to HCT by immunoadsorption, plasmapheresis (see also chapter 11), or slow infusions of incompatible donor-type RBC (Stussi et al. 2009). Both methods seem to be equally effective in reducing the isohemagglutinins titers lowering the pretransplant isohemagglutinins by five titer steps.

Center's experience and patient-related factors, such as difficulties with venous access, anticoagulant toxicity, vascular volume changes, mild platelet depletion, and the risk of infection with plasma exchange or immunoadsorption, might direct physicians rather to the second option, the pretransplant manipulation of the bone marrow product (Daniele et al. 2014) (see also chapter 10). RBC depletion from the stem cell product can be achieved by density centrifugation (sedimentation) and/or by bone marrow processing with a cell separator. While this technology has been used since many years in major ABO-incompatible bone marrow transplant recipients, it has partially lost its importance in the last decade due to the preferential use of peripheral blood stem cell products. However, with the renewed interest for bone marrow stem cell products in the context of haploidentical HCT, the processing of ABO-incompatible bone marrow products will be increasingly used again (Passweg et al. 2017).

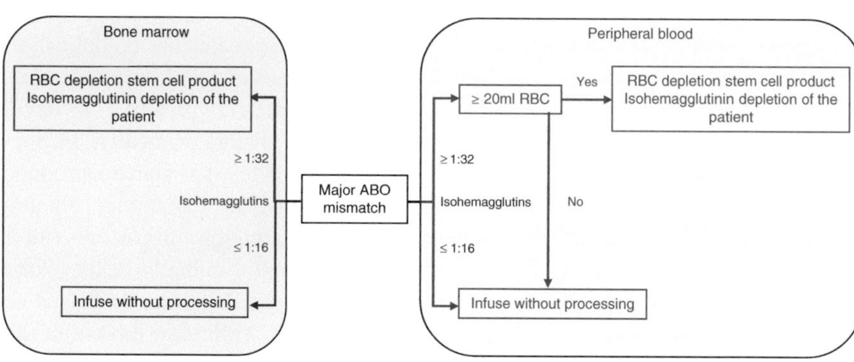

Fig. 12.3 Decision tree for processing stem cell products in major ABO-incompatible HCT

Table 12.2 Bone marrow processing devices

	Spectra Optia	Amicus	Fenwal CS3000	COBE Spectra
Volume reduction (%)	92	87	92	81
RBC depletion (%)	98	94	97	91
TNC recovery (%)	62	44	37	34
CD34 recovery (%)	94	70	84	91

Several separation devices and technologies have been applied in the past. For an historical overview of the developments in bone marrow processing of ABO-incompatible stem cell products, we recommend a review by Daniele and colleagues (Daniele et al. 2014). Recently, bone marrow processing with the Amicus, COBE Spectra, and Spectra Optia devices has been published with excellent results regarding RBC depletion. All devices have RBC depletion rates exceeding 90% (Table 12.2) (Sorg et al. 2015; Witt et al. 2011; Kim et al. 2016; Larghero et al. 2006). The loss of stem cells has become less of an issue since the recovery rates for $CD34^+$ positive cells in the newer generation of devices generally are more than 80%, and with the COBE Optia, the $CD34^+$ recovery is more than 90%. Nevertheless, in the context of accreditation, the procedure has to be validated.

The bone marrow processing program on the Spectra Optia was accepted by the FDA in 2015. The advantages of the Spectra Optia are clearly reduced manual handling during the process. A new single bag system for the Spectra Optia bone marrow processing program was developed allowing the bone marrow aspirate to be recirculated during the procedure, thereby eliminating the need for the operator to manually reverse flow multiple times, as required for bone marrow processing procedures on COBE Spectra system. The total number of operator adjustments was reduced from 23 per procedure on the COBE Spectra to four on the Spectra Optia. This led to a higher stability and reproducibility of the procedures.

12.5 Management of Delayed Hemolysis Due to Passenger Lymphocyte Syndrome

Passenger lymphocyte syndrome (PLS) is a rare and unpredictable complication after allogeneic HCT or solid organ transplantation (Hows et al. 1986; Shortt et al. 2008). It is characterized by a delayed hemolysis 1–4 weeks (typically 7–14 days) after minor or bidirectional ABO-incompatible HCT. Pathogenetically, PLS is caused by immunocompetent donor-derived B-lymphocytes that start to produce during the engraftment phase isohemagglutinins against the remaining patient's erythrocytes (Bolan et al. 2001; Booth et al. 2013). Although rare, it can cause severe hemolysis and may lead to multiorgan failure and eventually death (Watz et al. 2014). Hemolysis persists until the residual recipient RBCs are destroyed or replaced by donor or transfused RBC, which often occurs within few days after the onset of hemolysis. With the introduction of reduced-intensity conditioning regimen, an increased incidence of PLS has been observed. This is likely due to the higher lymphocyte content in the stem cell product and due to the higher percentage of remaining patient's erythrocytes. Risk factors for PLS include peripheral blood stem cells, a donor with blood group O, a recipient with blood group A, cyclosporine alone as GVHD prophylaxis, and reduced-intensity conditioning (Watz et al. 2014; Gajewski et al. 1992; Worel et al. 2007).

It is recommended that patients with minor ABO barrier should be regularly monitored for signs of hemolysis during the early posttransplant phase; however, there is no generally accepted strategy to prevent PLS. The reduction of remaining patient's erythrocytes by transfusing O-type RBC or by RBC exchange transfusions theoretically reduces the risk and the severity of delayed hemolysis with a therapeutic aim of less than 30% of residual patient's RBC. As some transplant centers routinely transfuse O-type and others donor- and/or recipient-type RBC in patients with minor ABO-incompatible HCT, the incidence of delayed hemolysis might be influenced by these different transfusion strategies among transplant centers (Worel et al. 2010). The concept of lowering patient's RBC content has been tested in a single-center study analyzing minor or bidirectional ABO-incompatible HCT receiving prophylactic RBC exchange transfusions with historical controls (Worel et al. 2007). All patients were transplanted with reduced intensity conditioning and mostly peripheral blood stem cells. To avoid immediate hemolysis, the bone marrow products were plasma depleted. The reason for starting the prophylactic RBC exchange program was that the incidence of PLS in this center among patients with reduced intensity conditioning was high (5/10 patients) with three patients dying of transplant-related mortality during the period of hemolysis. Thus, prophylactic RBC exchange transfusions were started prior to minor or bidirectional ABO-incompatible HCT replacing 1–1.5× the patient blood volume with a median of eight RBC concentrates. By this, the incidence of severe hemolysis and transplant-related mortality was reduced in minor ABO-incompatible HCT undergoing RBC exchange, while there was no difference in the incidence of GVHD and the overall survival.

A second retrospective single-center study analyzed prophylactic RBC exchange transfusion in minor and bidirectional ABO-incompatible HCT (Cunard et al. 2014). In contrast to the previous study, prophylactic RBC exchange was performed at day 4 after allogeneic HCT and only in patients deemed to be high risk according to the presence of predefined risk factors (minor or bidirectional ABO incompatibility, non-myeloablative conditioning, lack of prophylactic B cell-directed therapy (methotrexate)). It is of note that, in the RBC exchange group, a higher number of patients received reduced intensity conditioning regimens due to a change of the transplant practice in this period. The latter study showed a statistically not significant trend toward fewer severe hemolysis in the exchange group, while there was no difference in overall survival. Patients in the RBC exchange group required twice as many RBC transfusions compared to the historical group.

Taking this data together, there is no clear benefit of prophylactic RBC exchange to prevent PLS in patients with minor ABO-incompatible HCT resulting in a weak recommendation for RBC exchange in this clinical setting (2C) (Padmanabhan et al. 2019). Indeed, RBC exchange has not been widely accepted among transplant centers due to practical reasons and the relatively inefficient exchange procedure (Booth et al. 2013).

12.6 RBC Exchange for Treatment of Drug Overdoses

Some case reports have described RBC exchange as a treatment of drug intoxication with cyclosporine, tacrolimus, and sirolimus, alone or in combination with plasma exchange. The rationale for RBC exchange is that many drugs are not only bound to plasma proteins but also in the RBC compartment (Kurokawa et al. 1996; Hinderling 1997). Several case reports were published in patients with solid organ transplantation. In HCT, to the best of our knowledge, only two case reports are published. One case describes the successful treatment of cyclosporine intoxication (Moorman et al. 2011). Using sequential plasmapheresis and RBC exchange transfusions, the cyclosporine levels could be reduced to normal within 16 h. A second case describes the treatment of a sirolimus overdose (Galera et al. 2015). With four sessions of RBC exchange, the drug level could be reduced to normal levels; however, after stopping the RBC exchange, the sirolimus drug level rebounded due to redistribution of the drug from the extravascular compartment and the patient experienced renal failure.

12.7 Expert Point of View

RBC depletion in the context of major ABO-incompatible HCT is a standard procedure of bone marrow processing. The program on the Spectra Optia allows a standardized and efficient RBC depletion with an excellent recovery of CD34$^+$ positive cells. It should be preferred over manual depletion methods, as it requires less operator manipulations with its inherent risks.

The evidence for prophylactic RBC exchange in patients with minor ABO-incompatible HCT as well as in the setting of drug overdosing is insufficient for a general recommendation. Nevertheless, it might be indicated in some clinical high-risk situations. Given the rarity of the indication, it should be done in close collaboration with the apheresis medicine specialist.

References

Bolan CD, Childs RW, Procter JL, Barrett AJ, Leitman SF (2001) Massive immune haemolysis after allogeneic peripheral blood stem cell transplantation with minor ABO incompatibility. Br J Haematol 112(3):787–795

Booth GS, Gehrie EA, Bolan CD, Savani BN (2013) Clinical guide to ABO-incompatible allogeneic stem cell transplantation. Biol Blood Marrow Transplant 19(8):1152–1158

Cunard R, Marquez II, Ball ED et al (2014) Prophylactic red blood cell exchange for ABO-mismatched hematopoietic progenitor cell transplants. Transfusion 54(7):1857–1863

Daniele N, Scerpa MC, Rossi C et al (2014) The processing of stem cell concentrates from the bone marrow in ABO-incompatible transplants: how and when. Blood Transfus 12(2):150–158

Gajewski JL, Petz LD, Calhoun L et al (1992) Hemolysis of transfused group O red blood cells in minor ABO-incompatible unrelated-donor bone marrow transplants in patients receiving cyclosporine without posttransplant methotrexate. Blood 79(11):3076–3085

Galera P, Martin HC, Welch L et al (2015) Automated red blood cell exchange for acute drug removal in a patient with sirolimus toxicity. J Clin Apher 30(6):367–370

Hinderling PH (1997) Red blood cells: a neglected compartment in pharmacokinetics and pharmacodynamics. Pharmacol Rev 49(3):279–295

Holbro A, Passweg JR (2015) Management of hemolytic anemia following allogeneic stem cell transplantation. Hematology Am Soc Hematol Educ Program 2015(1):378–384

Hows J, Beddow K, Gordon-Smith E et al (1986) Donor-derived red blood cell antibodies and immune hemolysis after allogeneic bone marrow transplantation. Blood 67(1):177–181

Kim J, Joseph R, Matevosyan K, Sarode R (2016) Comparison of Spectra Optia and COBE Spectra apheresis systems' performances for red blood cell exchange procedures. Transfus Apher Sci 55(3):368–370

Klumpp TR (1991) Immunohematologic complications of bone marrow transplantation. Bone Marrow Transplant 8(3):159–170

Kuo KHM, Ward R, Kaya B, Howard J, Telfer P (2015) A comparison of chronic manual and automated red blood cell exchange transfusion in sickle cell disease patients. Br J Haematol 170(3):425–428

Kurokawa N, Kadobayashi M, Yamamoto K et al (1996) In-vivo distribution and erythrocyte binding characteristics of cyclosporine in renal transplant patients. J Pharm Pharmacol 48(6):553–559

Larghero J, Rea D, Esperou H et al (2006) ABO-mismatched marrow processing for transplantation: results of 114 procedures and analysis of immediate adverse events and hematopoietic recovery. Transfusion 46(3):398–402

Moorman MT, Epstein RB, Smith JW, O'Neal C, Holter JL (2011) Management of cyclosporine overdose in a hematopoietic stem cell transplant patient with sequential plasma exchange and red blood cell exchange. J Clin Apher 26(3):156–158

Padmanabhan A, Connelly-Smith L, Aqui N, Balogun RA, Klingel R, Meyer E et al (2019) Guidelines on the use of therapeutic apheresis in clinical practice—evidence-based approach from the Writing Committee of the American Society for Apheresis: the eighth special issue. J Clin Apher 34(3):171–354. https://doi.org/10.1002/jca.21705

Passweg JR, Baldomero H, Bader P et al (2017) Use of haploidentical stem cell transplantation continues to increase: the 2015 European Society for Blood and Marrow Transplant activity survey report. Bone Marrow Transplant 8:1–7

Rowley SD, Donato ML, Bhattacharyya P (2011) Red blood cell-incompatible allogeneic hematopoietic progenitor cell transplantation. Bone Marrow Transplant 46(9):1167–1185

Shortt J, Westall GP, Roxby D et al (2008) A "dangerous" group O donor: severe hemolysis in all recipients of organs from a donor with multiple red cell alloantibodies. Am J Transplant 8(3):711–714

Sokol RJ, Stamps R, Booker DJ et al (2002) Posttransplant immune-mediated hemolysis. Transfusion 42(2):198–204

Sorg N, Poppe C, Bunos M et al (2015) Red blood cell depletion from bone marrow and peripheral blood buffy coat: a comparison of two new and three established technologies. Transfusion 55(6):1275–1282

Stussi G, Halter J, Schanz U, Seebach JD (2006) ABO-histo blood group incompatibility in hematopoietic stem cell and solid organ transplantation. Transfus Apher Sci 35(1):59–69

Stussi G, Halter J, Bucheli E et al (2009) Prevention of pure red cell aplasia after major or bidirectional ABO blood group incompatible hematopoietic stem cell transplantation by pretransplant reduction of host anti-donor isoagglutinins. Haematologica 94(2):239–248

Swerdlow PS (2006) Red cell exchange in sickle cell disease. Hematology 2006(1):48–53

Watz E, Remberger M, Ringdén O et al (2014) Analysis of donor and recipient ABO incompatibility and antibody-associated complications after allogeneic stem cell transplantation with reduced-intensity conditioning. Biol Blood Marrow Transplant 20(2):264–271

Witt V, Beiglböck E, Fritsch G (2011) Bone marrow processing with the AMICUS™ separator system. J Clin Apher 26(4):195–199

Worel N (2016) ABO-mismatched allogeneic hematopoietic stem cell transplantation. Transfus Med Hemother 43(1):3–12

Worel N, Greinix HT, Supper V et al (2007) Prophylactic red blood cell exchange for prevention of severe immune hemolysis in minor ABO-mismatched allogeneic peripheral blood progenitor cell transplantation after reduced-intensity conditioning. Transfusion 47(8):1494–1502

Worel N, Panzer S, Reesink HW et al (2010) Transfusion policy in ABO-incompatible allogeneic stem cell transplantation. Vox Sang 98(3 Pt 2):455–467

Extracorporeal Photopheresis in Hematopoietic Cell Transplantation 13

Kristina Hölig and Hildegard Greinix

13.1 History and Methods of Action

Extracorporeal photopheresis (ECP), recently also referred to as extracorporeal photochemotherapy, was developed by the group of R. L. Edelson et al. (1987) in the 1980s. The method combines apheresis of mononuclear cells (MNC) with the principle of PUVA therapy, which is a well-known skin-directed therapeutic approach for a variety of skin diseases. Edelson adapted the PUVA principle treatment with psoralen followed by photoactivation with UVA light to leukocytes, particularly lymphocytes and monocytes. Psoralen, or 8-methoxypsoralen (8-MOP), is a naturally occurring photosensitizer that intercalates into the DNA. When exposed to UVA, it forms mono- and bifunctional adducts with the pyrimidine bases of DNA that result in irreversible cross-linking between the base-paired strands of DNA (Fig. 13.1). This process initiates apoptosis of the treated cells within different kinetics, depending on the cell types (Enomoto et al. 1997).

ECP had originally been developed for the treatment of Sézary syndrome, the leukemic variant of cutaneous T-cell lymphoma (CTCL). During the following decade, ECP had been applied for treatment of a range of autoimmune diseases and disorders with immune dysfunction after transplantation of solid organs and hematopoietic stem cells. The first reports of successful application of ECP in graft-versus-host disease (GvHD) date back to 1997 (Gerber et al. 1997; Besnier et al. 1997; Dall'Amico et al. 1997a).

K. Hölig (✉)
Clinic of Internal Medicine I, Department of Transfusion Medicine, University Hospital Carl Gustav Carus, TU Dresden, Dresden, Germany
e-mail: Kristina.hoelig@uniklinikum-dresden.de

H. Greinix
Division of Hematology, Medical University of Graz, Graz, Austria
e-mail: Hildegard.greinix@medunigraz.at

S. A. Abutalib et al. (eds.), *Best Practices of Apheresis in Hematopoietic Cell Transplantation*, Advances and Controversies in Hematopoietic Transplantation and Cell Therapy, https://doi.org/10.1007/978-3-319-55131-9_13

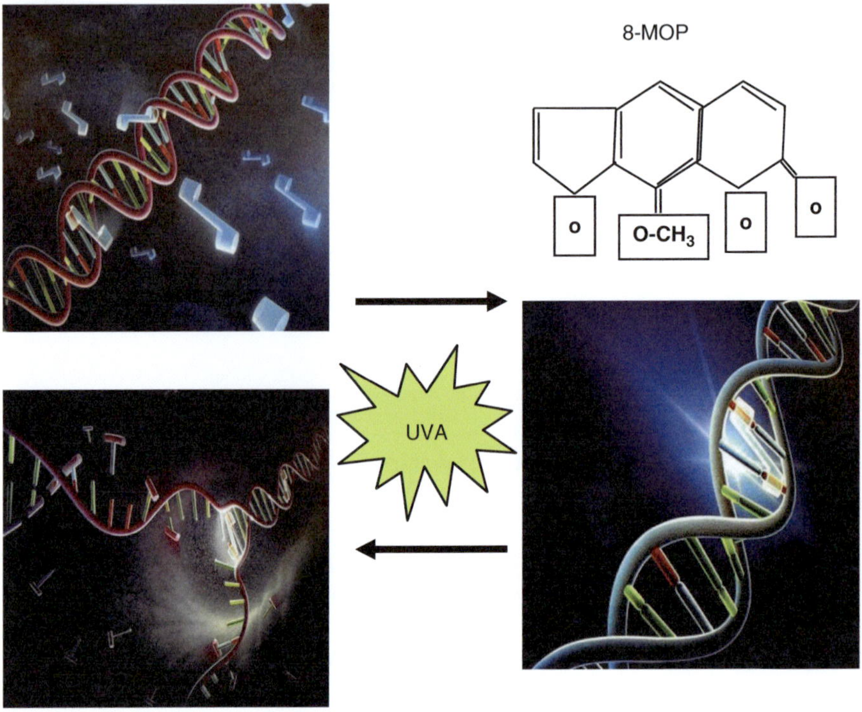

Fig. 13.1 Formation of cross-links of 8-MOP with pyrimidine bases of the DNA strands, resulting in apoptosis of the treated cells

13.2 Technologies of ECP Treatment

ECP has originally been developed as a single procedure, which combines the separation of the MNC from the whole blood with photoactivation of the 8-MOP-treated MNC products within a single device. Currently, the UVAR-XTS™ and CELLEX™ systems (both are from Mallinckrodt Pharmaceuticals, Bedminster, New Jersey) are used in parallel in the clinical praxis (Fig. 13.2). However, the UVAR-XTS™ is phasing out soon. The common features of these devices are a centrifuge bowl for blood cell separation and a photoactivation chamber. Upon completion of the photoactivation, the treated cells are reinfused into the patient. This technology represents the "closed system of ECP." Initially, the photosensitizer 8-MOP had to be taken orally by the patient 1–2 h prior to commencement of the ECP procedure. During the 1990s, liquid 8-MOP preparations became available which can be injected directly into the buffy coat bag (Knobler et al. 1993). This modification improved the tolerability of the procedure substantially by avoiding the gastrointestinal symptoms (mainly nausea) provoked by oral 8-MOP. This step of the procedure has to be performed manually by the operator in all types of ECP treatment. The photoactivation dosage is 1–2 J/cm^2; the intended 8-MOP concentration in the

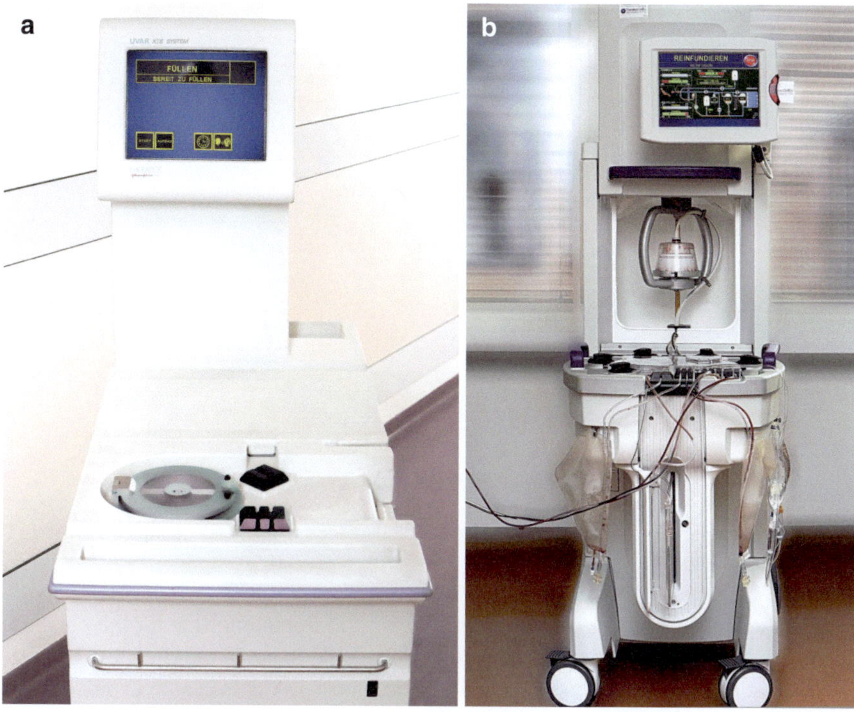

Fig. 13.2 Devices for online ECP currently in clinical use: UVAR-XTS™ (**a**) and CELLEX™ (**b**)

buffy coat is 200–300 ng/mL. The photoactivation time is automatically adjusted to the product's volume and hematocrit. Another way to perform ECP is using an "off-line technique" (Andreu et al. 1994). It includes as the first step cell separation with a standard blood cell separator that can also be used for the collection of donor lymphocytes or peripheral blood stem cells. The apheresis product is transferred into another disposable, and 8-MOP is added; subsequent photoactivation is performed with a separate device at a dosage of 2 J/cm^2. Various photoactivation devices are currently available in Europe, such as MacoGenic G2 (Macopharma, Mouvaux, France) (Del Fante et al. 2016a), PUVA Combi Light (Cell-Max GmbH, Munich, Germany) (Brosig et al. 2016), and UVA PIT System (MTS, Cadolzburg, Germany, Fig. 13.3) (Garban et al. 2014). After photoactivation, transfusion of the treated cells is carried out manually by a standard transfusion set.

A specific modification of the off-line ECP resembles the mini buffy coat photopheresis developed by Hackstein et al. (Hackstein et al. 2014). This procedure completely avoids apheresis of MNC. It starts with the collection of 5–8 mL/kg of whole blood into an umbilical cord blood collection bag (MacoPharma, Langen, Germany). Following centrifugation, the buffy coat is prepared with a separator for standard blood bags (Compomat G4, Fresenius, Bad Homburg, Germany). After adding 8-MOP, photoactivation is performed by the BS05 device (Gröbel, Ettlingen, Germany). Red cells, plasma, and the UVA-photoactivated buffy coat are returned

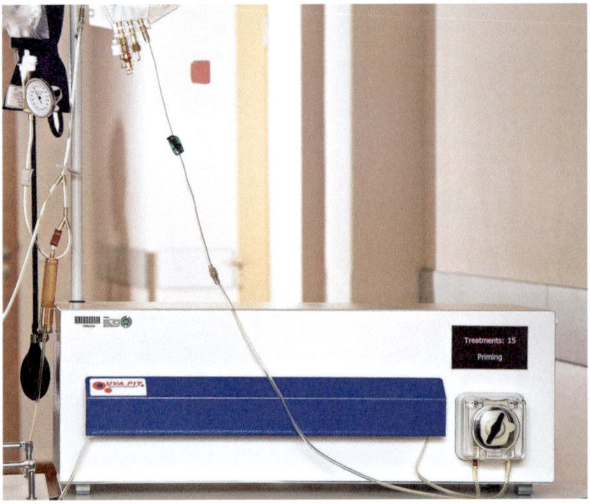

Fig. 13.3 Example for an irradiation device developed for off-line ECP treatment: UVA PIT System (MTS, Cadolzburg, Germany)

to the patients. This procedure minimizes stress and treatment time for the patients. Therefore, it can safely be applied directly at bedside in small children and in critically ill patients, and transfusion of allogeneic blood products can be avoided.

Both ECP techniques have demonstrated clinical efficacy, but most clinical studies have been undertaken using a single ECP technique. Studies comparing online and off-line treatment in the same patient population are almost completely lacking (Andreu et al. 1994; Brosig et al. 2016; Schooneman 2003).

Treatment parameters, amount, and subpopulations of the treated cells vary between the different techniques (Table 13.1), but the clinical significance of these differences remains elusive. Perseghin et al. reported a trend for better clinical outcome when a larger number of cells were treated (Perseghin et al. 2007), but very low cell doses can be clinically effective as evidenced by the favorable results of mini ECP treatment (Hackstein et al. 2014).

Comparing the one-step closed and the two-step open system, some practical features have to be underlined.

The closed system is a fixed treatment algorithm with few opportunities for modification by the user. Cell doses depend mainly on patient's condition and can only minimally be influenced by the operator. This apparent disadvantage gives rise to a good comparability of ECP treatments in different centers around the world. The only prospective, multicenter randomized trial on ECP in steroid-refractory, steroid-dependent, or steroid-intolerant chronic GvHD (cGvHD) published until now was certainly gained from this fact (Flowers et al. 2008). Furthermore, online ECP requires shorter working time for the operators and can be used both with single-needle and double-needle venous access. In patients with very difficult peripheral venous access, the single-needle option can also be used with apheresis port systems. One disadvantage of the online system is the rather high hematocrit needed

Table 13.1 Comparison of technical parameters of ECP technologies, adapted from Brosig et al. (2016)

Parameter	In-line system CELLEX® Therakos Inc.	Off-line system (various manufacturers)
Vascular access	Single or double needle (port system possible)	Double-needle or double-lumen CVC necessary
Anticoagulation	Heparin standard, ACD-A possible	ACD-A standard, additional heparin possible
Duration of treatment	1 h 30 min to 2 h	2 h 30 min to 3 h 30 min
Processed blood volume	1500 mL (adults), can be adapted/lowered in pediatric patients	1–2 × patient body blood volume
Number of leukocytes treated	$20–63 \times 10^8$	$57–220 \times 10^8$
MNCs in apheresis products	21–65%	68–99%
Platelets in apheresis products	$0.75–2 \times 10^{10}$	$0.5–6.3 \times 10^{11}$
Hematocrit of apheresis products	1.4–4%	1.3–12%
Sampling for process validation and quality control	Not required	Requested by regulatory authorities
Cleared by regulatory bodies in Europe (CE) and the United States (FDA)	Cleared for photopheresis in Europe and the United States for treatment of advanced CTCL	Cell separators are cleared for MNC collection in Europe and the United States; photoactivation devices are only cleared in Europe, not in the United States

CVC central venous catheter, *ACD-A* acid-citrate-dextrose-solution A, *MNC* mononuclear cells, *CTCL* cutaneous T-cell lymphoma

for successful treatment. The latter often leads to allogeneic red blood cell (RBC) transfusions in clinically asymptomatic patients that can worsen iron overload and, thus, liver toxicity. Another way is to blood prime the device, which can be performed in both double- and single-needle mode. The UVAR-XTS® had not been approved for treatment of patients with a body mass below 40 kg because of the high extracorporeal blood volume. The third-generation CELLEX® device has been developed for treatment of patients with small body weight but might require transfusion of two allogeneic RBC units per treatment depending on patient size.

A main advantage of the open system consists in the opportunity to change the technical parameters of the apheresis procedure and hereby influence the treated cell dose, the volume, and the hematocrit of the apheresis product. Due to the lower extra corporeal volume of up-to-date cell separators, the MNC collection can often be performed without RBC transfusion or RBC priming even in anemic patients. In young children below 25 kg body mass, priming of the disposable with allogeneic RBCs is also required, but a single RBC unit is always sufficient per treatment. ACD-A is routinely used as an anticoagulant for the apheresis procedures, thereby excluding the risk of heparin-induced thrombocytopenia (HIT) during ECP treatments. To date, only one case of HIT due to ECP treatment has been reported (Dittberner et al. 2002). One disadvantage of the open system is the requirement for double-needle access in all modern blood cell separators. Furthermore, the procedure is more time-consuming for the operators, and in some countries, a cell therapy unit is necessary for the photoactivation procedure as regulatory authority requirement.

13.3 Clinical Aspects of ECP

Similar to other apheresis procedures, well-working venous access is a necessary precondition for successful treatment. In contrast to hemodialysis, plasma exchange, and hematopoietic cell collection, ECP treatments can be performed with lower flow rates; e.g., Therakos devices are working well with collection rates of 20–40 mL/min. Thus, peripheral venous catheters or central lines with smaller lumen often allow satisfactory performance of ECP procedures. In patients with suitable peripheral veins, a 17G dialysis needle is appropriate for the collection in double-needle procedures and as the only access in single-needle procedures as well (Fig. 13.4). For the return line and in patients with less optimal peripheral veins, a 20G peripheral

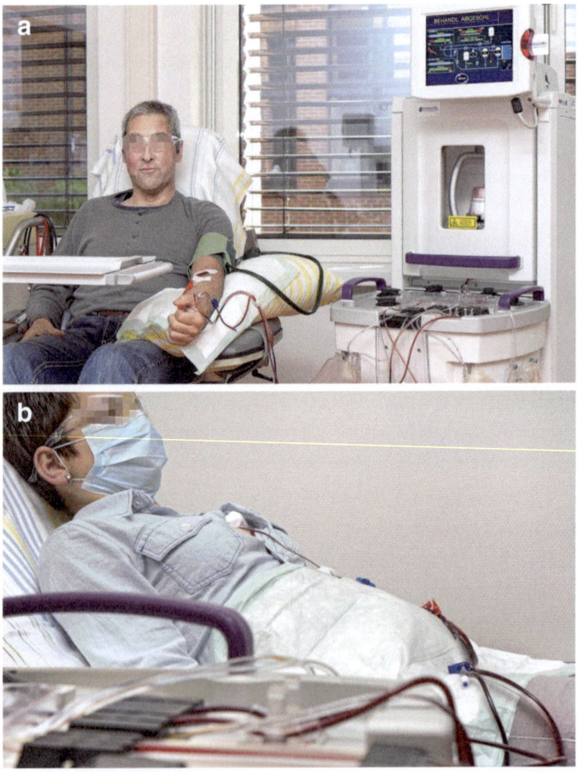

Fig. 13.4 Typical venous access devices in single-needle online ECP treatment (CELLEX™): 17G dialysis needle (**a**) and port system (**b**)

venous line is normally sufficient. In patients with central lines already in place, this access may be used for ECP. In an outpatient setting, individuals with very poor venous access can receive a special port system dimensioned for higher flow rate (Fig. 13.4). Our group has been using the Vortex™TR, SSDX-16-I (AngioDynamics Inc., Cambridge, the United Kingdom), for ECP treatment since 2007. These venous access devices allow only for single-needle procedures but provide the opportunity for therapies on a long-term basis (Cheung et al. 2009; Galloway and Bodenham 2004). Port systems have to be accessed with sufficiently large (18G) Huber-type needles and need to be blocked with anticoagulant-containing solutions (heparin or citrate). In general, the nursing team has to be well trained and experienced in all aspects of handling port systems, and the patients should be well informed about the basic rules of application and precautionary measures.

The first-line anticoagulant and recommendation of the manufacturer for in-line ECP procedures is heparinized saline (5000–15,000 IU heparin/500 mL saline). In thrombocytopenic patients (platelet counts less than 100×10^9/L), most centers use ACD-A for anticoagulation as a single agent (Del Fante et al. 2016a; Nedelcu et al. 2008) or in combination with heparin (Apsner et al. 2002), irrespectively of the ECP technology applied (Knobler et al. 2014). Possibly occurring paresthesia can be treated by intravenous infusion of calcium gluconate. In patients with normal or elevated platelet counts, the combination of ACD-A (ratio 1:10–1:18) and heparin (5000 IU) can be recommended for both off-line and in-line procedures. This approach minimizes citrate exposition and related paresthesia, and buffy coat collection can be improved and formation of thrombi within the system avoided, which specifically applies to the CELLEX™ in-line device. Whereas ACD-A does not interfere with systemic anticoagulation, the use of heparin during ECP causes elevated anti-factor Xa activity and prolongation of aPTT for about 3–4 h after treatment. This transient systemic anticoagulation should be considered by treating physicians (Ivancic et al. 2005).

The intervals of ECP treatments have been empirically defined, because underlying pathophysiological mechanisms are still largely unknown. In CTCL patients, the recommended schedule is one series (two consecutive treatments) every 2 weeks for the first 3 months, then once a month or every 3 weeks (Knobler et al. 2014). Chronic GvHD patients typically receive one ECP series every 1–2 weeks for 3 months. Thereafter, treatment intervals can be increased in responding patients. Patients with acute GvHD are usually treated on a weekly basis, with two to three treatments per week (Knobler et al. 2014; Greinix et al. 2006a).

13.4 Mechanism of Action of ECP: What Do We Know?

All concepts of the mechanism of action (MoA) of ECP are presented with the challenge to elucidate two different effects—the antineoplastic activity against Sézary syndrome and other T-cell lymphomas and the immunomodulatory efficacy in autoimmune diseases, GvHD, and solid organ rejection. Both fields of application of ECP have been in routine clinical use for nearly three decades, but systematic investigations of the underlying therapeutic principle have not been very successful until the turn of the millennium.

The starting point of all hypotheses regarding MoA of ECP is the induction of apoptosis in the collected mononuclear cells induced through covalent cross-links in DNA (Fig. 13.1). Lymphocytes are especially sensitive and undergo apoptosis within 24–48 h or even less time if activated (Enomoto et al. 1997; Garban et al. 2014; Heng et al. 2003; Lamioni et al. 2005). Monocytes are less susceptible and maintain their ability to differentiate for a few days after reinfusion (Setterblad et al. 2008). During ECP, monocytes are differentiating into dendritic cells (DCs), a process that is facilitated by the interaction with adherent platelets and plastic materials of the photopheresis system (Knobler et al. 2014; Berger et al. 2010; Edelson 2014).

After reinfusion, ECP-exposed apoptotic cells are phagocytosed by DCs which acquire an immature tolerogenic state, characterized by increased secretion of anti-inflammatory cytokines like TGFβ and IL-10. IL-10 plays a central role in tolerance induction by preventing DC maturation and generating regulatory T-cells (Tregs) (Flinn and Gennery 2017; Spisek et al. 2006). These data support the hypothesis that ECP at least in some circumstances induces immunological tolerance.

Current scientific standards require testing of novel therapeutic principles in animal models first before the implementation in human therapy. Unfortunately, animal models of CTCL and other major ECP indications are lacking (Garban et al. 2014). Ferrara and colleagues investigated ECP in a well-established and clinically relevant murine model of acute GvHD where donor and recipient were identical at the major histocompatibility (MHC) antigens but mismatched at multiple minor histocompatibility antigens and GvHD is mediated by donor $CD8^+$ T-cells (Gatza et al. 2008). Injections of ex vivo PUVA-treated splenocytes suppressed ongoing clinical GvHD, and 4 weekly injections improved both survival and GvHD clinical scores compared with controls injected with either untreated splenocytes or diluent. Mice receiving ECP-treated cells also showed significantly less histopathological damage in all GvHD target organs and improved immune reconstitution 56 days after transplant. The authors further investigated the role of different cell populations in this immunomodulatory process. They could show that $CD4^+$ $CD25^+$ $FoxP3^+$ Treg cells of donor origin were essentially required to reverse GvHD in this model since the beneficial effect could be completely abrogated by in vivo depletion of this cell population before and after the infusion of ECP-treated splenocytes. Of note, an increase in Treg cells has also been reported in GvHD patients responding to ECP treatment (Quaglino et al. 2009; Schmitt et al. 2009; Tsirigotis et al. 2012; Biagi et al. 2007).

Budde and colleagues confirmed in a mouse model with MHC class I and MHC class II mismatches where GvHD is mediated by both $CD4^+$ and $CD8^+$ T-cells that ECP is able to alleviate acute GvHD (Budde et al. 2014). However, ECP-treated cells from healthy mice with bone marrow donor's genetic background were not as effective as ECP-treated cells derived from GvHD mice. These experiments support the assumption that the MoA of ECP is not simply based on infusion of apoptotic cells but rather on a clonotypic response.

Florek and colleagues reported in another mouse model that a prophylactic effect could be observed when ECP-treated cells from recipient type had been administered in advance of the conditioning regimen (Florek et al. 2014). They found that phagocytosis of apoptotic cells reduced NF-κB activation and costimulatory molecule expression in host DCs and diminished trogocytosis, a phenomenon characterized by inflammation-dependent incorporation of cell surface proteins including MHC class II by T-cells (Joly and Hudrisier 2003) in donor T-cells. The authors hypothesize that the inhibition of trogocytosis by ECP contributes to reduce local inflammation. Host-type Foxp3$^+$ Treg cells and host IL-10 were required for the beneficial effect of ECP treatment in that model. Donor T-cell activation was significantly reduced, and the frequency of recipient DCs was lower in the ECP-treated group with an increase in apoptotic signals, thus reducing potential sites of donor T-cell priming.

Preemptive ECP treatment has also been shown to improve overall and disease-free survival and reduce the incidence of severe acute GvHD in clinical studies (Miller et al. 2004; Shaughnessy et al. 2009; Kitko and Levine 2015). In contrast to these experimental observations and clinical results, Bethge and colleagues were not able to show any protective effect of preemptive ECP treatment either alone or in connection with pentostatin on the prevention of acute GvHD in an allogeneic HLA nonidentical bone marrow transplant (BMT) model in dogs (Bethge et al. 2014). In these experiments, ECP had been performed on days 2 and 1 alone or on days 6 and 5 combined with 2 doses of pentostatin (days 4 and 3). The animals had been treated with the UVAR-XTS in an identical way to the human setting.

Another aspect of the MoA is highlighted by Rieber and colleagues who found an increase of neutrophilic myeloid suppressor cells (MDSCs) in GvHD patients treated with ECP (Rieber et al. 2014). MDSCs are innate immune cells characterized by their capacity to suppress T-cell proliferation. They resemble an intrinsic anti-inflammatory mechanism induced to dampen excessive T-cell activities and are thereby comparable to Treg cells. They exert their inhibitory effect on T-cells via arginase 1 activity, and the authors speculate that MDSC-derived arginase activity might contribute to the immunomodulatory effect of ECP in GvHD. An increase in arginase activity and secretion in neutrophils following ECP treatment has also been found by Franklin and colleagues (Franklin et al. 2015). This finding could be reproduced in neutrophils from blood samples of GvHD patients taken 24 h after ECP treatment, and these cells were still able to suppress CD4$^+$ and CD8$^+$ T-cell proliferation in a dose-dependent manner. The authors speculate that the anti-inflammatory modulation of neutrophil activity significantly adds to the MoA of ECP, because they resemble a significant amount of the treated cell population. This assumption holds especially true for the in-line ECP systems (see Table 13.1).

Apart from the cellular mechanisms, the soluble mediators released during ECP treatment are a matter of controversial discussion. Many reports relate to a more tolerogenic cytokine pattern induced by ECP treatment with decreased production of immunostimulatory cytokines such as TNF-α and IL-6 and an increase in IL-10 and IL-1Ra (Garban et al. 2014; Bladon and Taylor 1999; Merlin et al. 2011).

Recent studies using different in vitro models and analyzing clinical samples provided evidence that ECP markedly promotes bioactive IL-1β production (Yakut et al. 2015). IL-1β is a key immunostimulatory molecule that among other cytokines promotes full DC maturation. These findings support the hypothesis of Hannani, who interprets ECP as an immunogenic rather than a tolerogenic process (Hannani 2015). He assumes an immunogenic cell death (ICD) of ECP-treated pathogenic T-cells (either CTCL or autoreactive cells). The reinfusion of those T-cells undergoing ICD back into the patient could facilitate DC-mediated phagocytosis and DC maturation. Activated T-cells die more rapidly than resting T-cells; therefore, pathogenic cell clones might become the preferential source of antigens phagocytosed by DCs and presented to the immune system. This would lead to the induction of an anti-(oligo)clonotypic response against the pathogenic (oligo)clonal T-cell population (Fig. 13.5). This hypothesis very elegantly explains the therapeutic activity of ECP in CTCL, GvHD, solid organ rejection, and autoimmune diseases without inducing generalized immunosuppression.

Nevertheless, the wide range of clinical applications of ECP most likely will not be accommodated by a single MoA. Anyway the large body of experimental results and clinical data has brought us a huge step forward toward a deeper insight into the immunological mechanisms underlying the therapeutic and even prophylactic effects of ECP.

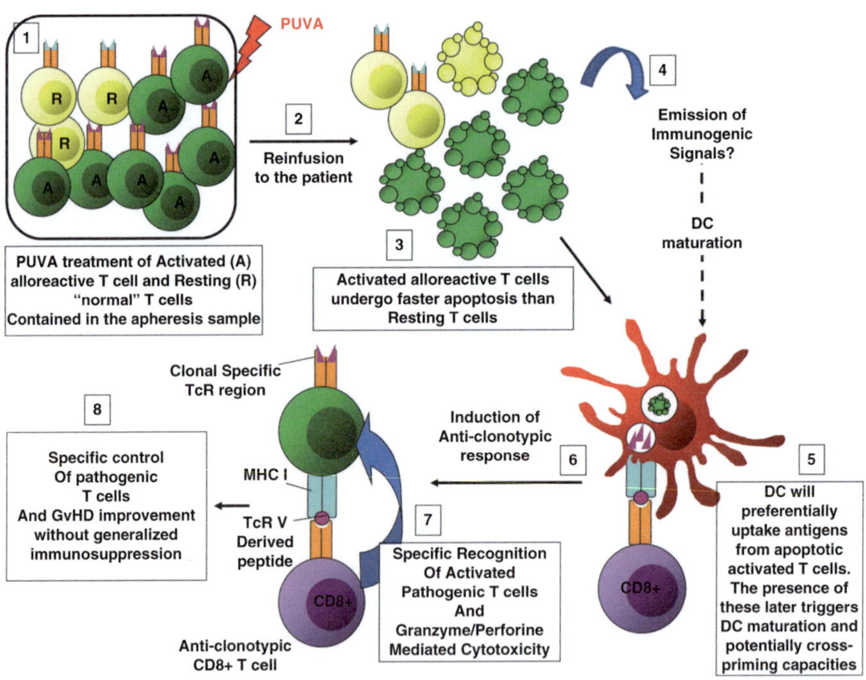

Fig. 13.5 ECP-induced anti-clonotypic response in GvHD. Kindly provided and reproduced with permission from Dr. Dalil HANNANI, Chargé de Recherche CNRS; Université Grenoble-Alpes—CNRS UMR 5525 Laboratoire TIMC-IMAG Equipe TheREx Faculté de Médecine de Grenoble Domaine de la Merci, 38,700, La Tronche, France

13.5 Results of ECP in Patients with Acute GvHD

Acute graft-versus-host disease (aGvHD) is a serious complication of allogeneic hematopoietic cell transplantation (HCT) affecting 20%–80% of patients and a main cause of transplant-related morbidity and mortality (TRM), mainly due to severe infections and organ toxicities (Martin et al. 2012). It occurs more frequently after HCT from an unrelated or HLA nonidentical $CD34^+$ cell donor or a female donor graft given to a male recipient (Flowers et al. 2011). In addition, conditioning intensity, use of total body irradiation, and graft source have an effect on risk of aGvHD (Jagasia et al. 2012). The development of aGvHD can be conceptualized in three sequential phases consisting of activation of antigen-presenting cells by the underlying disease and conditioning for HCT, donor T-cell activation, proliferation, differentiation, and migration leading to target tissue injury due to both cellular mediators such as cytotoxic T-cells (CTLs) and NK cells and soluble inflammatory mediators such as TNF-α, IFN-γ, IL-1, and nitric oxide (Ferrara et al. 2009). These soluble and cellular mediators synergize to amplify local tissue injury and further promote inflammation and target tissue destruction.

Currently, standard first-line therapy of aGvHD consists of corticosteroids at 1–2 mg/kg body weight (b.w.) resulting in complete response (CR) rates of 25%–54% (Martin et al. 2012; Wolff et al. 2013). Lack of response to first-line therapy reportedly is associated with significantly higher TRM and lower survival (Levine et al. 2010; Van Lint et al. 2006; MacMillan et al. 2010).

Currently, no consensus on the optimal choice of agents for secondary therapy of acute GvHD has been reached, and treatment decisions are based on risk of toxicity and potential exacerbation of preexisting comorbidity, interactions with other agents, physician's experience, and ease of use (Martin et al. 2012; Wolff et al. 2013). During the last years, ECP has been increasingly used as salvage treatment in patients with corticosteroid-refractory or corticosteroid-dependent aGvHD (Table 13.2) (Knobler et al. 2014; Greinix et al. 2006a, 2010; Messina et al. 2003; Salvaneschi et al. 2001; Dall'Amico and Messina 2002; Garban et al. 2005; Kanold et al. 2007; Calore et al. 2008; Gonzalez-Vicent et al. 2008; Perfetti et al. 2008; Perotti et al. 2010; Hautmann et al. 2013; Malagola et al. 2016; Berger et al. 2015).

Greinix and colleagues conducted a prospective phase II study of ECP in 59 adult patients with severe steroid-refractory or steroid-dependent aGvHD (Greinix et al. 2006a, 2010). CR rates for individual organs were 82% for skin involvement and 61% for gastrointestinal (GI) and liver involvement, respectively. Responses were highest in patients with only skin manifestations (87%) and lower for those who had two organs involved (62% for skin and liver involvement, 40% for skin and GI manifestations) or those who had all three organs affected (25%). Response rates were also higher for patients with less severe grades of aGvHD at the start of treatment. The administration of an intensified ECP schedule consists of two to three treatments per week on a weekly basis until maximum response led to improvements in CR rates in patients with grade 4 acute GvHD (60% vs. 12% in the pilot study with less intense treatment) and GI involvement (73% vs. 25%) as shown in Fig. 13.6. Best response to ECP was observed after a median of 1.3 (range, 0.5–6)

Table 13.2 Results of second-line treatment of acute GvHD using extracorporeal photopheresis

Author	No of patients	CR skin no (%)	CR liver no (%)	CR gut no (%)	OS%
Salvaneschi et al. (2001)	9	6/9 (67)	1/3 (33)	3/5 (60)	67
Dall'Amico and Messina (2002)	14	10/14 (71)	4/7 (57)	6/10 (60)	57
Messina et al. (2003)	33	25/33 (76)	9/15 (60)	15/20 (75)	69 at 5 yrs
Greinix et al. (2006a, 2010)	59	47/57 (82)	14/23 (61)	9/15 (60)	47 at 5 yrs
Garban et al. (2005)	12	8/12 (67)	0/2 (0)	2/5 (40)	42
Kanold et al. (2007)	12	9/10 (90)	5/9 (55.5)	5/6 (83)	75 at 8.5 mo
Calore et al. (2008)	15	12/13 (92)		14/14 (100)	85 at 5 yrs
Perfetti et al. (2008)	23	15/23 (65)	3/11 (27)	8/20 (40)	48 at 37 mo
Gonzalez-Vicent et al. (2008)	8	8/8 (100)	2/2 (100)	4/7 (57%)	37.5
Perotti et al. (2010)	50	39/47 (83)[a]	16/24 (67)[a]	8/11 (73)[a]	64 at 1 yr
Jagasia et al. (2013)	57	38/57 (67)[a]	38/57 (67)[a]	38/57 (67)[a]	59 at 2 yrs
Calore et al. (2015)	72	50/64 (78)	10/12 (84)	42/55 (76)	71 at 5 yrs

No number, *CR* complete resolution, *OS* overall survival, *yrs* years, *mo* months
[a]Results were provided as complete and partial resolution

months of treatment, and no flare-ups were seen after tapering and discontinuation of corticosteroids. In ECP-responding patients, steroids could be discontinued after a median of 55 days (range, 17–284) after the initiation of ECP. In univariate analysis, a lower grade of acute GvHD and fewer organs involved at the start of first-line therapy with corticosteroids and at start of ECP and a lower cumulative corticosteroid dose prior to ECP significantly increased the probability of CR to ECP. The cumulative incidence of TRM at 4 years was 14% in patients achieving a CR of steroid-refractory acute GvHD compared with 73% in patients without CR at 3 months after initiation of ECP ($p < 0.0001$). Patients achieving a CR to ECP had a significantly improved overall survival (OS) of 59% compared with 11% in patients without CR ($p < 0.0001$). Treatment with ECP was tolerated well, and no increase in rates of infection or relapse was observed.

These initial promising results have been confirmed in a larger number of patients with steroid-refractory aGvHD given ECP as second-line treatment and achieving high response rates and favorable OS after a median of 6 (range, 0.5–15) years of follow-up (Fig. 13.7).

Das-Gupta and colleagues performed a retrospective analysis including 128 patients with steroid-refractory aGvHD from three centers (Nashville, Nottingham, Vienna) treated with ECP with 2–3 treatments per week on a weekly basis between 1995 and 2011 (Das-Gupta et al. 2014). The median duration of ECP was 60 (range,

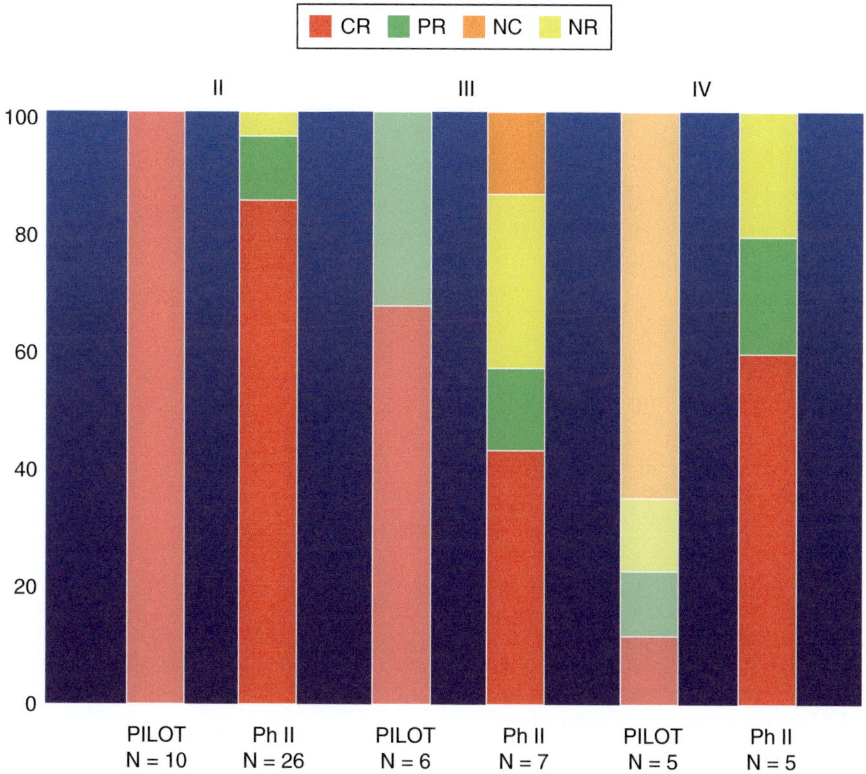

Fig. 13.6 Response of patients with steroid-refractory acute GvHD to extracorporeal photopheresis according to grade of graft-versus-host disease at initiation of ECP. The left columns show the responses in the pilot study (PILOT) and the right columns the responses of patients in the phase II study (Ph II) according to grade at initiation of ECP. *CR* complete resolution of GvHD defined as resolution of all organ manifestations, *PR* partial resolution of GvHD defined as greater than 50% response, *NC* no change of GvHD defined as stable organ involvement despite tapering of corticosteroids by at least 50%, *NR* no response of GvHD defined as progressive worsening of GvHD and the inability to taper corticosteroids. Modified according to reference (Greinix et al. 2006a)

0–324) days, and the median number of ECP treatments was 11 (range, 2–42). Of note, the median steroid dose at onset of ECP was 2 (range, 0.5–10) mg/kg b.w. The overall response rate (ORR) was 77% including 86 patients (87%) with CR and 13 patients (13%) with partial response (PR), respectively. Patients with stage 2 or less compared to stage 3–4 liver involvement (61.2% vs. 33.3%, $p = 0.005$), overall grade 2 or less compared to grade 3–4 aGvHD (65.7% vs. 36.2%, $p < 0.001$), and less than three organs compared to three organs affected (60.5% vs. 39.9%, $p = 0.007$) had significantly better 2-year OS. Furthermore, 2-year nonrelapse mortality (NRM) was significantly lower in patients with stage 2 or less compared to stage 3–4 liver involvement (27.3% vs. 61.7%, $p < 0.001$), overall grade 2 or less compared to grade 3–4 aGvHD (23.0% vs. 53.3%, $p < 0.001$), and less than three

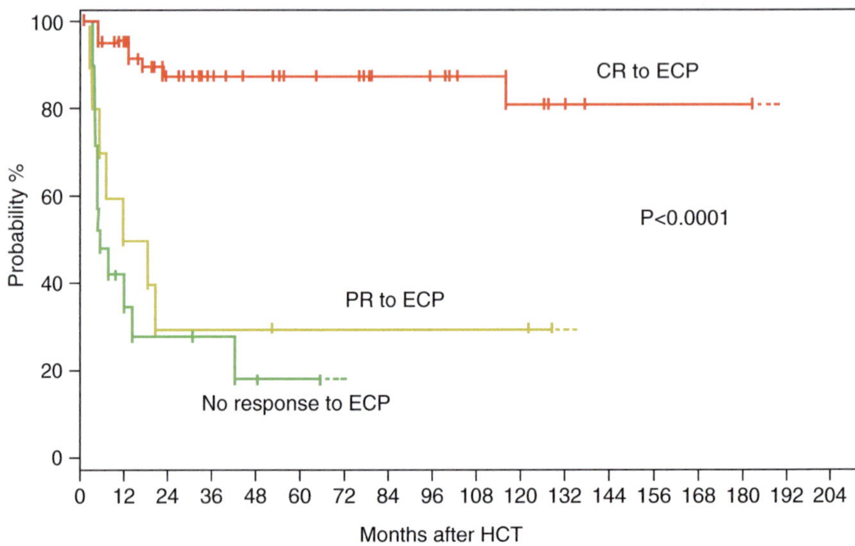

Fig. 13.7 Kaplan-Meier probability of overall survival of 96 patients with corticosteroid-refractory acute GvHD according to response to ECP. Overall survival is shown for patients with complete resolution of acute GvHD (CR to ECP), partial resolution of acute GvHD (PR to ECP), and no response to ECP (no response to ECP), respectively. According to De Gruyter Extracorporeal photopheresis. Eds Hildegard T. Greinix, Robert Knobler. 2012 Walter de Gruyter GmbH &Co KG, Berlin/Boston, with major modifications

organs compared to three organ involvement (27.4% vs. 50.6%, $p = 0.002$). Six-month freedom from treatment failure (6mFTF) was significantly better in patients with overall grade 2 or less compared to grade 3–4 aGvHD (79% vs. 52.6%, $p = 0.002$).

Calore and colleagues reported 72 consecutive pediatric patients given ECP for steroid-refractory ($n = 21$) and steroid-dependent ($n = 42$) acute GvHD or for first-line treatment ($n = 9$) of acute GvHD instead of steroids due to clinical contraindications (Calore et al. 2008). CR was obtained in 72% of patients, a PR in 11%, and no response in 17%. At day +180, TRM was 3% and 20% among responders and non-responders to ECP ($p < 0.0001$). The 5-year OS was 71% overall and was 78% and 30% in responders and nonresponders to ECP ($p = 0.0004$) confirming the beneficial impact of ECP on long-term outcome of responding patients.

In a systematic review of prospective studies, Abu-Dalle and colleagues included six studies with 103 patients given ECP for steroid-refractory aGvHD and achieving an ORR of 69% overall including ORR for cutaneous involvement with 84%, liver involvement with 55%, and GI manifestation with 65%, respectively (Abu-Dalle et al. 2014).

Jagasia and colleagues performed a retrospective analysis comparing different second-line treatment strategies in patients with steroid-refractory aGvHD grades 2–4 given HCT after 2005 and first-line therapy with corticosteroids of at least 1 mg/kg b.w. (Jagasia et al. 2013). Fifty-seven patients received ECP 2–3 times per week on a weekly basis and 41 anticytokine therapy consisting of either inolimumab or etanercept. ORR rates were 66% and 32% in the ECP and anticytokine cohort including CR rates of 54% and 20%, respectively. Results of both treatment strategies according to organ involvement and overall severity are shown in Fig. 13.8. ECP was an independent predictor of response (OR 3.42, $p = 0.007$) and survival (HR 2.12, $p = 0.018$). Furthermore, ECP was associated with superior survival (HR 4.6, $p = 0.016$) in patients with steroid-refractory grade 2 acute GvHD and was associated with lower NRM (HR 0.45, $p = 0.018$).

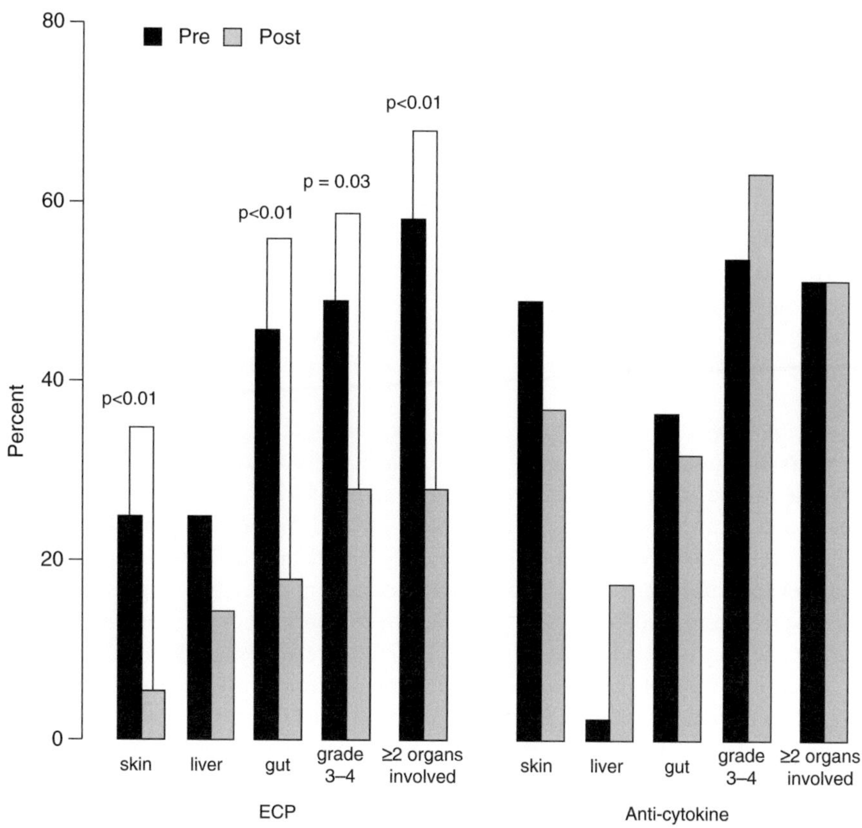

Fig. 13.8 Acute GvHD before and after therapy in the ECP and the anticytokine groups. Organ-specific involvement reflects stage 3–4 acute GvHD. P values reflect comparison of acute GvHD incidence before and after therapy. Categories without p values were statistically nonsignificant. Modified after reference (Jagasia et al. 2013)

13.6 Results of ECP in Patients with Chronic GvHD

Chronic GvHD (cGvHD) is associated with substantial morbidity and the major cause of NRM in patients surviving more than 2 years after allogeneic HCT (Lee et al. 2002; Socie et al. 1999; Jagasia et al. 2015). Infection from a broad array of pathogens is the major cause of death, followed by progressive organ failure from cGvHD involvement and/or GvHD treatment. It has features resembling autoimmune and other immunological disorders such as scleroderma, Sjogren's syndrome, primary biliary cirrhosis, wasting syndrome, bronchiolitis obliterans, immune cytopenias, and chronic immunodeficiency (Jagasia et al. 2015; Filipovich et al. 2005). Manifestations of cGvHD may be restricted to one organ or tissue or may be widespread. cGvHD can lead to debilitating consequences, e.g., joint contractures, loss of sight, end-stage lung disease, or death resulting from profound chronic immune suppression leading to recurrent or life-threatening infections. Reported incidence rates of cGvHD after allogeneic HCT range from 20% to 75% depending on recipient age, donor type, HCT source (peripheral blood, bone marrow, umbilical cord blood stem cells), graft manipulation (T-cell depletion), and use of posttransplant donor lymphocyte infusions (DLI) (Lee et al. 2002; Martin et al. 2004). During the past 30 years, survival of patients with high-risk cGvHD has not improved. Thus, new therapeutic approaches to improve treatment response of patients with chronic GvHD are urgently needed.

Recently, a three-step model for the initiation and the development of chronic GvHD has been proposed that involves early inflammation, tissue injury, dysregulated immunity, and aberrant tissue repair often with fibrosis (Cooke et al. 2017). Among other cellular components, B-cells reportedly have an important role in the development and the prolongation of chronic GvHD (Kuzmina et al. 2011; Greinix et al. 2015).

The most widely used first-line therapy for treatment of cGvHD is cyclosporine A (CSA) and prednisone. Thereby, approximately 50% of all patients with cGvHD are able to discontinue immunosuppressive treatment within 5 years after the diagnosis, and 10% require continued treatment beyond 5 years (Martin et al. 2004; Stewart et al. 2004; Wolff et al. 2010). Recently, Martin and colleagues reported that complete or partial response without secondary systemic immunosuppressive treatment or recurrent malignancy at 1 year after study enrolment provided clinical benefit in patients with cGvHD (Martin et al. 2017). Interestingly, success was observed in fewer than 20% of patients after initial systemic immunosuppressive therapy of cGvHD indicating the tremendous unmet clinical need for improvement of upfront treatment of cGvHD. If patients fail to respond or progress through steroid-based therapy, then secondary treatment is indicated. Steroid-refractory cGvHD is formally defined as either failure to improve after at least 2 months or progression after 1 month of standard immunosuppressive therapy, including corticosteroids and calcineurin inhibitors (CNI) (Wolff et al. 2011).

Although many therapeutic options have been reported for salvage treatment of steroid-refractory cGvHD, no single class of immunosuppressive agent has been established as standard therapy. ECP represents a frequently used therapeutic

Table 13.3 Results of use of extracorporeal photopheresis in chronic GvHD

	No of patients	CR/PR skin (%)	CR/PR liver (%)	CR/PR oral (%)	ORR (%)
Greinix et al. (1998)	15	80	70	100	na
Salvaneschi et al. (2001)	14	83	67	67	64
Messina et al. (2003)	44	56	60	–	57
Seaton et al. (2003)	28	48	32	21	36
Apisarnthanarax et al. (2003)	32	59	0	na	56
Foss et al. (2005)	25	64	0	46	64
Rubegni et al. (2005)	32	81	77	92	69
Greinix et al. (2006b)	47	93	84	95	83
Couriel et al. (2006)	71	57	71	78	61
Kanold et al. (2007)	15	75	82	86	50
Perseghin et al. (2007)	25	67	67	78	73
Flowers et al. (2008)	48	40	29	53	40
Jagasia et al. (2009)	43				65
Perotti et al. (2010)	23	96	100	80	69
Dignan et al. (2012)	82	92	na	91	74
Greinix et al. (2011)	29	31	50	70	na
Del Fante et al. (2012)	102	na	na	na	81
Ussowicz et al. (2013)	13	67	89	86	69
Hautmann et al. (2013)	32	59	100	60	44
Dignan et al. (2014)	38	65	–	29	50
Berger et al. (2015)	37	na	na	na	81

No number, *CR* complete resolution, *PR* partial resolution, *ORR* overall response rate, *na* not available

approach for treatment of cGvHD patients failing corticosteroids (Table 13.3) (Gerber et al. 1997; Dall'Amico et al. 1997a; Perseghin et al. 2007; Flowers et al. 2008; Knobler et al. 2014; Salvaneschi et al. 2001; Kanold et al. 2007; Gonzalez-Vicent et al. 2008; Perotti et al. 2010; Malagola et al. 2016; Berger et al. 2015; Greinix et al. 1998, 2006b, 2011; Couriel et al. 2006; Dignan et al. 2012; Apisarnthanarax et al. 2003; Del Fante et al. 2012). Most of the clinical experience in ECP treatment of steroid-refractory cGvHD patients is based on retrospective analyses with consistently high response rates in up to 80% of patients with cutaneous manifestations and substantial improvement in sclerodermatous skin involvement (Greinix et al. 1998; Couriel et al. 2006; Apisarnthanarax et al. 2003; Bisaccia et al. 2006). Couriel and colleagues reported in 71 patients with steroid-refractory severe chronic GvHD a response rate of 61% and in sclerodermatous skin manifestations a higher response rate than in lichenoid ones (Couriel et al. 2006). Of note, patients with thrombocytopenia had an inferior outcome. Del Fante and colleagues retrospectively analysed data on 102 patients with cGvHD given ECP at their center (Del Fante et al. 2012). Complete and partial responses to ECP were achieved in 16 (15.7%) and 38 (37.3%) of patients, and median time to response was 1.2 (range, 0.2–16.8) months. In multivariate analysis, only response to ECP was significantly

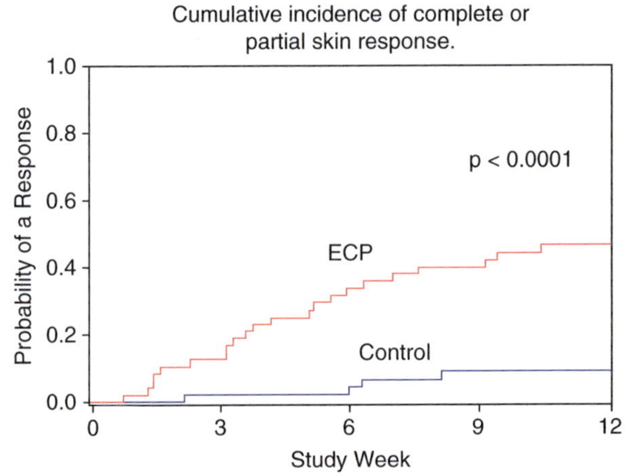

Fig. 13.9 Cumulative incidence of complete or partial skin response. Modified after reference (Flowers et al. 2008)

associated with survival. Improvements in quality of life and survival in ECP responders have also been reported by other investigators (Flowers et al. 2008; Messina et al. 2003; Greinix et al. 1998, 2006b).

Flowers and colleagues reported the first multicenter, randomized, controlled, prospective phase II study of ECP in 95 patients with steroid-refractory/dependent/intolerant cGvHD (Flowers et al. 2008). As primary efficacy endpoint of this study, a blinded quantitative comparison of percentage change from baseline in the total skin score (TSS) of 10 body regions at week 12 was defined. The median percentage improvement of TSS at week 12 was 15% and 9% for the ECP and the conventional therapy arm not significantly different. However, significantly, more patients in the ECP arm achieved a complete or partial response of cutaneous manifestations ($p < 0.001$, Fig. 13.9) as well as a 50% reduction in steroid dose and at least a 25% decrease in TSS ($p = 0.04$) by week 12, respectively. A steroid-sparing effect of ECP has also been reported by other investigators (Salvaneschi et al. 2001; Hautmann et al. 2013; Greinix et al. 1998, 2006b, 2011; Couriel et al. 2006; Foss et al. 2005; Jagasia et al. 2009).

In a subsequent prospective clinical study, 29 patients of the control arm not responding to conventional immunosuppressive therapy in the initial randomized trial were crossed over to open-label ECP in case of progression of cutaneous cGvHD or less than 15% improvement in the TSS by week 12 (Greinix et al. 2011). By week 24, 31% of patients achieved a complete or partial response of cutaneous manifestations to ECP treatment. Furthermore, responses to ECP in oral mucosa, eye, liver, and lung involvement were obtained in 70%, 47%, 50%, and 50% of patients, respectively (Fig. 13.10).

In a systematic review of prospective studies on the use of ECP in patients with cGvHD, Abu-Dalle and colleagues reported an ORR of 71% in cutaneous, 62% in gastrointestinal, 58% in hepatic, 63% in oral mucosal, and of 45% in musculoskeletal manifestations of cGvHD (Abu-Dalle et al. 2014). The rate of immunosuppression discontinuation was 23%, and ECP was tolerated excellently. In another meta-analysis, Malik and colleagues confirmed high response rates in cutaneous

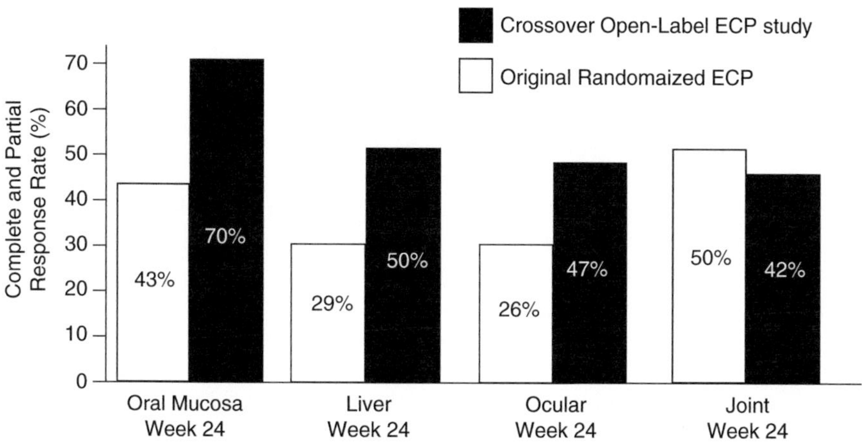

Fig. 13.10 Complete and partial response rates of extracutaneous manifestations of chronic GvHD to ECP: comparison of early versus late start of ECP. Early start represents patients given ECP in the initial randomized study, whereas late start of ECP represents patients initially given 12 weeks of non-ECP standard treatment and then crossed over to ECP therapy. Modified after reference (Greinix et al. 2011)

and extracutaneous manifestations of cGvHD including 48% of responses in lung involvement (Malik et al. 2014).

Use of ECP is limited in patients with pulmonary manifestations of cGvHD with around 135 reported patients achieving a response rate of 56% including complete and partial remissions, improvements, and stabilization of patients' pulmonary function (Flowers et al. 2008; Messina et al. 2003; Greinix et al. 2011; Couriel et al. 2006; Child et al. 1999; Dall'Amico et al. 1997b; Lucid et al. 2011; Brownback et al. 2016; Del Fante et al. 2016b). In view of the dismal prognosis of lung GvHD and the limited therapeutic options available for these patients, results of ECP in lung involvement by cGvHD are encouraging and support further prospective studies to determine its efficacy in a larger well-defined patient cohort.

ECP is a safe and efficacious treatment for patients with cGvHD with steroid-sparing capacity. Prospective clinical studies are warranted to assess the efficacy of ECP in well-defined cohorts of cGvHD patients treated earlier in the course of their disease. Recently, Jagasia and colleagues reported first results of a randomized, controlled multicentre study in NIH-defined moderate/severe cGvHD patients given ECP in the study arm in combination with standard of care immunosuppression (Jagasia et al. 2017). Besides an ORR of 74% and, thus, promising efficacy, ECP was demonstrated to be safe and tolerated well.

13.7 ECP for Prophylaxis of GvHD

Preliminary studies have investigated the use of ECP as part of the conditioning regimen prior to HCT in an attempt to reduce the incidence of aGvHD. Miller and colleagues reported a lower incidence of severe aGvHD when ECP was included in a novel reduced intensity conditioning (RIC) regimen with no negative impact on hematopoietic engraftment or recurrence of underlying malignant disease (Miller et al. 2004).

When ECP was incorporated into standard myeloablative conditioning in a phase II study and combined with cyclosporine A and methotrexate for GvHD prophylaxis, the incidence of aGvHD observed was similar to that found in studies without ECP (Shaughnessy et al. 2009). When the ECP-treated cohort was compared to historical controls, a lower incidence of grade 2 to 4 aGvHD and a longer OS was observed after use of ECP during conditioning. However, these data have to be confirmed in a larger patient number with a longer duration of follow-up.

In a prospective phase II clinical study, Kitko and colleagues investigated the combination of GvHD prophylaxis with tacrolimus, mycophenolate mofetil (MMF), etanercept, and ECP in 48 patients undergoing RIC unrelated donor transplantation (Kitko et al. 2016). Etanercept was given subcutaneously twice weekly from day 0 until day 56 after HCT for a total of 16 doses. ECP was started on day 28 on a weekly basis until day 70 and then tapered to every other week for another two treatments and then monthly until day 18 for a total of 11 or 12 ECP procedures. All patients engrafted neutrophils after a median of 12 days. The cumulative incidence of aGvHD grades 2–4 at day 100 was 46% and 84% of patients achieved a complete or partial response to first-line therapy with corticosteroids by day 56. Overall survival at 1 year was 73% with low rates of NRM (21%) and relapse (19%). However, cumulative incidences of NIH-defined moderate-to-severe cGvHD at 1 and 2 years were 42% and 58%, negatively impacting OS at 2 years that declined to 56%. Thus, this combination strategy was not able to efficiently prevent cGvHD. It is currently unclear whether more intense and/or prolonged ECP treatments might produce improved prophylactic efficacy and whether the combination of etanercept and ECP is an ideal one for this purpose.

Recently, Michallet and colleagues reported results of a prospective multicenter phase II study evaluating the safety and efficacy of prophylactic ECP in adult patients with hematological malignancies after RIC HCT starting ECP on day 21 after HCT twice per week for 2 weeks followed by once weekly for another 4 weeks for a total of eight courses of ECP (Michallet et al. 2018). Seventeen of twenty patients (85%) enrolled into the study received eight courses of ECP and tolerated these well and had uneventful hematopoietic engraftment. Seven patients developed aGvHD with 15% grade 2 or more by day 100. The cumulative incidence of cGvHD at 2 years was 22%, and OS and progression-free survival (PFS) at 2 years were 84% and 74%, respectively. This study showed promising results with low incidence rates of both acute and chronic GvHD and should be confirmed in a larger patient number.

13.8 Conclusions

ECP has been used for over 30 years in the treatment of CTCL, acute and chronic GvHD, and solid organ transplant rejection. Multiple scientific organizations recommend its use due to ECP's efficacy and excellent safety profile (Dittberner et al.

2002; Knobler et al. 2014; Martin et al. 2012; Kanold et al. 2007; Wolff et al. 2011; Schwartz et al. 2013; Pierelli et al. 2013; Alfred et al. 2017). Due to the lack of interactions with other agents and the avoidance of general immunosuppression, ECP compares favorably with other immunosuppressive strategies, supporting its increasingly frequent use as second-line therapy of steroid-refractory/dependent acute and chronic GvHD. Of note, the corticosteroid-sparing potential of ECP has been confirmed in numerous retrospective and prospective studies and translates into immediate clinical benefit for patients with GvHD as well as a reduction of transplant-associated morbidity and mortality.

No general recommendation can be made on treatment schedule due to missing evidence. Ideally, ECP treatment should be initiated as early as possible after the indication is confirmed. Especially in patients with steroid-refractory aGvHD, earlier treatment onset and an intensified ECP schedule resulted in improved response rates and patients' outcome. Prospective studies on the use of ECP as upfront treatment in GvHD are warranted as well as its investigation for prophylactic/preemptive use during allogeneic HCT.

References

Abu-Dalle I, Reljic T, Nishihori T et al (2014) Extracorporeal photopheresis in steroid-refractory acute or chronic graft-versus-host disease: results of a systematic review of prospective studies. Biol Blood Marrow Transplant 20:1677–1686

Alfred A, Taylor PC, Dignan F et al (2017) The role of extracorporeal photopheresis in the management of cutaneous T-cell lymphoma, graft-versus-host disease and organ transplant rejection: a consensus statement update from the UK Photopheresis Society. Brit J Haematol 177:287–310

Andreu G, Leon A, Heshmati F et al (1994) Extracorporeal photochemotherapy: evaluation of two techniques and use in connective tissue disorders. Transfus Sci 15:443–454

Apisarnthanarax N, Donato M, Korbling M et al (2003) Extracorporeal photopheresis therapy in the management of steroid-refractory or steroid-dependent cutaneous chronic graft-versus-host disease after allogeneic stem cell transplantation: feasibility and results. Bone Marrow Transplant 31:459–465

Apsner R, Uenver B, Sunder-Plassmann G et al (2002) Regional anticoagulation with acid citrate dextrose-A for extracorporeal photoimmunochemotherapy. Vox Sang 83:222–226

Berger C, Hoffmann K, Vasquez JG (2010) Rapid generation of maturationally synchronized human dendritic cells: contribution to the clinical efficacy of extracorporeal photochemotherapy. Blood 116:4838–4847

Berger M, Albiani R, Sini B, Fagioli F (2015) Extracorporeal photopheresis for graft-versus-host disease: the role of patient, transplant, and classification criteria and hematologic values on outcome-results from a large single-center study. Transfusion 55:736–747

Besnier DP, Chabannes D, Mahe B et al (1997) Treatment of graft-versus-host disease by extracorporeal photochemotherapy. Transplantation 64:49–54

Bethge W, Kerbauy FR, Santos EB (2014) Extracorporeal photopheresis combined with pentostatin in the conditioning regimen for canine hematopoietic cell transplantation does not prevent GVHD. Bone Marrow Transplant 49:1198–1204

Biagi E, Di Biaso I, Leoni V et al (2007) Extracorporeal photochemotherapy is accompanied by increasing levels of circulating CD4 + CD25 + GITR+Foxp3 + CD62L+ functional regulatory T-cells in patients with graft-versus-host disease. Transplantation 84:31–39

Bisaccia E, Palangio M, Gonzalez J et al (2006) Treatment of extensive chronic graft-versus-host disease with extracorporeal photochemotherapy. J Clin Apher 21:181–187

Bladon J, Taylor PC (1999) Extracorporeal photopheresis induces apoptosis in the lymphocytes of cutaneous T-cell lymphoma and graft-versus-host disease patients. Br J Haematol 107:707–711

Brosig A, Hähnel V, Orsó E et al (2016) Technical comparison of four different photopheresis systems. Transfusion 56:2510–2519

Brownback KR, Simpson SQ, Pitts LR et al (2016) Effect of extracorporeal photopheresis on lung function decline for severe bronchiolitis obliterans syndrome following allogeneic stem cell transplantation. J Clin Apher 31:347–352

Budde H, Kolb S, Salinas Tejedor L et al (2014) Modified extracorporeal photopheresis with cells from a healthy donor for acute graft-versus-host disease in a mouse model. PLoS One 9:e105896

Calore E, Calo A, Tridello G et al (2008) Extracorporeal photochemotherapy may improve outcome in children with acute GVHD. Bone Marrow Transplant 42:421–425

Calore E, Marson P, Pillon M et al (2015) Treatment of acute graft-versus-host disease in childhood with extracorporeal photochemotherapy/photopheresis: the Padova experience. Biol Blood Marrow Transplant 21:1963–1972

Cheung E, Baerlocher MO, Asch M et al (2009) Venous access. A practical review for 2009. Can Fam Physician 55:494–496

Child FJ, Ratnavel R, Watkins P et al (1999) Extracorporeal photopheresis (ECP) in the treatment of chronic graft-versus-host disease (GVHD). Bone Marrow Transplant 23:881–887

Cooke KR, Luznik L, Sarantopoulos S et al (2017) The biology of chronic graft-versus-host disease: a task force report from the National Institutes of Health consensus development project on criteria for clinical trials in chronic graft-versus-host disease. Biol Blood Marrow Transplant 23:211–234

Couriel DR, Hosing C, Saliba R et al (2006) Extracorporeal photochemotherapy for the treatment of steroid-resistant chronic GVHD. Blood 107:3074–3080

Dall'Amico R, Messina C (2002) Extracorporeal photochemotherapy for the treatment of graft-versus-host disease. Ther Apher 6:296–304

Dall'Amico R, Rosetti F, Zulian F et al (1997a) Photopheresis in pediatric patients with drug-resistant chronic graft-versus-host disease. Br J Hematol 97:848–854

Dall'Amico R, Rossetti F, Zulian F et al (1997b) Photopheresis in pediatric patients with drug-resistant chronic graft-versus-host disease. Brit J Haematol 97:848–854

Das-Gupta E, Greinix H, Jacobs R et al (2014) Extracorporeal photopheresis as second-line treatment for acute graft-versus-host disease: Impact on six month freedom from treatment failure. Haematologica 99:1746–1752

Del Fante C, Scudeller L, Virengo G et al (2012) Response and survival of patients with chronic graft-versus-host disease treated by extracorporeal photochemotherapy: a retrospective study according to classical and National Institutes of Health consensus. Transfusion 52:2007–2015

Del Fante C, Scudeller L, Martinasso A et al (2016a) Comparison of two automated mononuclear cell collection systems in patients undergoing extracorporeal photopheresis: a prospective crossover equivalence study. Transfusion 56:2078–2084

Del Fante C, Galasso T, Bernasconi P et al (2016b) Extracorporeal photopheresis as a new supportive therapy for bronchiolitis obliterans syndrome after allogeneic stem cell transplantation. Bone Marrow Transplant 51:728–731

Dignan FL, Greenblatt D, Cox M et al (2012) Efficacy of bimonthly extracorporeal photopheresis in refractory chronic mucocutaneous GVHD. Bone Marrow Transplant 47:824–830

Dignan FL, Aguilar S, Scarisbrick JJ et al (2014) Impact of extracorporeal photopheresis on skin scores and quality of life in patients with steroid-refractory chronic GVHD. Bone Marrow Transplant 49:704–708

Dittberner T, Schöttler E, Ranze O et al (2002) Heparin-induced thrombocytopenia: a complication in extracorporeal photochemotherapy (photopheresis). J Am Acad Dermatol 47:452–453

Edelson RL (2014) Mechanistic insights into extracorporeal photochemotherapy: efficient induction of monocyte-to-dendritic cell maturation. Transfus Apher Sci 50:322–329

Edelson R, Berger C, Gasparro F et al (1987) Treatment of cutaneous T-cell lymphoma by extracorporeal photochemotherapy. Preliminary results. N Engl J Med 316:297–303

Enomoto DNH, Schellekens PTA, Yong S-L et al (1997) Extracorporeal photochemotherapy (photopheresis) induces apoptosis in lymphocytes: a possible mechanism of action of PUVA therapy. Photochem Photobiol 65:177–180

Ferrara JL, Levine JE, Reddy P, Holler E (2009) Graft-versus-host disease. Lancet 373:1550–1561

Filipovich AH, Weisdorf D, Pavletic S et al (2005) National Institutes of Health Consensus Development Project on criteria for clinical trials in chronic graft-versus-host disease: I. Diagnosis and Staging Working Group Report. Biol Blood Marrow Transplant 11:945–955

Flinn AM, Gennery AR (2017) Treatment of pediatric acute graft-versus-host disease-lessons from primary immunodeficiency? Front Immunol 8:328–338

Florek M, Sega EI, Leveson-Gower DB et al (2014) Autologous apoptotic cells preceding transplantation enhance survival in lethal murine graft-versus-host models. Blood 124:1832–1842

Flowers MED, Apperley J, von Besien K et al (2008) A multicenter prospective phase 2 randomized study of extracorporeal photopheresis for treatment of chronic graft-versus-host disease. Blood 112:2667–2674

Flowers MED, Inamoto Y, Carpenter PA et al (2011) Comparative analysis of risk factors for acute graft-versus-host disease and for chronic graft-versus-host disease according to National Institute of Health consensus criteria. Blood 117:3214–3219

Foss FM, DiVenuti GM, Chin K et al (2005) Prospective study of extracorporeal photopheresis in steroid-refractory or steroid-resistant extensive chronic graft-versus-host disease: analysis of response and survival incorporating prognostic factors. Bone Marrow Transplant 35:1187–1193

Franklin C, Cesko E, Hillen U et al (2015) Modulation and apoptosis of neutrophil granulocytes by extracorporeal photopheresis in the treatment of chronic graft- versus-host disease. PLoS One 10(8):e0134518. https://doi.org/10.1371/journal.pone.0134518

Galloway S, Bodenham A (2004) Long-term central venous access. Br J Anaesth 92:722–734

Garban F, Drillat P, Makowski C et al (2005) Extracorporeal chemophototherapy for the treatment of graft-versus-host disease: hematologic consequences of short-term, intensive courses. Haematologica 90:1096–1101

Garban F, Makowski C, Carras S et al (2014) Extracorporeal photopheresis: scientific and technical considerations for improving clinical management of patients. J Stem Cell Res Ther 4:232–236

Gatza E, Rogers CE, Clouthier SG et al (2008) Extracorporeal photopheresis reverses experimental graft-versus-host disease through regulatory T cells. Blood 112:1515–1521

Gerber M, Gmeinhart B, Volc-Platzer B et al (1997) Complete remission of lichen-planus-like graft-versus-host-disease (GVHD) with extracorporeal photochemotherapy (ECP). Bone Marrow Transplant 19:517–519

Gonzalez-Vicent M, Ramirez M, Perez A et al (2008) Extracorporeal photochemotherapy for steroid-refractory graft-versus-host disease in low-weight pediatric patients. Immunomodulatory effects and clinical outcome. Haematologica 93:1278–1280

Greinix HT, Volc-Platzer B, Rabitsch W et al (1998) Successful use of extracorporeal photochemotherapy in the treatment of severe acute and chronic graft-versus-host disease. Blood 92:3098–3104

Greinix HT, Knobler RM, Worel N et al (2006a) The effect of intensified extracorporeal photochemotherapy on long-term survival in patients with severe acute graft-versus-host disease. Haematol 91:405–408

Greinix HT, Socie G, Bacigalupo A et al (2006b) Assessing the potential role of photopheresis in hematopoietic stem cell transplant. Bone Marrow Transplant 38:265–273

Greinix HT, Worel N, Knobler R (2010) Role of extracorporeal photopheresis (ECP) in treatment of steroid-refractory acute graft-versus-host disease. Biol Blood Marrow Transplant 16:1747–1748

Greinix HT, van Besien K, Elmaagacli AH et al (2011) Progressive improvement in cutaneous and extracutaneous chronic graft-versus-host disease after a 24-week course of extracorporeal photopheresis–results of a crossover randomized study. Biol Blood Marrow Transplant 17:1775–1782

Greinix HAT, Kuzmina Z, Weigl R et al (2015) $CD19^{+}CD21^{low}$ B cells and $CD4^{+}CD45RA^{+}CD31^{+}$ T cells correlate with first diagnosis of chronic graft-versus-host disease. Biol Blood Marrow Transplant 21:250–258

Hackstein H, Amoros JJV, Bein G et al (2014) Successful use of miniphotopheresis for the treatment of graft-versus-host disease. Transfusion 54:2022–2027

Hannani D (2015) Extracorporeal photopheresis: tolerogenic or immunogenic cell death? Beyond current dogma. Front Immunol 6:349–352

Hautmann AH, Wolff D, Hahn J et al (2013) Extracorporeal photopheresis in 62 patients with acute and chronic GVHD: Results of treatment with the COBE Spectra system. Bone Marrow Transplant 48:439–445

Heng AE, Sauvezie B, Genestier L et al (2003) PUVA apoptotic response in activated and resting human lymphocytes. Transfus Apher Sci 28:43–50

Ivancic E, Knobler R, Quehenberger P et al (2005) The course of anticoagulation after extracorporeal photochemotherapy. Photoderm Photoimmunol Photomed 21:150–151

Jagasia MH, Savani BN, Stricklin G et al (2009) Classic and overlap chronic graft-versus-host disease (cGVHD) is associated with superior outcome after extracorporeal photopheresis (ECP). Biol Blood Marrow Transplant 15:1288–1295

Jagasia M, Arora M, Flowers MED et al (2012) Risk factors for acute GVHD and survival after hematopoietic cell transplantation. Blood 119:296–307

Jagasia M, Greinix H, Robin M et al (2013) Extracorporeal photopheresis versus anticytokine therapy as a second-line treatment for steroid-refractory acute GVHD: A multicentre comparative analysis. Biol Blood Marrow Transplant 19:1124–1133

Jagasia MH, Greinix HT, Arora M et al (2015) National Institutes of Health Consensus Development Project on criteria for clinical trials in chronic graft-versus-host disease: I. The 2014 Diagnosis and Staging Working Group Report. Biol Blood Marrow Transplant 21:389–401

Jagasia M, Greinix H, Scheid C et al (2017) A randomized controlled study of extracorporeal photopheresis (ECP) therapy with UVADEX (methoxsalen) for National Institutes of Health (NIH)-graded moderate to severe chronic graft-versus-host disease (cGvHD). Blood 130:1970

Joly E, Hudrisier D (2003) What is trogocytosis and what is its purpose? Nat Immunol 4:815

Kanold J, Merlin E, Halle P et al (2007) Photopheresis in pediatric graft-versus-host disease after allogeneic marrow transplantation: clinical practice guidelines based on field experience and review of the literature. Transfusion 47:2276–2289

Kitko CL, Levine JE (2015) Extracorporeal photopheresis in prevention and treatment of acute GVHD. Transfus Apher Sci 52:151–156

Kitko CL, Braun T, Couriel DR et al (2016) Combination therapy for graft-versus-host disease prophylaxis with etanercept and extracorporeal photopheresis: results of a phase II clinical trial. Biol Blood Marrow Transplant 22:862–868

Knobler RM, Trautinger F, Graninger W et al (1993) Parenteral application of 8-methoxypsoralen during photopheresis. J Am Acad Dermatol 28:580–584

Knobler R, Berlin G, Calzavara-Pinton P et al (2014) Guidelines on the use of extracorporeal photopheresis. J Eur Acad Dermatol Venereol 28(Suppl 1):1–37

Kuzmina Z, Greinix HT, Weigl R et al (2011) Significant differences in B-cell subpopulations characterize patients with chronic graft-versus-host disease-associated dysgammaglobulinemia. Blood 117:2265–2274

Lamioni A, Parisi F, Isacchi G et al (2005) The immunological effects of extracorporeal photopheresis unraveled: induction of tolerogenic dendritic cells in vitro and regulatory T-cells in vivo. Transplantation 79:846–850

Lee SJ, Klein JP, Barrett AJ et al (2002) Severity of chronic graft-versus-host disease: association with treatment-related mortality and relapse. Blood 100:406–414

Levine JE, Logan B, Wu J et al (2010) Graft-versus-host disease treatment: predictors of survival. Biol Blood Marrow Transplant 16:1693–1699

Lucid CE, Savani BN, Engelhardt BG et al (2011) Extracorporeal photopheresis in patients with refractory bronchiolitis obliterans developing after allo-SCT. Bone Marrow Transplant 46:426–429

MacMillan M, DeFor TE, Weisdorf DJ (2010) The best endpoint for acute GVHD treatment trials. Blood 115:5412–5417

Malagola M, Cancelli V, Skert C et al (2016) Extracorporeal photopheresis for treatment of acute and chronic graft versus host disease: an Italian multicentric retrospective analysis on 94 patients on behalf of the Gruppo Italiano Trapianto di Midollo Osseo. Transplantation 100:e147–e155

Malik MI, Litzow M, Hogan W et al (2014) Extracorporeal photopheresis for chronic graft-versus-host disease: a systematic review and meta-analysis. Blood Res 49:100–106

Martin PJ, Carpenter PA, Sanders JE, Flowers ME (2004) Diagnosis and clinical management of chronic graft-versus-host disease. Int J Hematol 79:221–228

Martin PJ, Rizzo JD, Wingard JR et al (2012) First-and second-line systemic treatment of acute graft-versus-host disease: recommendations of the American Society of Blood and Marrow Transplantation. Biol Blood Marrow Transplant 18:1150–1163

Martin PJ, Storer BE, Inamoto Y et al (2017) An endpoint associated with clinical benefit after initial treatment of chronic graft-versus-host disease. Blood 130:360–367

Merlin E, Goncalves-Mendes N, Hannani D et al (2011) Extracorporeal photochemotherapy induces arginase 1 in patients with graft versus host disease. Transplant Immunol 24:100–106

Messina C, Locatelli F, Lanino E et al (2003) Extracorporeal photochemotherapy for paediatric patients with graft-versus-host disease after haematopoietic stem cell transplantation. Br J Haematol 122:118–127

Michallet M, Sobh M, Garban F et al (2018) Extracorporeal photopheresis for GVHD prophylaxis after reduced intensity conditioning allogeneic hematopoietic stem cell transplantation: a prospective multicenter phase 2 study. Leuk Lymph 59:372–380

Miller KB, Roberts TF, Chan G et al (2004) A novel reduced intensity regimen for allogeneic hematopoietic stem cell transplantation associated with a reduced incidence of graft-versus-host disease. Bone Marrow Transplant 33:881–889

Nedelcu E, Ziman A, Fernando LP et al (2008) Exclusive use of acid citrate dextrose for extracorporeal photopheresis in patients with contraindications to heparin: an effective protocol. J Clin Aph 23:66–73

Perfetti P, Carlier P, Strada P et al (2008) Extracorporeal photopheresis for the treatment of steroid refractory acute GVHD. Bone Marrow Transplant 42:609–617

Perotti C, Del Fante C, Tinelli C et al (2010) Extracorporeal photochemotherapy in graft-versus-host disease: a longitudinal study on factors influencing the response and survival in pediatric patients. Transfusion 50:1359–1369

Perseghin P, Galimberti S, Balduzzi A et al (2007) Extracorporeal photochemotherapy for the treatment of chronic graft-versus-host disease: trend for a possible cell dose-related effect? Ther Apher Dial 11:85–93

Pierelli L, Perseghin P, Marchetti M et al (2013) Extracorporeal photopheresis for the treatment of acute and chronic graft-versus-host disease in adults and children: best practice recommendations from an Italian Society of Hemapheresis and Cell Manipulation (SIdEM) and Italian Group for Bone Marrow Transplantation (GITMO) consensus process. Transfusion 53:2340–2352

Quaglino P, Comessatti A, Ponti R et al (2009) Reciprocal modulation of circulating CD4+CD25+bright T cells induced by extracorporeal photochemotherapy in cutaneous T-cell lymphoma and chronic graft-versus-host-disease patients. Int J Immunopathol Pharmacol 22:353–362

Rieber N, Wecker I, Neri D et al (2014) Extracorporeal photopheresis increases neutrophilic myeloid-derived suppressor cells in patients with GvHD. Bone Marrow Transplant 49:545–552

Rubegni P, Cuccia A, Sbano P et al (2005) Role of extracorporeal photochemotherapy in patients with refractory chronic graft-versus-host disease. Br J Haematol 130:271–275

Salvaneschi L, Perotti C, Zecca M et al (2001) Extracorporeal photochemotherapy for treatment of acute and chronic GVHD in childhood. Transfusion 41:1299–1305

Schmitt S, Johnson TS, Karakhanova S et al (2009) Extracorporeal photopheresis augments function of CD4 + CD25 + FoxP3 + regulatory T cells by triggering adenosine production. Transplantation 88:411–416

Schooneman F (2003) Extracorporeal photopheresis technical aspects. Transfus Apher Sci 28:51–61

Schwartz J, Winters JL, Padmanabhan A et al (2013) Clinical applications of therapeutic apheresis: an evidence based approach, 6th edition. J Clin Apheresis 28:145–284

Seaton ED, Szydlo RM, Kanfer E et al (2003) Influence of extracorporeal photopheresis on clinical and laboratory parameters in chronic graft-versus-host disease and analysis of predictors of response. Blood 102:1217–1223

Setterblad N, Garban F, Weigl R et al (2008) Extracorporeal photopheresis increases sensitivity of monocytes from patients with graft-versus-host disease to HLA-DR-mediated cell death. Transfusion 48:169–177

Shaughnessy PJ, Bolwell BJ, van Besien K et al (2009) Extracorporeal photopheresis for the prevention of acute GVHD in patients undergoing standard myeloablative conditioning and allogeneic hematopoietic stem cell transplantation. Bone Marrow Transplant 45:1068–1076

Socie G, Stone JV, Wingard JR et al (1999) Long-term survival and late deaths after allogeneic bone marrow transplantation. Late effects working committee of the International bone marrow transplant registry. N Engl J Med 341:14–21

Spisek R, Gasova Z, Bartunkova J (2006) Maturation state of dendritic cells during the extracorporeal photopheresis and its relevance for the treatment of chronic graft-versus-host disease. Transfusion 46:55–65

Stewart BL, Storer B, Storek J et al (2004) Duration of immunosuppressive treatment for chronic graft-versus-host disease. Blood 104:3501–3506

Tsirigotis P, Kapsimalli V, Baltadakis I et al (2012) Extracorporeal photopheresis in refractory chronic graft-versus-host disease: the influence on peripheral blood T cell subpopulations. A study by the Hellenic Association of Hematology. Transfus Apher Sci 46:181–188

Ussowicz M, Musiał J, Mielcarek M et al (2013) Steroid-sparing effect of extracorporeal photopheresis in the therapy of graft-versus-host disease after allogeneic hematopoietic stem cell transplantation. Transplant Proc 45:3375–3380

Van Lint MT, Milone G, Leotta S et al (2006) Treatment of acute graft-versus-host disease with prednisolone: significant survival advantage for day +5 responders and no advantage for nonresponders receiving anti-thymocyte globulin. Blood 107:4177–4181

Wolff D, Gerbitz A, Ayuk F et al (2010) Consensus Conference on clinical practice in chronic graft-versus-host disease (GVHD): first-line and topical treatment of chronic GVHD. Biol Blood Marrow Transplant 16:1611–1628

Wolff D, Schleuning M, von Harsdorf S et al (2011) Consensus conference on clinical practice in chronic GVHD: second-line treatment of chronic graft-versus-host disease. Biol Blood Marrow Transplant 17:1–17

Wolff D, Ayuk F, Elmaagacli A et al (2013) Current practice in diagnosis and treatment of acute graft-versus-host disease: Results from a survey among German-Austrian-Swiss hematopoietic stem cell transplant centers. Biol Blood Marrow Transplant 19:767–776

Yakut E, Jakobs C, Peric A et al (2015) Extracorporeal photopheresis promotes IL-1beta production. J Immunol 194:2569–2577

Prevention and Management of Apheresis Complications

14

Marleen M. Neyrinck and Hans Vrielink

14.1 Introduction

The majority of apheresis procedures performed for both therapeutic and collection purpose are completed without complications. However, both expected and unexpected side effects can occur anytime. Furthermore, various factors may increase the risk of adverse events during apheresis therapy. These examples include, but are not limited to, environment, staff, and type of apheresis procedure, replacement fluids, anticoagulation, and the comorbidities of the donor or the patient. Furthermore, adverse events can occur during or after apheresis procedure and may not specifically be related to the apheresis procedure itself (e.g., hematomas or infection from access). However, all adverse events must be appropriately treated and documented to prevent future events. Thus, anticipation of potential adverse events and, therefore, earlier recognition and possibilities to diminish the severity need a thorough understanding by the apheresis practitioner. In this chapter, many variations of side effects that can occur during an apheresis procedure are discussed.

14.2 An Overview of Types and Severity of Complications

The complications can be of immunologic (e.g., hemolytic or anaphylactic transfusion reactions and reaction to ethylene oxide) or non-immunologic (hematomas, bleeding complications, and vasovagal reactions) origins. Side effects can also be

M. M. Neyrinck
Department of Hematology, AZ Delta, Roeselare, Belgium
e-mail: marleen.neyrinck@azdelta.be

H. Vrielink (✉)
Unit of Transfusion Medicine, Sanquin Blood Supply, Amsterdam, The Netherlands
e-mail: h.vrielink@sanquin.nl

S. A. Abutalib et al. (eds.), *Best Practices of Apheresis in Hematopoietic Cell Transplantation*, Advances and Controversies in Hematopoietic Transplantation and Cell Therapy, https://doi.org/10.1007/978-3-319-55131-9_14

categorized as systemic and/or local and acute or delayed as some side effects may occur many days after the therapeutic apheresis procedure. The severity of adverse events is typically categorized as mild, moderate, or severe. Mild and moderate reactions are much more common than severe reactions. Mild reactions are usually limited to mild paresthesia, pallor, weakness, intermittent dizziness, sweating, nausea, and/or an episode of vomiting, transient hypotension, light-headedness, hyperventilation, and asymptomatic bradycardia. Moderate reactions may be defined as mild reaction with symptoms that do not respond to routine nursing interventions (per standard operating procedure [SOP]) and require clinician at the bedside and might require termination, either briefly or permanently, of apheresis procedure. Severe reactions require immediate termination of procedure. Severe reactions may be characterized by long-lasting unconsciousness, convulsions, tetany due to severe hypocalcemia, incontinence, and, in rare occasions, death. Surveillance and acknowledgment of such side effects require well-trained apheresis staff, nursing, and clinicians.

14.2.1 Reactions of Immunologic Origin

14.2.1.1 Etiology, Identification, and Prevention

The majority of immunologic reactions seen by the apheresis practitioner are transfusion reactions secondary to the use of blood components during the procedure, as either a priming or replacement fluid. Transfusion reactions can be seen after transfusion of all blood components and can be acute (occurring within 24 h of transfusion), delayed (within 3–14 days), or late (after many years, such as transfusion-transmitted viral infection). Typically, institutional transfusion protocols shall be followed with at least vital signs recorded at regular intervals to monitor for reactions. The frequency of such monitoring depends on the type of procedure performed, the patient's hemodynamic condition and comorbidities, and institutional policies.

Based on the international hemovigilance reports, hemolytic transfusion reaction can be caused by human errors. Around 1 in 13,000 blood component units is transfused to the wrong patient (not always with adverse consequences), and up to 1 in 1300 pre-transfusion blood samples is taken from the wrong patient (http://www.transfusionguidelines.org.uk/transfusion-handbook/5-adverse-effects-of-transfusion n.d.). The error can be made by the health-care staff collecting the tubes for laboratory testing (misidentification of the patient, mislabeling on tubes), in the laboratory or immediately prior to the transfusion (misidentification of the patient to be transfused). When in apheresis procedures blood components are used for replacement fluid all good nursing practices associated with blood administration must be performed. All individuals involved need to be alert. All blood handling (labeling, sampling) needs to be checked carefully based on institutional policy to prevent clerical errors that may lead to adverse event(s). In addition to clerical errors, the majority of transfusion reactions are related to acute hemolysis, sepsis due to bacterial contamination of blood products, transfusion-associated circulatory overload (TACO), and transfusion-related acute lung injury (TRALI). Less common but more severe are allergic reactions, posttransfusion purpura, and transfusion-associated graft-versus-host disease (Ta-GvHD).

When a patient develops new signs and symptoms during or after the administration of a blood component, a transfusion reaction should be suspected, and blood administration shall be stopped immediately. All suspected transfusion reactions, including those during an apheresis procedure, should be reported to the hospital transfusion service, and it is advised also to report to a regional and/or national hemovigilance system depending on the regulations. Posttransfusion blood samples need to be drawn from the patient for laboratory tests used to investigate the cause of the observed transfusion reaction, especially to rule out hemolytic transfusion reaction. It is also advisable to notify the physician covering the transfusion service.

14.2.1.2 Immune-Mediated Hemolytic Transfusion Reaction: Early Versus Delayed Reaction

The most severe and feared immune-mediated hemolytic transfusion reaction is an intravascular destruction of red blood cells (i.e., hemolysis), which can be either acute or delayed and can lead to mortality or significant morbidity. Acute reactions are usually caused by IgM antibodies present in the patient's plasma directed against the ABO-incompatible or IgG antibodies directed against other red blood cell antigen-incompatible donor erythrocytes. Less commonly, the acute hemolysis is caused by antibodies present in transfused donor plasma directed against the patient's RBCs. This intravascular hemolysis may normally occur during or immediately after the transfusion and may be seen during therapeutic apheresis procedures. Other causes of hemolysis include thermal effects (storage and/or heating during administration by incorrectly working blood warmers), infusion of hypotonic or hypertonic solutions with a blood product, or rarely by contamination by microorganisms.

During intravascular hemolysis, the RBCs lyse, and hemoglobin is released into the circulation. Free hemoglobin protein is bound to haptoglobin and removed from circulation by the reticuloendothelial system. Massive intravascular hemolysis may overwhelm hemoglobin clearance mechanisms leading to accumulation of excess of free hemoglobin. The circulating free hemoglobin may result in acute kidney injury resulting from direct proximal tubular cell toxicity through generation of radical oxygen species, cast formation and subsequent tubular obstruction, and vasoconstriction resulting from free hemoglobin scavenging of nitric oxide. Symptoms associated with intravascular hemolysis include fever, chills, hypotension (can lead to shock), tachycardia, back pain, headache, nausea, and hemoglobinuria and can lead to disseminated intravascular coagulation (DIC) and multi-organ failure causing mortality. Treatment includes immediate discontinuation of the transfusion, fluid administration, and catecholamine support with continuous vital monitoring. Laboratory evaluation in these cases should include a direct antiglobulin test (DAT), repeated compatibility testing (e.g., crossmatching donor units with pre- and post-transfusion blood from the patient), complete blood count, lactate dehydrogenase

(LDH), bilirubin, haptoglobin levels, and an urine analysis for the presence of hemoglobinuria.

Delayed hemolytic transfusion reactions are frequently unnoticed but may occur 1–4 weeks after transfusion and usually appear as extravascular hemolysis. In extravascular hemolysis, red blood cells are phagocytized by macrophages in the spleen and liver and are therefore less clinically significant. Delayed reactions result from either development of a new red blood cell antibody (IgG) or the anamnestic response of a preformed antibody following antigen re-exposure through transfusion. The majority of patients with delayed hemolytic reactions only require close monitoring of the hemoglobin, however, anamnestic response due to anti-Kidd antibody may cause intravascular hemolysis.

14.2.1.3 Transfusion-Related Acute Lung Injury (TRALI)

Another acute complication after transfusion is TRALI. TRALI is usually caused by donor antibodies to the patient's human leukocyte antigens (HLA) and/or human neutrophilic antigens (HNA). These antibodies result in activation of the patient's neutrophils, which damage pulmonary endothelium and lead to pulmonary edema. According to the international consensus (Kleinman et al. 2004), a diagnosis of TRALI requires new acute lung injury occurring within 6 h of transfusion, evidenced by hypoxia and bilateral pulmonary infiltrates on the chest X-ray, as well as the absence of preexisting acute lung injury or other risk factors for pulmonary edema. Treatment for TRALI is supportive with the symptoms usually resolving within 48–96 h from onset. It's often difficult to distinguish TRALI from transfusion-associated circulatory overload (TACO) which is also a frequent complication seen during or after transfusion. The patients with TACO are usually hypertensive and have tachycardia. Treatment of TACO is diuresis and/or slowing the infusion rate (or possibly terminating the transfusion and the therapeutic apheresis procedure), while in TRALI, diuresis is contraindicated.

14.2.1.4 Transfusion-Associated Graft-Versus-Host Disease (Ta-GvHD)

A severe delayed complication of transfusion of cellular blood components in immunocompromised patients is the Ta-GvHD. Ta-GvHD arises when transfused alloreactive T lymphocytes (in the graft) attack the patient's cells (the host). Since the patient is immunosuppressed, the patient's immune systems fail to eliminate the transfused T-cells. Instead, the surviving donor's T-cells attack recipient cells that have mismatched HLA antigens. Ta-GvHD can be seen in patients with congenital or acquired immunodeficiency and patients who undergo intensive chemotherapy or transplantation (need for immunosuppressive drugs) and receive blood components with viable T lymphocytes. Symptoms will start usually 1–2 weeks after the transfusion. Target organs are the skin, intestine, liver, and bone marrow. Characteristics for the Ta-GvHD are fever, skin rash, and diarrhea. Laboratory tests reveal signs of bone marrow failure (pancytopenia due to donor's T-cell alloreactivity) and liver malfunction. Ta-GvHD is associated with high mortality rate since there is no effective treatment.

As leukocyte-reduced cellular components contain sufficient T-cells to cause Ta-GvHD, leukocyte reduction of the blood components is not an optimal strategy to prevent such complication. Only irradiation of cellular blood products can prevent Ta-GvHD. Following irradiation of cellular blood components with at least 25 Gy, the T-cells in these blood components are no longer able to divide and, therefore, unable to cause Ta-GvHD. Hence, established guidelines for irradiation of blood products in these patients shall be followed. In case of peripheral blood $CD34^+$ cell donation, all persons (donating autologous or allogeneic $CD34^+$ cells) in need of transfusion of cellular blood components should solely receive irradiated blood components from a period of 3 months before donation until end of donation. Also when the apheresis machine needs to be primed with blood in case of pediatric or small-size donors, irradiated blood must be used.

14.2.1.5 Other Immunologic Reactions

If plasma-containing blood products are transfused during apheresis, allergic and anaphylactic reactions are also potential complications caused by plasma proteins. Symptoms of a mild allergic transfusion reaction include vasodilatation, edema, and erythema. Additional symptoms can include pruritus, urticaria, and headache. Localized allergic reactions may be treated with antihistamines and/or steroids and, if necessary, a short interruption of the procedure. Rarely, allergic reactions during an apheresis procedure can be caused by ethylene oxide (ETO), a gas used for the sterilization of the disposable. Symptoms of an anaphylactic reaction include dyspnea, wheezing, severe hypotension, bronchospasm, bronchospasm, and shock. The specific allergen causing the anaphylaxis is often unknown, but these patients should be worked up for IgA deficiency and IgA antibodies, and it may be worthwhile gathering other history in regard to allergies from the patient. It is also important to obtain the history of medication that the patient may take prior to or during the procedure since the reaction may be related to the medication and not the procedure itself. Treatment of an anaphylactic reaction includes immediate discontinuation of the procedure and immediate aggressive resuscitation support. Significant allergic reactions may warrant premedication with antihistamines and/or steroids prior to future apheresis procedures, but this may be nowadays routine in procedures with blood component infusion in many centers. In case of significant allergic reactions in donor apheresis procedures, it is advised to refrain from donation.

14.2.2 Reactions of Non-immunologic Origin

14.2.2.1 Bacterial Infections and Sepsis

Blood components can be contaminated from many sources. In developed countries, traditional transfusion-transmitted infections as human immunodeficiency virus (HIV) and the hepatitis viruses are extremely rare. On the contrary, bacterial infections are rather common and can lead to severe morbidity and mortality. Bacterial contaminations of blood components are most often derived from the collection line especially if the skin decontamination prior to venipuncture is not done properly. The normal skin flora, such as the coagulase-negative staphylococci, rarely produces severe infections, although febrile reactions may occur. Different pathogenic bacteria can be derived from an asymptomatic infection present in the donor during donation. Some of them may lead to life-threatening reactions. Other sources of bacteria include incorrect sterilization of the collection bags and contamination during the preparation of the blood components. Transfusion-related sepsis is more common with platelet transfusions than with other blood products because of their storage temperature at 20–24 °C. However, red blood cell unit can also be contaminated with bacteria, such as gram-negative ones. Symptoms include rapid onset of fever, rigors, abdominal cramping, and hypotension (even septic shock) and may be indistinguishable for many causes of immunologic reactions described above. Disseminated intravascular coagulopathy (DIC) can also occur. It is important to immediately stop the apheresis procedure to limit the amount of possibly contaminated blood. The needle should be kept intravenously and open with saline in the likely event that medications may need to be rapidly administered. Fluid resuscitation is also useful to treat hypotension and stimulate urine production. Further treatment includes supportive care, including intravenous fluids, as well as administration of appropriate antimicrobial agents. It is important to note that similar “transfusion bacterial contamination type” reactions can be observed if the infected central venous line (mostly in patients if the line is already inserted for a long time) is used. Therefore, it is important to culture both the patient (before antibiotics is given) and the blood product, when available, if transfusion-related sepsis is suspected. Usually the organisms grew must be identical between the infected unit and the patient’s blood in order to confirm bacterial contamination from the transfused unit.

14.2.2.2 Reactions Related to Volume Shifts During Apheresis

Volume shifts normally occur during any apheresis procedure. It is critical to consider the patient’s total blood volume, the extracorporeal blood volume during the apheresis procedure, and the hemodynamic changes during the procedure. For example, it is important to ensure that the extracorporeal volume (ECV) and red cell volume is within the 15% of the patient’s total blood volume and total red cell volume during the procedure, respectively. If the volume removed is more than 15% of the patient’s blood volume, then crystalloid or colloid fluids shall be given to avoid hypotension. It should be noted that in certain patients (older age, vasoactive medication, sepsis), the compensatory mechanisms may be less effective, and in pediatric apheresis where the disposable is primed with blood components prior to the procedure, no rinse back should be performed after the procedure to avoid extra fluid being given.

Hypotension during an apheresis procedure may be associated with a vasovagal reaction, citrate toxicity, anaphylaxis, or hypovolemia secondary to volume loss. Contemporary apheresis machines are designed to use less extracorporeal volume (ECV) than earlier versions, which helps to minimize the risk of a hypovolemic side effect. However, especially in small children, the ECV of the apheresis circuit can be relatively high.

Hypotension due to hypovolemia is characterized by a hypotension with tachycardia and tachypnea. In contrast, vasovagal reactions, which are also associated with hypotension, are characterized by concurrent bradycardia. In patients of low total blood volume (TBV) (low body weight or pediatric patient), it may be necessary to prime the extracorporeal circuit with 5% albumin or RBCs to avoid adverse events. To treat hypotension due to intravascular volume depletion, the procedure is usually paused temporarily, and the patient is given a fluid bolus and assessed by the supervising physician.

At the end of the apheresis procedure, the apheresis operator must calculate the patient's net fluid balance. Fluid delivery varies depending on the apheresis device utilized and the type of procedure performed. Volume lost secondary to vomiting, diarrhea, and perspiration should also be taken into account. The net difference between these total "remove" and "replace" volumes should be calculated, documented, and communicated to the clinical service to include in tracking of the patient's fluid intake and output.

14.2.3 Hypotension During Apheresis While on ACE Inhibitors

Hypotension during apheresis procedures can also be seen in individuals taking angiotensin-converting enzyme (ACE) inhibitors 48–72 h prior to the procedure. These medications are used primarily for the treatment of hypertension by inhibiting the vasoconstriction. Besides that, ACE inhibitors also decrease the ability to inactivate bradykinin. Bradykinin triggers an increased vascular permeability and dilatation of the blood vessels resulting in decreasing the blood pressure. Release of bradykinin is caused by the activation of the kinin system, and activation of this system can be initiated by apheresis due to contact with negatively charged plastic disposable kits or the LDL apheresis column, as well as activation of pre-kallikrein-activating factor which is present in albumin. Hypotensive reactions, bradycardia, flushing, and dyspnea have been reported in patients receiving blood products and therapeutic plasma exchanges (TPE). Since apheresis is an elective procedure, ACE inhibitor should be held approximately 24 h prior to the procedure. Angiotensin receptor blockers are acceptable alternative to ACE inhibitors during the treatment period. If the procedure is emergent and the patient has taken an ACE within 24 h, plasma may be used as a replacement fluid to avoid the potential refractory hypotension caused by this medication.

14.2.4 Vasovagal Reaction During Apheresis

A vasovagal reaction is a reflex of the parasympathetic nervous system (vagal nerve), usually following activation of the sympathetic nervous system which can be triggered by anxiety, pain (from line placement) associated with the procedure, hypocalcemia during the procedure (discussed below), or hypovolemia from volume shift as described above. Overcompensation of the parasympathetic response leads to cardioinhibitory response, characterized by negative chronotropic and inotropic effects leading to a decrease in cardiac output. Such phenomena may cause hypotension and sometimes syncope. Concomitantly, the overcompensation of the parasympathetic nervous system leads to vasodilatation resulting in marked hypotension (blood pressure can be as low as 50/20 mmHg) without reflex tachycardia. This should be distinguished from the tachycardia usually associated with hypovolemia. In addition to changes in vital signs, clinical symptoms of a vasovagal reaction include pallor, diaphoresis, nausea and vomiting, syncope, and possibly convulsions. Sometimes there is incontinence of urine and/or feces. The situation can be very similar to epileptic seizures.

Nursing interventions shall start when observing a pale person starting to yawn during apheresis with attempting to calm the donor/patient with deep breathing exercises, coughing, laughing, or repositioning to reduce pain and increase comfort which may be sufficient to treat a vasovagal reaction. If necessary, these reactions can also be treated by stopping (in donors) or temporarily pausing the procedure (in patients), placing the donor/patient in the Trendelenburg position, and providing a fluid bolus.

14.2.5 Anticoagulation in Apheresis with Citrate and Heparin

14.2.5.1 Citrate

Citrate is being used very frequently in routine life, especially in the food industry as flavoring and buffering agent in drinks and food. Citrate is also used as anticoagulant in medical procedures. Its use as anticoagulant in the transfusion medicine has been since 1913. Citrate works through chelation of divalent cations such as calcium and magnesium. By binding the ionized calcium, various steps within the coagulation system are inhibited, and thus, clotting can be avoided in the extracorporeal circuit. During apheresis, in continuous-flow procedures, citrate is reinfused continuously, while in intermittent flow devices, citrate is returned intermittently. Consequently, this citrate infusion during apheresis may result in decreased serum levels of ionized calcium and magnesium. Ionized calcium levels can decrease 25% or more during apheresis procedure. The decrease of ionized calcium will lead to an increased production of parathyroid hormone (PTH), aiming to increase ionized calcium level (Buchta et al. 2003). Within 15 minutes after the start of the procedure, PTH levels are elevated.

Besides being an essential cofactor in the coagulation cascade, calcium also plays an important role in the conduction of nerve impulses and in the contraction of muscles. Because of a decrease in ionized calcium, an increased excitability of neurons to the point of spontaneous depolarization can be achieved and, thus, is responsible for some of the symptoms of hypocalcemia.

14.2.5.2 Citrate Toxicity: Citrate-Induced Hypocalcemia

Symptoms of hypocalcemia can be separated into minor, moderate, and severe (see Table 14.1) (Lee and Arepally 2012). With minor reactions, the donor or patient

Table 14.1 Citrate-induced hypocalcemia

Severity	Clinical presentation
Mild	Acral and/or perioral paraesthesia Flushing Shivering Headaches Sneezing Light-headedness
Moderate	Nausea and vomiting Abdominal pain Nervousness Irritability Tremor Muscle spasms Involuntary muscle contractions Tetany Drop in blood pressure
Severe	Cardiac arrhythmia Seizures

may experience a metallic taste, as well as perioral and/or acral paraesthesia. With moderate reactions, the symptoms remain, despite nursing interventions such as slowing down the whole blood flow rate, increasing the anticoagulant to whole blood ratio (AC/WB ratio) if possible, and/or administering calcium supplementation. The donor or patient may suffer from nausea, vomiting, abdominal pain, shivering, light-headedness, tremors, and hypotension mimicking hypovolemia and vasovagal reactions. With severe reactions, symptoms may progress to carpopedal spasm, tetany seizure, and cardiac arrhythmia, specifically prolonging the QT interval. Special attention is needed for patients under sedation or in coma and for pediatric patients, who may not be able to verbally alert the apheresis staff of citrate toxicity symptoms.

Patients receiving blood components as replacement fluid or with a preexisting baseline hypocalcemia prior to apheresis procedure may be at greater risk of citrate-related complications. Similarly, patients with severe liver or kidney disease are also at higher risk of citrate toxicity due to their inability to adequately metabolize citrate. A periodic check of ionized calcium levels and prophylactic calcium supplementation may be warranted in these patients.

14.2.5.3 Citrate Toxicity: Citrate-Induced Metabolic Acidosis and Subsequent Hypokalemia

Various other cofactors should also be mentioned as an effect of citrate infusion during an apheresis procedure. Alkalosis will decrease the ionized calcium levels and therefore increase the effects of citrate. It should be noted that bicarbonate is produced during citrate metabolism, increasing the pH in the blood. In patients with reduced renal bicarbonate excretion, such as those with renal failure or on diuretic medication, bicarbonate accumulation influences the pH considerably. These patients may require monitoring of their acid-base status, especially since metabolic alkalosis increases the potassium intake into the cells, leading to hypokalemia, possibly also leading to cardiac arrhythmias. Besides the additional bicarbonate production, hyperventilation can also cause alkalosis.

14.2.5.4 Citrate Toxicity: Citrate-Induced Hypomagnesemia

Besides the chelation of calcium, ionized magnesium is also bound to citrate. Significant drops in magnesium levels during apheresis procedures are measured. For example, during a plateletapheresis procedure, a decrease of 30% of the magnesium level is demonstrated. The decrease of magnesium is also more pronounced, and it recovers more slowly than calcium. Magnesium influences the electrical activity of myocardial cells because of changes in the stabilization of the axons and the release of neurotransmitters needed to activate the muscles. The symptoms of hypomagnesaemia are rather similar to the effects of hypocalcemia. As calcium and magnesium both bind to proteins, especially albumin (competitive inhibition), in case of hypocalcemia, more magnesium will be bound, leading to hypomagnesaemia. If citrate toxicity is suspected and calcium supplementation does not resolve symptoms, hypomagnesemia and magnesium supplementation should be considered.

14.2.5.5 Prevention and Management of Citrate Toxicity and Use of Heparin as an Alternative Anticoagulation

If citrate toxicity is suspected, the apheresis operator or nurse may elect to slow the flow rate, adjust the citrate infusion ratio if possible, or temporarily pause the procedure. Modern apheresis devices often will not allow infusion rates of citrate that exceed 1.2 mL/min/L blood volume in order to prevent citrate toxicity and hypocalcemia. Some apheresis devices will reduce the whole blood flow rate automatically in order to maintain the citrate infusion rate even lower. Oral (calcium carbonate) and intravenous (calcium chloride or calcium gluconate) calcium supplementation are additional treatment options. In therapeutic apheresis procedures, especially in patients with low baseline ionized calcium levels or procedures where a high amount of citrate will be needed (large volume of stem cell collection), prophylactic calcium administration should be considered. If significant citrate toxicity persists, use of an alternative anticoagulant, such as heparin, or a mixture of heparin and citrate may be used. However, it should be noted that heparin is also associated with adverse events, such as bleeding secondary to persistence in patient plasma several hours after the apheresis therapy and association with heparin-induced thrombocytopenia (HIT). Therefore, it is best to use heparin-only anticoagulation in individuals with citrate allergy and/or in patients with severe renal and hepatic dysfunction.

14.3 Hypothermia

In apheresis techniques, whole blood is separated in the apheresis machine. The desired blood component is collected, and the remaining blood components are returned to the donor or patient. By measuring the temperature of the circulating blood, the hypothalamus can keep up to the mark of the body temperature. When the blood temperature decreases, e.g., because of cooling down of the blood to be returned from the apheresis machine, or reinfusion of colder fluids, the hypothalamus will react by sending impulses to the skin resulting in chills leading to a discomfort in the donor/patient. To avoid cooling down during the apheresis procedure, the use of blood warmers needs to be considered.

14.3.1 Local Adverse Events

None of the apheresis procedures can be performed without venous access, in the form of either peripheral or a central venous catheter. A few apheresis procedures can be performed using single needle access, however, the majority of procedures require double needle access with an acceptable drawn and return flow. For donor procedures, the cubital fossa is usually used for access, however, there is a relatively complex anatomy there. The vein, artery, and nerve are next to each other. Anatomic variances can be the cause that in some persons frequently arterial punctures are performed instead of venous. In such case, an adequate pressure after removing the needle is needed to avoid large hematomas.

When peripheral access is used, phlebotomy may be associated with bruising, hematoma, nerve injury, infections, phlebitis, and/or deep venous thrombosis. Bueno et al. (2006) studied almost 5200 apheresis procedures in 1373 donors and found that in 3.3% of the procedures, hematomas were seen, related to the experience of the operator (<500 procedures performed, more hematomas), prior donations with apheresis machines (experienced donors, more hematomas), and the vein where the venipuncture was made. The basilic vein showed a higher rate of hematoma than cephalic and median veins and others due to various causes such as anatomy and elasticity. Surprisingly, low diastolic blood pressure was also correlated to more hematomas. A clear explanation for this isn't possible. There were no correlations with age, previous hematomas, and gender.

Another problem is nerve injury caused by the needle. The donor or patient will observe a burning shooting electrical pain during the time that the needle is in place. In some cases, the pain starts hours after the venipuncture. In a study from Horowitz (2000), 24 patients with causalgia after venipuncture were analyzed. In a follow-up of 1.5–3 years, only three improved spontaneously, six showed no change, and 15 worsened. However, in a study published by Newman and Waxman (1996), 52 of 56 individuals showed full recovery, and four had mild residual complaints. In the study from Horowitz, however, 70% of the persons involved had also a hematoma worsening the pressure on the nerve.

Risks associated with central venous catheters include infection, thrombosis, hemorrhage, air embolism, pneumothorax, hematothorax, and/or arrhythmias. Even in very experienced clinicians, the puncture to insert a subclavian catheter is complicated by a pneumothorax in 1.5–3% of the patients. Thus, before connecting an apheresis device to a central venous line, the position of the line has to be assured by adequate means (e.g., X-ray). In all procedures, the apheresis operator must regularly evaluate the site of venous access, checking for signs of hematoma, infection, thrombosis, bleeding, and correct insertion.

14.4 Medication Adverse Events

Donors for peripheral hematopoietic progenitor cell collections need to be mobilized prior to the apheresis procedure with medication as G-CSF and/or plerixafor. This medication has its own series of side effects (discussed in Chapts. 5 and 6). Some of these side effects can be difficult to differentiate between the medications and apheresis procedure. Examples are not only gastrointestinal disorders as nausea and vomiting but also headaches, musculoskeletal pains, and fatigue. These can be caused by mobilization and medication and yet, at the same time, can be a side effect from the apheresis procedure, for instance, citrate intoxication.

14.5 Prevention of Apheresis Complications in Children

Indications for performing apheresis procedures in adults also apply to children. However, children are not little adults, so special considerations are required. Children undergo complex development of physiology, psychology, cognition, and behavior. For example, there are few opportunities for an adequate venous access (small vessels), the relatively small TBV in combination with the ECV of the apheresis device and the collected volume and increased sensitivity to hypocalcemia. Also, pediatric patients may also have difficulty in concentration and have increased mobility, and these factors can affect the success of an apheresis procedure.

Depending on the specific apheresis procedure, the ECV can be as high as about 300 mL. This ECV is unacceptable in (very) young children. In adolescents and adults without significant comorbidities, an extracorporeal volume of 15% is well tolerated. In very small children or hemodynamically unstable patients, the maximum tolerable ECV may be lower, such as 10%. If the expected ECV is not acceptable, a blood or albumin prime of the apheresis disposable may be needed. With this, isovolemia can be maintained throughout the procedure.

Because of the small peripheral veins in (very) young children, they may be not large enough to maintain the blood flow rates needed for apheresis. The adequacy of vascular access will vary according to the age, gender, and size of the child. Normally, a 16–17-gauge needle is needed for the drawn line and a 19–22-gauge needle for the return line. A double-lumen central venous catheter can be preferred in younger children with its own risks and considerations as discussed above. Sedation may also be needed for central line placement or in conjunction with muscular paralysis in a patient on mechanical ventilation. The effect of sedatives and other medication administered before apheresis may wear off during a procedure, perhaps partly as a result of drug removal. Thus, for patients requiring sedation during apheresis, repeated dosing during the procedure may be needed.

In children, the burden of the anticoagulant, such as citrate, used in the apheresis procedure is relatively large. For example, relatively more citrate per kilogram of body weight per minute is administrated, and together with the limited metabolic capacity of the pediatric liver and/or kidney, there is an increased risk of hypocalcemia. Symptoms of hypocalcemia and hypomagnesemia in children are difficult to recognize. They may be subtle and difficult to assess, especially in young or sedated children. In children, clinical manifestations of citrate toxicity can consist of acute abdominal pain (with or without vomiting), agitation, pallor, and sweating, followed by tachycardia and hypotension. Hypotension in very sick or unconscious children during apheresis should be assumed to be due to citrate toxicity and treated appropriately.

Toxic effects of citrate anticoagulation can be avoided in children by carefully monitoring the ionized serum calcium levels pre-, during, and post procedure and providing calcium supplementation if necessary. In adolescents and older children, minor symptoms of hypocalcemia can be treated with oral calcium supplementation. Calcium can also be administered intravenously; in many apheresis centers, intravenous calcium supplementation is given routinely.

In colder conditions, humans lose heat via the head and the trunk. The body shape of a child differs from that of an adult. The head and trunk can be over 60% of the total body length. Therefore, smaller children can lose greater heat. This is something an apheresis physician must think of, especially when also colder fluids are returned as is the situation during apheresis procedures. Therefore, the room temperature needs to be high, and the use of blood warmers needs to be considered.

14.6 Expert Point of View

Apheresis procedures are generally safe, and serious adverse events occur very rarely. However, we must learn from each other's adverse events in an attempt to avoid it as much as possible. Since side effects occur only rarely, registration at least in regional but preferably in global registries (e.g., apheresis registration of the World Apheresis Association) of all procedures and their side effects is of high importance. With all gathered data, the frequency, the probable cause of specific side effects, and their management options can be evaluated. These lessons can make apheresis safer in the future.

References

Buchta C, Macher M, Bieglmayer C, Höcker P, Dettke M (2003) Reduction of adverse citrate reactions during autologous large-volume PBPC apheresis by continuous infusion of calcium-gluconate. Transfusion 43(11):1615–1621

Bueno JL, Castro E, García F, Barea L, González R (2006) Hematomas in multicomponent apheresis: searching for related factors. Transfusion 46:2184–2191

Horowitz SH (2000) Venipuncture-induced causalgia: anatomic relations of upper extremity superficial veins and nerves, and clinical considerations. Transfusion 40:1036–1040

http://www.transfusionguidelines.org.uk/transfusion-handbook/5-adverse-effects-of-transfusion

Kleinman S, Caulfield T, Chan P, Davenport R, McFarland J, McPhedran S, Meade M, Morrison D, Pinsent T, Robillard P, Slinger P (2004) Toward an understanding of transfusion-related acute lung injury: statement of a consensus panel. Transfusion 44:1774–1789

Lee G, Arepally GM (2012) Anticoagulation techniques in apheresis: from heparin to citrate and beyond. J Clin Apher 27:117–125

Newman BH, Waxman DA (1996) Blood donation-related neurologic needle injury: evaluation of 2 years' worth of data from a large blood center. Transfusion 36:213–215

Challenges and Optimization of Apheresis Procedures in Resource-Limiting Environments

15

Mickey B. C. Koh, Senarath Banda Abeykoon Jayasekara, and Rajeeka Lakmali Morawakage

15.1 Introduction

The acquisition and development of apheresis technology, knowledge, and capabilities in resource limited countries are usually driven by essential clinical needs. These include the need for safe and sufficient blood transfusion and the collection of hematopoietic stem/progenitor cells (HPCs) for transplants or as effective treatment in a wide variety of medical conditions including sickle cell disease, acquired thrombotic thrombocytopenia purpura, and/or selected demyelinating neurological diseases. In the majority of resource limited nations, provision of an adequate and safe blood supply is a major challenge due to scarcity of voluntary blood donors and resources. Fortunately, many of those countries now have systems in place for obtaining and testing the blood provided by volunteer donors to ensure a safe blood supply. This is fundamental in improving health outcomes. The establishment of a clinical HPC transplant program is also another area of essential development for many resource limited countries. This is because of the increasing effectiveness and improved safety of hematopoietic cell transplantation (HCT) in the treatment of a variety of hematological malignancies as well as other congenital conditions. Professional training needs form a key component of quality systems, and all apheresis programs should have an embedded quality system from the onset. In this

M. B. C. Koh (✉)
Department of Haematology, St George's University Hospital Hospitals, London, UK

Blood Services Group, Health Sciences Authority, Singapore, Singapore
e-mail: mickey.koh@stgeorges.nhs.uk

S. B. A. Jayasekara
National Blood Centre, National Blood Transfusion Service of Sri Lanka, Colombo, Sri Lanka

R. L. Morawakage
Regional Blood Centre, National Cancer Institute of Sri Lanka, Maharagama, Sri Lanka

S. A. Abutalib et al. (eds.), *Best Practices of Apheresis in Hematopoietic Cell Transplantation*, Advances and Controversies in Hematopoietic Transplantation and Cell Therapy, https://doi.org/10.1007/978-3-319-55131-9_15

chapter, we also highlighted the country-specific examples with an overview of the unique challenges and opportunities that exist for setting up a viable apheresis service as well as an in-depth focus on the developmental pathways.

15.1.1 Setting Up an Apheresis Program

In the majority of resource limited nations, provision of an adequate and safe blood supply is a major challenge due to scarcity of voluntary blood donors and resources. It is estimated that about 80% of the world population has access to only 20% of the world blood supply (McCullough 2013). The imperative for safe blood has been a WHO priority with various guidelines, and documents have been developed to assist countries in achieving this goal (WHO 2011). Fortunately, many countries now have systems in place for provision of blood provided by volunteer donors and test them for infectious disease markers as part of the provision of safe blood. This is fundamental in improving health outcomes. It allows for complex diseases, such as hematological malignancy, to be treated with advanced therapy, which in turn results in a greater demand for the transfusion services to supply more specialized blood components. Apheresis capabilities can help to meet that demand while also providing the impetus for training specialized staff.

The establishment of a clinical HCT program is another area of important development for many resource limited countries. This is because of the increasing effectiveness and improved safety of HCT in treating a variety of hematological malignancies as well as other congenital conditions, both of which are often disproportionately more common in these resource limited countries (Koh et al. 2018). One of the minimal requirements for establishing such HCT programs is the ability to collect donor or patient's HPCs via apheresis as well as the ability to process the collected product in the HPC processing laboratory (Koh 2017). As such, this could provide the driving force for the establishment of an apheresis service. Sometimes, this interfaces and relies on the already established apheresis capabilities within the transfusion service (or blood bank). A good example is the recent developments in Myanmar. A dedicated and forward-thinking team of transfusion specialists developed stepwise improvements in their blood supply through increased voluntary donations, infectious disease testing, and appropriate use of blood resources. This was partially facilitated by external agencies including the WHO, Japanese Red Cross, and a volunteer team of Singaporean hematologists. These experts provided hands on training and quality management as well as seminars and lectures. The improvement in the blood supply and better hematology knowledge led to the initiation of an HPC transplant program that has in turn leveraged on the resources of the blood service. The blood service was able to provide special blood components (platelets and plasma) via apheresis, and there was cross-training of staff allowing the hospitals to develop the apheresis capabilities to harvest HPCs. To date, several successful clinical transplants have taken place (Gyi et al. 2017).

It is not unusual for the transfusion service to take on the role of HPC collection. This remains a common practice in the many developed countries where the hospitals provide their own HPC apheresis services while the blood banks provide the apheresis support for the hospital HCT programs, thereby rationalizing and maximizing precious resources including equipment as well as trained staff (Leemhuis et al. 2014). Furthermore, the transfusion service is often in a better position to be funded due to it being a vital and necessary national investment as it is considered an essential part of the basic medical care. International agencies are sometimes also instrumental in helping these services develop as well as international agencies (e.g., PFAR in Ethiopia, WHO in Myanmar). On the other hand, hospitals, already having to consider the considerable investment needed to establish a clinical HCT program, would often prefer to delegate that responsibility to the transfusion services. Ethiopia is also currently following this example by leveraging on the improvements made in the transfusion service, the progressive capabilities for apheresis (equipment purchase, training) in supporting their proposed HCT program in Addis Ababa (personal communication).

Variations of this model exist due to several factors which are critical in the establishment of an apheresis service. This includes financial considerations, physical location, existing infrastructure, and the presence of trained specialist staff that can operate the equipment. For instance, an apheresis program can also be initiated and developed via the need from clinicians for effective treatment of their patients, such as red cell exchange for sickle cell disease or therapeutic plasma exchange (TPE) for many neurological conditions. However, in these instances, the transfusion services, being already equipped to provide specialized blood components, would often already have an apheresis capability and, thus, can be utilized in the cross-training and knowledge exchange for development of a therapeutic apheresis (TA) program.

In order to set up any apheresis program, the key considerations are the following:

- Financial: government, aid agencies, and hospital. Evaluate for the affordability and cost-effectiveness for having an apheresis service.
- Physical location: transfusion service vs. hospital based.
- Clinical needs: provision of blood components, stem cell collection, or therapeutic apheresis.
- Trained apheresis operators as well as training for venous access.
- Reliable hardware/device, including validation, maintenance, and backup.
- Quality systems and standard operating procedures (SOPs).
- Projected growth and sustainability of the service. It is not advisable to implement donor apheresis programs with considerable capital cost without a long-term plan for sustainability of financial and technological support.

15.1.2 Training Needs and Quality Systems

With the availability of instruments and hardware, training needs should be identified by careful analysis of the present situation and the expected future plan with the respective health sector development. Professional training services, such as international consultancy services in Sanquin Blood Center, access to professional apheresis organizations like ASFA (American Society for Apheresis), and basic technical support provided by majority of instrument suppliers, would be the available options for training requirements.

Training needs form a key component of quality systems, and all apheresis programs should have an embedded quality system from the beginning. This quality system can be quite basic initially and will evolve as the apheresis program matures. SOPs, appropriate standardization with guidelines, quality control, and internal and external quality assurances are all part of this quality system and are essential for an effective and sustainable practice.

The importance of training and access to systematic training has been highlighted in a cooperative project between Indonesia and the Sanquin Blood Service (Triyono and Vrielink 2015). Two hundred and four leukocytapheresis procedures were performed in 137 patients and 71 TPE procedures in 17 patients. These procedures were safe and thought to be cost-effective. A training program for apheresis nurses in HPC collection by leukocytapheresis and therapeutic apheresis was developed by the Joint Task Force for Apheresis Education and Certification. This is a modular program with theoretical and practical information and knowledge. On the request of the Indonesian authorities, a certification course for apheresis nurses/operators based on the training program was organized consisting of modules related to apheresis, such as hematology, anatomy, physiology, calculations, adverse events, basics of apheresis, nursing aspects, quality, collection of cells for cellular therapies, pediatrics, and therapeutic collections (cell reductions and exchange procedures). A pre-test and post-test regarding the knowledge and judgment in the themes described were taken. In total, 38 apheresis nurses and 32 physicians participated in the course. In the post-test, the nurses scored an average of 72% and the physicians 77%, which was significantly better than the results of the pre-test (54% and 53%, respectively ($P < 0.0001$ for both)) (Neyrinck et al. 2015).

In India, formal continuing medical education (CME) was provided to transfusion medicine physicians in therapeutic apheresis (TA) according to the guidelines by the American Society for Apheresis (ASFA). Seventy-three physicians participated in this educational activity, and it was demonstrated that there was significant improvement in performing TA by the correct indications and there was a significant reduction in the number of TAs done for non-recommended categories. There was also a change in practice observed in the duration of therapy and the replacement fluid used (Tiwari et al. 2016).

The Alliance for Harmonisation of Cellular Therapy Accreditation (AHCTA) conducted a survey worldwide for practices in apheresis and cord blood collection for HPC transplantation. It was recognized that as HCT expands globally, identification of the key elements that make up high-quality training programs will become more important to optimizing collection practices and the quality of HPC products. Multiple-choice and open-ended questions to identify training practices were distributed via an electronic survey tool worldwide. Respondents from more than 50 countries representing transplant centers or transfusion services participated. For the majority of staff performing HPC collections by apheresis (50%), initial training required as many procedures as necessary to be done until competency was achieved. Competency was evaluated by direct observation comparing performance to written procedures or protocol steps (47%), combination of written assessment and observation (45%), evaluation of product quality (40%), and written assessment alone (12%). Staff retraining was customized on a case-by-case basis (42%) (Celluzzi et al. 2014).

15.1.3 Examples of Setting up Apheresis Programs Worldwide

The following country-specific examples aim to provide an illustration, an overview, as well as the unique challenges and opportunities that exist for setting up a viable apheresis service.

15.2 Therapeutic Apheresis in India

Manual techniques for plasma exchange were used until 1985 when a membrane filtration was first introduced. Centrifugation using cell separators (Haemonetics MCS 2P), as a method for plasma exchange, was later introduced in 1992. By 1998, the main therapeutic centers in India were New Delhi, Mumbai, Chennai, Hyderabad, and Lucknow (Srivastava et al. 1998). Normal saline was the main replacement fluid used followed by albumin (Srivastava 2002; Sharma et al. 2011).

By 2005, the Indian Society for Apheresis recognized the importance of therapeutic apheresis in medical care and promoted therapeutic apheresis for medical tourism citing cost efficiency as the main advantage compared to the USA and Europe—the cost for procedure being around 25% compared to the cost in the USA at the time (Srivastava 2006). Moreover, there are well-established HCT programs across India, and these have provided the clinical need for establishing peripheral blood stem cell collection via apheresis.

15.3 Donor Apheresis for Blood Transfusion in India

The most common apheresis procedure in resource limited countries like India remains plateletpheresis from blood donors to meet the demand and supplied mainly for hemato-oncology patients (Chaudhary et al. 2005). The difficulty in recruiting apheresis donors was felt to be due to the perceived increased commitment, longer time for procedure, various cultural beliefs, and other unknown fears among Indian donors due to lack of proper awareness (Agarwal and Verma 2009). In addition, lack of dietary iron due to a vegetarian diet of the majority of the population has added more burden to an already low donor pool. A significant number of donors were deferred due to low hemoglobin (<12.5 g/dL) (Agarwal and Verma 2009). It was also suggested that lower threshold recommendations of single donor platelet (SDP) yield of 2×10^{11}/unit by the Council of Europe recommendation may be more suitable than the AABB recommended yield of 3×10^{11} in the Indian scenario (Agarwal and Verma 2009).

15.4 Apheresis in Malaysia

Clinical and therapeutic aphereses are managed by the respective clinicians and departments in hospitals. HCT centers have been established, and this incorporates an HPC collection service provided by apheresis.

An average of 4.6% of the annual collection in Malaysia comes from apheresis donations, and the cost of running an apheresis center remains the main obstacle to increasing activity, and it is mostly driven by clinical need or special request by clinicians to avoid any wastage.

In Malaysia, the protocols for apheresis are standardized, and training programs have been implemented. However, there is still a need for further strengthening of quality assurance of apheresis and awareness programs for donors (Eichbaum et al. 2014).

15.5 Donor Apheresis in African Countries

Apheresis technology plays an important role in only a limited number of African countries even though there is a considerable potential and benefits for its application. By 2013, the main users of apheresis in the African continent were Egypt, Libya, Algeria, and South Africa (Eichbaum et al. 2014).

In Africa where there is no availability or poor quality of whole blood-derived platelets and high incidence of transfusion-transmitted infections exist, apheresis platelet collection can play an important role in minimizing donor exposure and in the provision of a product of consistently high quality. For example, a fixed-site center in Pretoria, South Africa, provides approximately 5000 products annually with only a 350 donor panel, using 8 apheresis devices, mostly collecting high-yield units which could be divided into 2–3 adult therapeutic doses of at least 3×10^{11}/unit platelets (Eichbaum et al. 2014).

The majority of apheresis facilities available are operated by national or regional blood services, and most of the donors are voluntary donors except in few countries where replacement donors are still enrolled (Eichbaum et al. 2014).

In addition to financial constraints, some countries in the region do not have the proper infrastructure facilities for a successful and reliable apheresis operation, such as a dependable power supply. Moreover, they have to face other problems such as political instability and military conflicts. Easy accessibility to medical and technical support and the need for professional development with continuous training are other barriers faced to setting up apheresis programs (Eichbaum et al. 2014).

With regard to HCT programs, South Africa, Algeria, Tunisia, and Egypt have well-established centers with apheresis capabilities; however, HCT is lacking in the majority of the other African countries.

TPE is neither readily available nor affordable in many parts of Africa. Arogundade et al. described the challenges of starting a TPE program in a resource-constrained economy. A survey in Nigeria revealed that 56.7% of respondents had very little or no knowledge of TPE, 40.5% had moderate knowledge, and only 2.7% admitted to having a good knowledge of this procedure. Only 18.9% of respondents have ever participated or observed a TPE procedure with the remaining 81.1% not having any exposure to the procedure. A vast majority of the respondents (97.3%) felt they needed better exposure and training in TPE and its applications. Among the consultants, 56% had little knowledge, 88% had never participated or observed the TPE procedure, and 94% felt they needed better exposure and training. The author concluded that efforts should be concentrated on improving the knowledge and availability of TPE in resource-constrained economy, such as Nigeria, and apheresis centers that are able to manage cases requiring TA should be developed (Arogundade et al. 2014).

15.6 Apheresis in Brazil

Brazil is the largest collector of apheresis platelets in South America followed by Colombia, Peru, and Argentina. Apheresis procedures in Brazil are overseen by hematologists in both private and public blood banks. Although it is a common practice in Brazil to request for replacement donations, over 60% of the donors are motivated to donate voluntarily. Under TA, TPE is the most common therapeutic apheresis procedure in Brazil with albumin being the commonest replacement fluid. Extracorporeal photopheresis is in place in few hospitals.

The main challenges of these apheresis programs are cost recovery, which is partly covered by reimbursement from public health system, and the lack of structured training programs covering relevant technical and clinical professionals (Eichbaum et al. 2014).

15.7 Apheresis in Sri Lanka

Sri Lanka is a small island with a land area of 62,705 km^2 and a population of approximately 21 million (2015) with a per capita income of $3836 in 2015. The National Blood Transfusion Service (NBTS) of Sri Lanka is centrally coordinated under the Ministry of Health and has its headquarters in Colombo, which is the capital of the country. Patient care services, including blood and blood products, for patients in the state sector hospitals are provided free of charge.

Since 2013, 100% of blood units collected by the NBTS are from voluntary nonremunerated donors. Sri Lanka has a low prevalence of transfusion-transmitted infections among blood donors, and it also has an active quality assurance program.

Apheresis was first introduced to the country in the late 1980s with the purchase of a COBE Spectra apheresis machine. The machine, located at the "Central Blood Bank" within the premises of the National Hospital of Sri Lanka, was used only for TPEs.

Although there was an attempt to start a HCT program at the National Cancer Institute of Sri Lanka with HPC collection using the COBE Spectra, the program ended after a few autologous HPC transplants in the early 1990s.

Renewed interest in apheresis resurfaced in the late 1990s although it was limited to the collection of platelets using a Baxter Amicus automated cell separator at the Central Blood Bank in Colombo to cater to the increasing demand for platelets. Collection of platelets by apheresis saw a gradual increase with the procurement of additional Amicus and Haemonetics (MCS 3P and MCS+) cell separators. In addition to Colombo, some of these were located in larger hospital-based blood banks all over the country. Although the Amicus was used exclusively for the collection of platelets, additional capabilities of the Haemonetics cell separators saw the reintroduction of automation to TPEs.

Two parallel programs, one for capacity building with assistance from the WHO and the Japanese Bank for International Cooperation (JBIC) and the other a postgraduate diploma training program in transfusion medicine, commenced in 1998. It was in 2006 when the diploma training program extended to a full-fledged MD training program in transfusion medicine. These developments led to renewed interest in starting an HPC transplant program in Sri Lanka. By this time, the NBTS developed the capability of supporting a comprehensive transplant program, including the training of personnel in overseas centers, such as the St. Vincent's Hospital in Sydney, Australia, and postgraduate training to the National Blood Service in Singapore, which included training in transplants, cell therapy, and apheresis.

The clinical drive and commitment to establish an HPC transplant program resulted in NBTS procuring two Spectra Optia cell separators for a new facility for HPC collection and processing at the Blood Bank of the National Cancer Institute, the tertiary care hospital for patients with oncology and hematological malignancies. Since then, successful peripheral HPC collections have been undertaken with the expertise of the transfusion medicine specialists associated with capabilities in processing and cryopreservation of the cells. This has resulted in successful and durable engraftments and transplants in patients with multiple myeloma. The initial transplants were performed under the guidance of a team of medical experts from Australia. Currently, as of early 2018, within 1 year since the commencement of the program, peripheral HPC collections have been performed in thirty patients leading to twenty-five successful transplants.

The success at the National Cancer Institute has led to plans for an expansion of the HPC transplant program in other parts of the country, such as at the Kandy and Kurunegala, as well as inclusion of the nonmalignant pediatric diseases. Parallel to the developments in the state sector, some leading private hospitals in Sri Lanka also have started their own transplant programs, catering mainly to many pediatric patients with thalassaemia.

The donor apheresis program in Sri Lanka is overseen by transfusion medicine specialists attached to blood centers in major hospitals. In 2016, there were 1737 apheresis platelet donations from regular donors, collecting approximately 3015 units. An HLA-typed donor pool is also maintained to provide transfusion support for patients with immune-mediated platelet refractoriness.

15.8 Therapeutic Apheresis in Sri Lanka

TA is available since the late 1980s at the National Hospital of Sri Lanka—the main tertiary care hospital of the country. It expanded rapidly to the periphery with the availability of equipment and the presence of transfusion medicine specialists in major hospitals. TPE is the most common procedure and is most commonly done for demyelinating neurological disorders, pre- or post-renal transplant complications, and acquired thrombotic thrombocytopenic purpura. There had been several cases of TPE for acute renal injuries, autoimmune encephalopathy, and rare cases of nonresponsive HELLP syndrome and snake bites. Varity of apheresis machines, such as Haemonetics MCS+, COBE Spectra, Spectra Optia, and Fresenius Kabi Comtec, are available for selection. Upon the request of the clinicians, procedures are performed by the blood bank staff under the direct supervision of the transfusion medicine specialist who is also involved in the patient management. In 2016, there were 2538 TPEs performed for 671 patients with majority of them being performed in Colombo, Kandy, and Karapitiya (Galle). Recently, there have been significant TA prcedures performed for leptospirosis with pulmonary haemorrhage with some success.

15.8.1 Guidelines and Resources for Apheresis

Numerous national and international guidelines exist for the appropriate use of blood and blood products. This is critical in rationalizing and managing blood use.

With regard to the practice of collection of products by apheresis, the WHO has some guidance (WHO document: technical report series no. 961) (WHO 2011). It states that for collection by apheresis, the operational parameters of the apheresis system should be implemented in compliance with the instructions of the equipment manufacturer and in compliance with any specified safety requirements of the National Regulatory Authorities (NRA). It also recommends that the volume of the component collected from the donor during one procedure and over a period of time should be regulated by internal policies based on current medical knowledge and on national regulations set by the NRA. An adequately trained physician should be available during apheresis sessions. The donor apheresis collection process should be followed at all times using validated methods and SOPs. Any deviations from the established procedures and processes may result in products not meeting specifications and, therefore, should be considered as nonconforming products and must not be automatically released for distribution.

International HPC transplant organizations, such as the Worldwide Network for Blood and Marrow Transplantation (WBMT), also provide essential guidelines for starting a clinical transplant service, and this includes the requirements needed for apheresis procedures for collection of HPCs (Leemhuis et al. 2014).

The British Society for Haematology provides useful guidelines for TA (which includes exchange transfusions). These outline the available evidence for efficacy of TPE in various conditions and also grades these conditions according to the level of evidence (Howell et al. 2015). Similarly, the American Society for Apheresis

(ASFA) provides forums for discussions including webinars and chat groups which members can log onto. The ASFA guidelines are again concentrated mainly on the evidence of the use of therapeutic apheresis in certain diseases and conditions, and it is updated every 3 years. It is currently in the 7th edition (published in 2016) (Schwartz et al. 2016). Furthermore, the Qualification in Apheresis certificate is offered by ASFA which is partnered with the board of certification by the American Society for Clinical Pathology for apheresis practitioners. Other official publications by ASFA include the *Principles of Apheresis Technology Textbook, 6th Edition.* Other useful resources which resource limited countries can refer to are the various international organizations for apheresis including the ISFA (International Society for Apheresis), which publishes the Therapeutic Apheresis and Dialysis Journal.

There are considerably less resources available for the practical aspects of starting an apheresis program, and international societies should perhaps take on that task. In this respect, the International Society of Blood Transfusion (ISBT) has a specific focus and mission on resource limited apheresis in less-experienced countries. The webpage link to the Apheresis Working Party of ISBT states, "We focus on the various apheresis technologies; assess new equipment, collection methods and materials in order to improve the current methods. We are also interested in the quality, safety and storage of blood components collected by apheresis methods. We are setting up various educational and training programs related to the latest apheresis technologies with a special focus on resource limited countries or inexperienced blood banks."

15.9 Conclusion

In conclusion, apheresis programs are increasingly part of the essential infrastructure of national health systems in resource limited countries. Although there are initial capital costs for starting such a program, there has been confirmation of its cost-effectiveness. Guidelines as well as systematic training and qualification have been consistently identified as important areas to focus upon in resource limited countries.

References

Agarwal P, Verma A (2009) Automated platelet collection using the latest aphaeresis devices in an Indian setting. Transfus Apheres Sci 41:135–138

Arogundade FA, Sanusi AA, Oguntola SO, Omotoso BA, Abdel-Rahman EM, Akinsola A, Balogun RA (2014) Benefits and challenges of starting a new therapeutic apheresis service in a resource-constrained setting. J Clin Apher 29(4):194–198. https://doi.org/10.1002/jca.21328

Celluzzi CM, Keever-Taylor C, Aljurf M, Koh MB, Rabe F, Rebulla P, Sacchi N, Sanders J, McGrath E, Loper K, Alliance for Harmonisation of Cellular Therapy Accreditation (AHCTA) (2014) Training practices of hematopoietic progenitor cell-apheresis and -cord blood collection staff: analysis of a survey by the Alliance for harmonisation of cellular therapy accreditation. Transfusion 54(12):3138–3144. https://doi.org/10.1111/trf.12753

Chaudhary R, Das SS, Agarwal P, Shukla JS (2005) Quality systems in automated plateletpheresis in hospital based blood transfusion service in North India. J Clin Apher 20:81–85

Eichbaum Q, Smid MW, Crookes R, Naim M, Mendrone A Jr, Marques JFC Jr, Marques MB (2014) Apheresis in developing countries around the world. J Clin Apher 30(4):238–246
Gyi AA, Mra R, Nyein HL, Aung T, Win N, Khin PT, Issaragrisil S, Srivastava A, Ma D, Koh M (2017) Where there's a will, there's a way: establishing hematopoietic stem cell transplantation in Myanmar. Poster presented at 59th annual meeting & exposition of American Society of Hematology Atlanta GA, December 9–12, 2017
Howell C, Douglas K, Cho G, El-Ghariani K, Taylor P, Potok D, Rintala T, Watkins S (2015) Guideline on the clinical use of apheresis procedures for the treatment of patients and collection of cellular therapy products. Transfus Med 25(2):57–78. https://doi.org/10.1111/tme.12205
Koh MBC (2017) Considerations in setting up and planning a graft processing facility. Hematol Oncol Stem Cell Ther 10(4):195–197
Koh MBC, Lowdell M, Leemhuis T (2018) Essential requirements for setting up a stem cell processing laboratory. In: Gluckman É, Niederwieser D, Aljurf M (eds) Establishing a hematopoietic stem cell transplantation unit. Springer, Cham, pp 155–169
Leemhuis T, Padley D, Keever-Taylor C, Niederwieser D, Teshima T, Lanza F, Chabannon C, Szabolcs P, Bazarbachi A, Koh MBC on behalf of the Graft Processing Subcommittee of the Worldwide Network for Blood and Bone Marrow Transplantation (WBMT) (2014) Essential requirements for setting up a stem cell processing laboratory. Bone Marrow Transplant 49:1098–1105
McCullough TK, McCullough J (2013) Strengthening blood programs in developing countries. Transfus Apher Sci 49(3):408–415
Neyrinck M, Vrielink H, Joint Task Force for Apheresis Education and Certification (2015) Apheresis training for nurses and physicians around the World. J Clin Apher 30(1):32–37. https://doi.org/10.1002/jca.21345
Schwartz J, Padmanabhan A, Aqui N, Balagun RA, Conelly-Smith L, Delaney M, Dunbar NM, Witt V, Wu Y, Shaz BH (2016) Guidelines on the use of therapeutic apheresis in clinical practice: evidence-based approach from the writing committee of the American Society for Apheresis: the seventh special issue. J Clin Apher 31(3):149–162
Sharma RR, Saluja K, Jain A, Dhawan HK, Thakral B, Marwaha N (2011) Scope and application of therapeutic apheresis: experience from a tertiary care hospital in North India. Transfus Apher Sci 45:239–245
Srivastava R (2002) Changing perspectives of apheresis in India in the twentieth century. Transfus Apher Sci 26:97–101
Srivastava R (2006) Indian Society for Apheresis and apheresis tourism in India – is there a future? Transfus Apher Sci 34:139–144
Srivastava R, Gupta RC, Khatri PC, Lalchandani A (1998) Changing scenario of therapeutic apheresis in India in last 14 years. Ther Apheres 2(4):317–319
Tiwari AK, Dara RC, Pandey P, Arora D, Rawat G, Raina V (2016) Change in therapeutic apheresis practices: role of continuing medical education (CME). J Clin Apher 31(1):16–21. https://doi.org/10.1002/jca.21397
Triyono T, Vrielink H (2015) Therapeutic apheresis in Asia: an Indonesia single center experience. J Clin Apher 30(3):139–140. https://doi.org/10.1002/jca.21350
WHO (2011) Expert Committee on specifications for pharmaceutical preparations. (WHO technical report series (2011) no. 961)

References for Sri Lanka Demographic Data

Area 65,610 km^2. http://www.statistics.gov.lk/Pocket%20Book/chap01.pdf
GDP LKR 11,183,220 million (US$ bn 82.3) http://www.cbsl.gov.lk/pics_n_docs/10_pub/_docs/statistics/other/Socio_Econ_Data_2016_e.pdf
Per Capita Income (2015)—USD 3836. http://www.cbsl.gov.lk/pics_n_docs/10_pub/_docs/statistics/other/Socio_Econ_Data_2016_e.pdf